The Nation's Health

Edited by

Philip R. Lee
Carroll L. Estes

Institute for Health Policy Studies
School of Medicine
University of California,
San Francisco

JONES AND BARTLETT PUBLISHERS
BOSTON

Editorial, Sales, and Customer Service Offices

Jones and Bartlett Publishers
20 Park Plaza
Boston, MA 02116

Printed in the United States of America
10 9 8 7 6 5 4 3 2 1

Library of Congress Cataloging-in-Publication Data

Lee, Philip R., and Carroll L. Estes, eds.
  The Nation's health.

   Includes bibliographical references.
   1. Public health--United States. I. Lee, Philip R. (Philip Randolph). II. Estes, Carroll L.
RA445.N36 1990   362.1'0973--dc20   90-33128

ISBN: 0-86720-428-1

Text photographs: pp. 2, 360, Harold M. Lambert; pp. 68, 172, Camerique Stock Photography; p. 120, Dennis DeSilva; pp. 202, 294, 336, Rafael Millán.

Cover photographs: Camerique (1); Rafael Millán.

Table of Contents

Acknowledgments

Chapter One

Thomas McKeown. "Determinants of Health." Abridged from *Human Nature, April 1978*. Copyright © 1978 by Human Nature, Inc. Reprinted by permission of the publisher.

Lois M. Verbrugge. "Longer Life but Worsening Health? Trends in Health and Mortality of Middle-Aged and Older Persons." Abridged from the *Milbank Quarterly*, Volume 62, Number 3, 1984. Copyright © 1984 by Milbank Quarterly. Reprinted by permission of the publisher.

James J. Fries. "An Introduction to the Compression of Morbidity." Abridged from *Gerontologica perspecta*, Volume 1, 1987. Copyright © 1987 in Canada by Gerontologica perspecta. Reprinted by permission of the publisher.

Jack M. Guralnik and Edward L. Schneider. "The Compression of Morbidity: A Dream Which May Come True, Someday!" Abridged from *Gerontologica perspecta*, Volume 1, 1987. Copyright © 1987 in Canada by Gerontologica perspecta. Reprinted by permission of the publisher.

S. M. Miller. "Race in the Health of America." Abridged from *Milbank Quarterly*, Volume 65, Supplement 2, 1987. Copyright © 1987 by Milbank Quarterly. Reprinted by permission of the publisher.

Chapter Two

Dorothy P. Rice. "The Medical Care System: Past Trends and Future Projections." Abridged from *The New York Medical Quarterly*. Copyright © 1986 by The New York Medical Quarterly. Reprinted by permission of the publisher.

Arnold S. Relman. "The New Medical Industrial Complex." Abridged from *New England Journal of Medicine*, Volume 303, Number 17, 1980. Copyright © 1980 by New England Journal of Medicine. Reprinted by permission of the publisher.

Uwe E. Reinhardt. "Rationing the Health-Care Surplus: An American Tragedy." Abridged from *Nursing Economic$*, Volume 4, Number 3, 1986. This article originally appeared in *The New Physician*, Volume 34, Number 7, 1985, as "Economics, Ethics and the American Health Care System." Copyright © 1985 by the American Medical Student Association. Reprinted by permission of the publisher.

Robert J. Haggarty. "The Boundaries of Health Care." Reprinted from *The Pharos* of Alpha Omega Alpha, July 1972, Volume 35, Number 3, pp. 106–111, with the permission of the editor. Copyright © 1972 by The Pharos of Alpha Omega Alpha.

Chapter Three

Richard D. Lamm. "The Ten Commandments of Health Care." This article first appeared in *The Humanist* issue of May/June 1987 and is reprinted by permission. Copyright © 1987 by the American Humanist Association.

Philip R. Lee and Lynn Etheredge. "Clinical Freedom: Two Lessons for the U.K. from U.S. Experience with Privatization of Health Care." Abridged from *The Lancet,* February 4, 1989. Copyright © 1989 in the United Kingdom by The Lancet. Reprinted by permission of the publisher.

Theodor J. Litman. "Government and Health: The Political Aspects of Health Care — A Sociopolitical Overview." Abridged from *Health Politics and Policy in Perspective.* Copyright © 1984 by John Wiley & Sons, Inc. Reprinted by permission of John Wiley & Sons, Inc.

Vicente Navarro. "Federal Health Policies in the United States: An Alternative Explanation." Abridged from *Milbank Quarterly,* Volume 65, Number 1, 1987. Copyright © 1987 by Milbank Quarterly. Reprinted by permission of the publisher.

Theodore R. Marmor. "American Medical Policy and the 'Crisis' of the Welfare State: A Comparative Perspective." Abridged from *Journal of Health Politics, Policy and Law,* Volume 11, Number 4, 1986. Copyright © 1986 by Duke University Press. Reprinted with permission of the publisher.

Chapter Four

U.S. Department of Health and Human Services, "Secretary's Commission on Nursing, Executive Summary, Final Report," Volume 1, December 1988.

Linda H. Aiken and Connie Flynt Mullinix. "The Nurse Shortage: Myth or Reality?" Abridged from *New England Journal of Medicine,* Volume 317, Number 10, 1987. Copyright © 1987 by New England Journal of Medicine. Reprinted by permission of the publisher.

Claire M. Fagin. "The Visible Problems of an Invisible Profession: The Crisis and Challenge for Nursing." Reprinted with permission from the Blue Cross and Blue Shield Association, from *Inquiry,* Volume 24, Number 2, pp. 119–126. Copyright © 1987 by Blue Cross and Blue Shield Association. All rights reserved.

Chapter Five

Division of National Cost Estimates, Office of the Actuary, Health Care Financing Administration. "National Health Care Expenditures 1986–2000." *Health Care Financing Review,* Volume 8, Number 4. HCFA Publication Number 03239. Office of Research and Demonstrations, Health Care Financing Administration. Washington. U.S. Government Printing Office, August 1987.

Physician Payment Review Commission. *1988 Annual Report to Congress.* Washington, D.C. March 1988.

Philip R. Lee, Paul Ginsburg, Lauren LeRoy, and Glenn Hammons. "The Physician Payment Review Commission Report to Congress — 1989." Abridged from *JAMA,* Volume 261, Number 16, 1989.

Eli Ginzberg. "A Hard Look at Cost Containment." Abridged from *New England Journal of Medicine,* Volume 316, Number 18, 1987. Copyright © 1987 by New England Journal of Medicine. Reprinted by permission of the publisher.

Victor R. Fuchs. "Has Cost Containment Gone Too Far?" Abridged from *Milbank Quarterly,* Volume 64, Number 3, 1986. Copyright © 1986 by Milbank Quarterly. Reprinted by permission of the publisher.

Chapter Six

Victor R. Fuchs. "The 'Competition Revolution' in Health Care." Abridged from *Health Affairs,* Volume 7, Number 3, 1988. Copyright © 1988 Health Affairs Project Hope. Reprinted by permission of the publisher.

Bruce C. Vladeck. "The Market vs. Regulation: The Case for Regulation." Abridged from *Milbank Quarterly,* Volume 59, Number 2, 1981. Copyright © 1981 by Milbank Quarterly. Reprinted by permission of the publisher.

Alain C. Enthoven. "Health Care Costs: Why Regulation Fails, Why Competition Works, How to get There from Here." Condensed from *National Journal.* Copyright © 1979 by National Journal. Reprinted by permission of the publisher.

Chapter Seven

Karen Davis and Diane Rowland. "Uninsured and Underserved: Inequalities in Health Care in the United States." Abridged from *Milbank Quarterly,* Volume 61, Number 2, 1983. Copyright © 1983 by Milbank Quarterly. Reprinted by permission of the publisher.

Howard E. Freeman, Robert J. Blendon, Linda H. Aiken, Seymour Sudman, Connie Flynt Mullinix, and Christopher R. Corey. "Americans Report on Their Access to Health Care." Abridged from *Health Affairs,* Volume 6, Number 1, 1987. Copyright © 1987 Health Affairs Project Hope. Reprinted by permission of the publisher.

Gail R. Wilensky. "Solving Uncompensated Hospital Care: Targeting the Indigent and the Uninsured." Abridged from *Health Affairs,* Volume 3, Number 4, 1985. Copyright © 1985 Health Affairs Project Hope. Reprinted by permission of the publisher.

Lawrence S. Lewin and Marion Ein Lewin. "Financing Charity Care in an Era of Competition." Abridged from *Health Affairs,* Volume 6, Number 1, 1987. Copyright © 1987 Health Affairs Project Hope. Reprinted by permission of the publisher.

Chapter Eight

Robert H. Brook. "Health Services Research: Is It Good for You and Me?" Abridged from *Academic Medicine,* Volume 64, 1989. Copyright © 1989 by Association of American Medical Colleges. Reprinted by permission of the publisher.

David M. Eddy. "Variations in Physician Practice: The Role of Uncertainty." Abridged from *Health Affairs,* Volume 3, Number 2, 1984. Copyright © 1984 Health Affairs Project Hope. Reprinted by permission of the publisher.

Peter E. Dans. "The Health Care Revolution: A Preliminary Report from the Front." Abridged from *New England Journal of Medicine,* Volume 259, Number 23, 1988.

Chapter Nine

Robert N. Butler. "The Tragedy of Old Age in America." Excerpts from *Why Survive? Being Old in America* by Robert N. Butler, M.D. Copyright © 1975 by Robert N. Butler, M.D. Reprinted by permission of Harper & Row, Publishers, Inc.

Carroll L. Estes and Juanita B. Wood. "The Non-profit Sector and Community-based Care for the Elderly in the U.S.: A Disappearing Resource?" Abridged from *Social Science & Medicine,* Volume 23, Number 12, 1986. Copyright © 1986 by Pergamon Press, Inc. Reprinted by permission from the publisher.

Anne A. Scitovsky and Alexander M. Capron. "Medical Care at the End of Life: The Interaction of Economics and Ethics." Quoted with permission, from the *Annual Review of Public Health,* Volume 7. Copyright © 1986 by Annual Reviews, Inc.

Anne R. Somers and Victoria D. Weisfeld. "Improving the Elderly 'Healthspan' and Postponing 'Old Age.'" Abridged from *Clinical Report on Aging,* Volume 2, Number 3, 1988. Copyright © 1988 by American Society on Geriatrics. Reprinted by permission from the publisher.

Chapter Ten

Philip R. Lee. "AIDS: Allocating Resources for Research and Patient Care." Abridged from *Issues in Science and Technology,* Volume 2, 1986. Copyright © 1986 by the National Academy of Sciences, Washington, D.C. Reprinted with permission from the publisher.

Allan M. Brandt. "AIDS in Historical Perspective: Four Lessons from the History of Sexually Transmitted Diseases." Abridged from the *American Journal of Public Health,* Volume 78, Number 4, 1988. Copyright © 1988 by the American Public Health Association. Reprinted with permission from the publisher.

John K. Iglehart. "Financing the Struggle Against AIDS." Abridged from *New England Journal of Medicine,* Volume 317, Number 3, 1987. Copyright © 1987 by New England Journal of Medicine. Reprinted by permission of the publisher.

Anne A. Scitovsky. "The Economic Impact of AIDS in the United States." Abridged from *Health Affairs,* Fall 1988. Copyright © 1988 Health Affairs Project Hope. Reprinted by permission of the publisher.

Preface

THE THIRD EDITION of *The Nation's Health* represents part of a multidisciplinary program for advanced training and education in health policy, which has been undertaken by the Institute for Health Policy Studies, School of Medicine, and the Institute for Health and Aging, School of Nursing, University of California, San Francisco, and is funded by the Pew Memorial Trust. The editors would like to acknowledge the valuable support of the Pew Memorial Trust, which provided the funds for the editorial and clerical efforts required to prepare the new edition.

A number of people have provided invaluable assistance in the production of this book. Members of the Institute for Health Policy Studies administrative staff have cooperated on every stage of this project. Special appreciation goes to Nancy Ramsay for her critical role in the entire process, from review and selection of articles to final publication; to Ida Red for assistance in developing Chapters 4 and 9; and to Steve Guinn, who shepherded the manuscript through each stage of production. In addition we wish to thank the administration of the Institute for Health and Aging for their contributions.

Although *The Nation's Health* is a project of the Institute for Health Policy Studies, the Institute for Health and Aging, and the Pew Memorial Trust, the views expressed are those of the authors only and do not necessarily reflect those of the funding agency or the University of California.

Philip R. Lee
Carroll L. Estes

Introduction

IN THIS VOLUME, we have attempted to provide a clear view of the factors affecting the health of people who live in the United States. The emphasis of this third edition of *The Nation's Health* is the peculiar set of circumstances faced by the nation's health care system as the 1990s begin to unfold. We intend this textbook to represent a range of views about factors affecting health status, the current state of health care, and the future of the health care system.

During the 1980s there was a revolution in the organization and financing of health care. It still is difficult, if not impossible, to fully assess this revolution. Certain aspects are clear; others are still in the process of evolution. Certainly a major element on the spectrum is technological progress coupled with dramatic growth in scientific knowledge; this combination has altered the way health care is delivered and generally the way medicine is practiced in the United States. This and a number of market factors vastly affected the price paid for health care services, and in the decade of the 1980s costs became a central issue.

The market's response to soaring costs and the meaning of this response in terms of health care quality and access to services comprise a large proportion of this book. The debate about competition and regulation of those who deliver health care services rages on. Many economists and policymakers characterize the decade as a period of increased competition and deregulation. Nevertheless, government still looms large in the health care arena, and its shadow falls heavily in certain areas, particularly as a purchaser of services through Medicare and Medicaid. Most strongly felt in recent years was the institution of the prospective payment system for hospital services provided to Medicare beneficiaries.

Many sick people see medicine as the key to life and well-being, and thus doctors and hospitals become the arbiters of our most precious commodities. This, coupled with the high cost of services and the cushion provided by insurance, particularly first-dollar coverage, makes health care an atypical economic market. The result is that in a free, unfettered market with little or no regulation, those who can afford it receive care of the highest quality, others find health care to be a great financial burden, and still others are unable to obtain medical services at all. The most vulnerable fare poorest in a competitive market. Costs dictate access and quality, and the tradeoff is increasingly

problematic. In addition, those who hold the pursestrings — third party payers — have come to dictate treatment plans.

The issue most central to the nation's health is the effort to provide and
finance adequate health care services equitably for all citizens. The country's
failure to develop a comprehensive health plan to control costs and insure
access to services culminated in the 1980s in vastly inferior health care for
millions of Americans. Soaring costs and the depletion of financial support for
the uninsured and underinsured are a deadly combination existing side by
side with the world's most sophisticated and high-priced health care technology. Thus, infant mortality, which is related to access to prenatal and maternity care, is considerably higher for blacks than for whites. It is higher for the
poor than the rich, and it is higher in the United States than in 19 other
countries. Sophisticated treatments such as coronary artery bypass graft surgery, coronary angioplasty, and total hip replacement are unavailable to many
poor people who could benefit from them. Countless such discrepancies exist.

A number of our contributors argue that the nation is confronted by an
outmoded system that is the result of failed policies, abdication of government
responsibilities, and runaway technological expansion at the expense of the
provision of sound basic care for all and effective nationwide programs of
prevention and health promotion. The 1980s saw many institutions attempt to
abdicate responsibility for footing the bill for the care of the nation's neediest.
Leading the exodus was the federal government, followed closely by private
insurance companies, state government, hospitals, and other health care
providers.

Expenditures for medical care surpassed $540 billion in 1988, representing
a record 11.3 percent of the gross national product. In order to control costs,
the federal government has devised ingenious schemes to limit spending, most
notably through the Medicare prospective payment system. The repercussions
of these schemes have dramatically affected hospitals and patients alike
through reducing hospital stays and, temporarily, reducing admissions as well.

Throughout the decade, the nation also saw a rapid emergence of corporate
for-profit medicine. This hotly debated phenomenon has resulted in the
ownership for profit of many hospitals, surgicenters, urgent care centers,
clinical laboratories, and x-ray facilities. The effects of this trend are just
beginning to be understood.

The irony is that at a time when the poor have been reconciled to society's
disparities, a large segment of society has come to expect unlimited medical
care. Along with the benefits of high-priced care come the pitfalls of overtreatment, overprescribing, unnecessary surgery, and neglect of emphasis on sound
preventive measures. Thus, issues related to quality of care are being examined
anew. Measuring the effects of medical interventions is a complex and imprecise science. Increasingly, physicians are asked to interpret medical findings
that they are ill-equipped to evaluate. This causes treatment modes that differ

vastly from one physician to another, and the end result is that new issues related to inappropriate care are being addressed by investigators today.

In 1981, AIDS — acquired immune deficiency syndrome — came to the attention of public health officials in the United States. By December of that year, some 200 cases had been identified, and many of those stricken with *Pneumocystis carinii* pneumonia or other diseases that are the hallmark of infection with the human immunodeficiency virus (HIV) had already died. The number of cases reported in the United States increased to epidemic proportions in the decade that followed, and the disease has now been reported in more than 113 countries on six continents. In 1983, the U. S. Department of Health and Human Services declared AIDS to be the nation's "number one health priority." By January 1990, around the nation almost 120,000 cases had been reported. Although the period from diagnosis to death may be several years or even longer (particularly with the advent of a host of new drugs), no one is known to have recovered from the disease. The crisis of the AIDS epidemic has stimulated responses from all levels of government as well as from the private sector. Because of the nature and magnitude of this epidemic and its implications for public health and health care, AIDS occupies an important chapter here.

In this book, the role of modern medicine is critically examined. Rather than merely emphasizing its many contributions in the care of the sick and in improving the health of the population, we have looked at the complex web of issues, policies, controversies, problems, and solutions that surround the health care system. While acknowledging the inevitability of death, we would like to explore a means to greater health and longevity for everyone. Despite the quantum advances of science, a dramatic decline in infant mortality, a rapid decline in mortality due to infectious disease, and a substantial increase in life expectancy, twentieth century America still faces critical issues at the dawn of its ultimate decade.

The Jones and Bartlett Series in Health Sciences

PART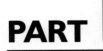

Health
and
Health Care

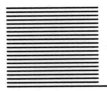

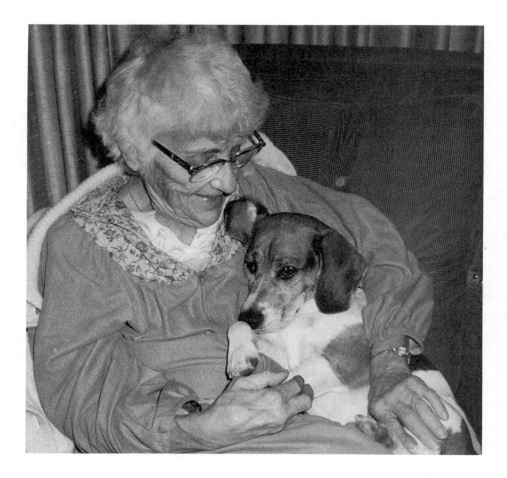

I

Health Status and Its Determinants

SINCE THE EIGHTEENTH CENTURY, there has been a dramatic improvement in the health and life span of Americans. This largely reflects a decline in the infectious diseases that once claimed the lives of many children. After dramatic declines in mortality from some infectious diseases following the introduction of the sulfanilamides in the 1930s, penicillin in the 1940s, and broad-spectrum antibiotics in the 1940s and early 1950s, progress slowed in the mid-1950s. From the mid-1950s to the mid-1960s, little progress was made in reducing infant mortality or increasing life expectancy. Beginning in the mid-1960s, however, and continuing into the 1980s, America's health improved. Infant deaths dropped to about one-half the 1965 level. The life expectancy of those born in 1979 rose more than three years over that of 1965.

In the 1980s, the leading causes of death were heart disease, cancer, strokes, accidents, homicides, and suicides. In some metropolitan areas, toward the end of the decade, AIDS became a leading cause of death among males. These causes result in part from the ways we choose to live and the environments we create. Management of these problems requires different strategies than for the infectious diseases that were the leading killers of the early part of the century. We often cannot rely on the cures of modern medicine or collective public health measures. Today, more than ever, assuring good health, or the control of disease, requires a focus on individual behavior and the factors that influence health-related behaviors. The role of health professionals has changed. When cures cannot be effected, medical care can facilitate and encourage healthy behaviors, provide treatment and rehabilitation, offer

[3]

reassurance, and help us to function as well as possible in the face of serious disease. Current technologies allow people to live many years after contracting an incurable chronic illness, thus prolonging life in a state of compromised health.

The authors in this chapter analyze trends in morbidity and mortality during the twentieth century with a view toward understanding the impact of modern medicine and public health on the human life span and on the quality of lives. These trends are of interest to policymakers and analysts as a means to understand the role of medicine and point the direction for future policy decisions. All analysts however do not draw the same conclusions from available data, and thus the conclusions drawn and the forecasts for future generations vary.

Using primary data on death rates (mortality), the late British physician Thomas McKeown, in "Determinants of Health," discusses the reasons for the dramatic decline in the death rate since the eighteenth century. He notes that much of the decline in mortality took place before the introduction of specific medical interventions, such as antibiotics. Therefore, McKeown argues, improved nutrition, a safer, cleaner environment, and a change in sexual behavior (smaller family size) were more significant determinants of health than improvements in medical care. He also suggests that for improvements in health we should look more toward changing our ways of living and personal health habits than to continued reliance on modern medicine.

Lois M. Verbrugge, in her article "Longer Life but Worsening Health? Trends in Health and Mortality of Middle-aged and Older Persons," chronicles health trends for people over the age of 45 during a 25-year period. This material gives us an opportunity to observe indicators of acute and chronic morbidity for this age group and their fluctuations through the critical periods of the 1960s and 1970s and to consider possible explanations for trends in medical and social conditions. Dr. Verbrugge analyzes such indicators as incidence of acute and chronic conditions, disability days, limitations in activity, prevalence of specific chronic and acute conditions, mortality trends, and quality of life, and she looks at the meaning of these findings for the health of future cohorts. She concludes that individuals will continue to live longer in the coming years, with a growing burden of chronic illness because of our longer life span, but that we will experience less severe chronic conditions and that medical science will become more focused on the causes and cures of chronic conditions as they continue prominence in the lives of older people.

James F. Fries outlines the basis for his theory that there is an average human life span of approximately 85 years, and that old age brings us inevitably toward death but not necessarily a greater morbidity in old age due to chronic illness. In his article, "An Introduction to the Compression of Morbidity," Dr. Fries postulates the probability that chronic illness can be postponed until late in life as a result of modern treatment modes and modifications in lifestyle, but he maintains that, although morbidity can be compressed into a shorter portion of an individual's life span, the life span itself is genetically fixed.

Jack M. Guralnik and Edward L. Schneider take issue with Fries's predictions concerning the compression of morbidity, seeing it more as a distant dream than a short-term reality. They also fail to see evidence that life expectancy is approaching its upper limit, thereby narrowly compressing mortality. These authors survey the evidence concerning incidence of morbidity and mortality and predict that in the foreseeable future prolonged life will continue to bring with it the burden of age-related chronic disease.

In the article "Race in the Health of America," S. M. Miller looks at differential health data between black and white Americans and concludes that, while considerable progress has been made in social and economic conditions for blacks, "to be poor and black is to run the risk of ill health." The author reviews current data on biological, social, economic, and cultural factors as they affect health to explore reasons why differences persist between blacks and whites in both morbidity and mortality rates. He also reviews major policy issues that affect the health of black Americans, not least the question of whether the emphasis should be on improving medical treatment or on raising the standard of living of the poor.

All our lives long, every day and every hour, we are engaged in the process of accommodating our changed and unchanged selves to changed and unchanged surroundings; living, in fact, is nothing else than a process of accommodation.

SAMUEL BUTLER

Thomas McKeown

Determinants of Health

Modern medicine is not nearly as effective as most people believe. It has not been effective because medical science and service are misdirected and society's investment in health is misused. At the base of this misdirection is a false assumption about human health. Physicians, biochemists, and the general public assume that the body is a machine that can be protected from disease primarily by physical and chemical intervention. This approach, rooted in 17th-century science, has led to widespread indifference to the influence of the primary determinants of human health — environment and personal behavior — and emphasizes the role of medical treatment, which is actually less important than either of the others. It has also resulted in the neglect of sick people whose ailments are not within the scope of the sort of therapy that interests the medical professions.

An appraisal of influences on health in the past suggests that the contribution of modern medicine to the increase of life expectancy has been much smaller than most people believe. Health improved, not because of steps when we are ill, but because we become ill less often. We remain well, less because of specific measures such as vaccination and immunization than because we enjoy a higher standard of nutrition, we live in a healthier environment, and we have fewer children.

For some 300 years an engineering approach has been dominant in biology, and medicine and has provided the basis for the treatment of the sick. A mechanistic concept of nature developed in the 17th century led to the idea that a living organism, like a machine, might be taken apart and reassembled if its structure and function were sufficiently understood. Applied to medicine, this concept meant that understanding the body's response to disease would allow physicians to intervene in the course of disease. The consequences of the engineering approach to medicine are more conspicuous today than they were in the 17th century, largely because the resources of the physical and chemical sciences are so much greater. Medical education begins with the study of the structure and function of the body, continues with examination of disease processes, and ends with clinical instruction on selected sick people. Medical service is dominated by the image of the hospital for the acutely ill, where

The late Thomas McKeown, M.D., was professor emeritus, Department of Social Medicine, University of Birmingham, England, and author of *The Role of Medicine: Dream, Mirage, or Nemesis?*

[6]

technological resources are concentrated. Medical research also reflects the mechanistic approach, concerning itself with problems such as the chemical basis of inheritance and the immunological response to transplanted tissues.

No one disputes the predominance of the engineering approach in medicine, but we must now ask whether it is seriously deficient as a conceptualization of the problems of human health. To answer this question, we must examine the determinants of human health. We must first discover why health improved in the past and then go on to ascertain the important influences on health today, in the light of the change in health problems that has resulted from the decline of infectious diseases.

It is no exaggeration to say that health, especially the health of infants and young children, has been transformed since the 18th century. For the first time in history, a mother knows it is likely that all her children will live to maturity. Before the 19th century, only about three out of every 10 newborn infants lived beyond the age of 25. Of the seven who died, two or three never reached their first birthday, and five or six died before they were six. Today, in developed countries fewer than one in 20 children die before they reach adulthood.

The increased life expectancy, most evident for young children, is due predominantly, to a reduction of deaths from infectious diseases. Records from England and Wales (the earliest national statistics available) show that this reduction was the reason for the improvement in health before 1900 and it remains the main influence to the present day.

But when we try to account for the decline of infections, significant differences of opinion appear. The conventional view attributes the change to an increased understanding of the nature of infectious disease and to the application of that knowledge through better hygiene, immunization, and treatment. This interpretation places particular emphasis on immunization against diseases like smallpox and polio, and on the use of drugs for the treatment of other diseases, such as tuberculosis, meningitis, and pneumonia. These measures, in fact, contributed relatively little to the total reduction of mortality; the main explanation for the dramatic fall in the number of deaths lies not in medical intervention. but elsewhere.

Deaths from the common infections were declining long before effective medical intervention was possible. By 1900, the total death rate had dropped substantially, and over 90 percent of the reduction was due to a decrease of deaths from infectious diseases. The relative importance of the major influences can be illustrated by reference to tuberculosis. Although respiratory tuberculosis was the single largest cause of death in the mid-19th century, mortality from the disease declined continuously after 1938, when it was first registered in England and Wales as a cause of death.

Robert Koch identified the tubercle bacillus in 1882, but none of the treatments used in the 19th or early 20th centuries significantly influenced the course of the disease. The many drugs that were tried were worthless; so, too, was the practice of surgically collapsing an infected lung, a treatment introduced about

1920. Streptomycin, developed in 1947, was the first effective treatment, but by this time mortality from the disease had fallen to a small fraction of its level during 1848 to 1854. Streptomycin lowered the death rate from tuberculosis in England and Wales by about 50 percent, but its contribution to the decrease in the death rate since the early 19th century was only about 3 percent.

Deaths from bronchitis, pneumonia, and influenza also began to decline before medical science provided an effective treatment for these illnesses. Although the death rate in England and Wales increased in the second half of the 19th century, it has fallen continuously since the beginning of the 20th. There is still no effective immunization against bronchitis or pneumonia, and influenza vaccines have had no effect on deaths. The first successful treatment for these respiratory diseases was a sulfa drug introduced in 1938, but mortality, attributed to the lung infections was declining from the beginning of the 20th century. There is no reason to doubt that the decline would have continued without effective therapeutic measures, if at a far slower rate.

In the United States, the story was similar: Thomas Magill noted that "the rapid decline of pneumonia death rates began in New York State before the turn of the century and many years before the 'miracle drugs' were known." Obviously, drug therapy was not responsible for the total decrease in deaths that occurred since 1938, and it could have had no influence on the substantial reduction that occurred before then.

The histories of most other common infections such as whooping cough, measles, and scarlet fever, are similar. In each of these diseases, mortality had fallen to a low level before effective immunization or therapy became available.

In some infections, medical intervention *was* valuable before sulfa drugs and antibiotics became available. Immunization protected people against smallpox and tetanus; antitoxin treatment limited deaths from diphtheria; appendicitis, peritonitis, and ear infections responded to surgery; Salvarsan was a long-sought "magic bullet" against syphilis, intravenous therapy saved people with severe diarrheas; and improved obstetric care prevented childbed fever.

But even if such medical measures had been responsible for the whole decline of mortality from these particular conditions after 1900 (and clearly they were not), they would account for only a small part of the decrease in deaths attributed to all infectious diseases before 1935. From that time, powerful drugs came into use and they were supplemented by improved vaccines. But mortality would have continued to fall even without the presence of these agents; and over the whole period since cause of death was first recorded, immunization and treatments have contributed much less than other influences.

The substantial fall in mortality was due in part to reduced contact with microorganisms. In developed countries an individual no longer encounters the cholera bacillus, he is rarely exposed to the typhoid organism, and his contact with the tubercle bacillus is infrequent. The death rate from these infections fell continuously from the second half of the 19th century when

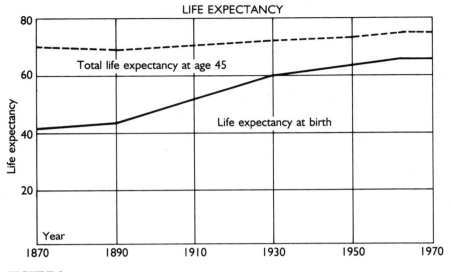

FIGURE 1

basic hygienic measures were introduced: purification of water, efficient sewage disposal, and improved food hygiene—particularly the pasteurization of milk, the item in the diet most likely to spread disease.

Pasteurization was probably the main reason for the decrease in deaths from gastroenteritis and for the decline in infant mortality from about 1900.

In the 20th century, these essential hygienic measures were supported by improved conditions in the home, the work place, and the general environment. Over the entire period for which records exist, better hygiene accounts for approximately a fifth of the total reduction of mortality.

But the decline of mortality caused by infections began long before the introduction of sanitary measures. It had already begun in England and Wales by 1838, and statistics from Scandinavia suggest that the death rate had been decreasing there since the first half of the 18th century.

A review of English experience makes it unlikely that reduced exposure to microorganisms contributed significantly to the falling death rate in this earlier period. In England and Wales that was the time of industrialization, characterized by rapid population growth and shifts of people from farms into towns, where living and working conditions were uncontrolled. The crowding and poor hygiene that resulted provided ideal conditions for the multiplication and spread of microorganisms, and the situation improved little before sanitary measures were introduced in the last third of the century.

A further explanation for the falling death rate is that an improvement in nutrition led to an increase in resistance to infectious diseases. This is, I believe, the most credible reason for the decline of the infections, at least until the late 19th century, and also explains why deaths from airborne diseases like

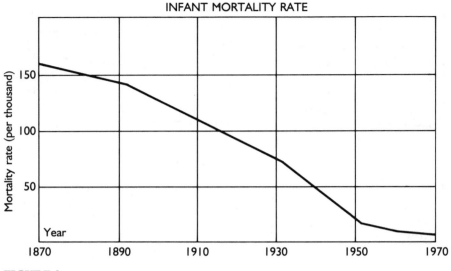

FIGURE 2

scarlet fever and measles have decreased even when exposure to the organisms that cause them remains almost unchanged. The evidence demonstrating the impact of improved nutrition is indirect, but it is still impressive.

Lack of food and the resulting malnutrition were largely responsible for the predominance of the infectious diseases, from the time when men first aggregated in large population groups about 10,000 years ago. In these conditions an improvement in nutrition was necessary for a substantial and prolonged decline in mortality.

Experience in developing countries today leaves no doubt that nutritional state is a critical factor in a person's response to infectious disease, particularly in young children. Malnourished people contract infections more often than those who are well fed and they suffer more when they become infected. According to a recent World Health Organization report on nutrition in developing countries, the best vaccine against common infectious diseases is an adequate diet.

In the 18th and 19th centuries, food production increased greatly throughout the Western world. The number of people in England and Wales tripled between 1700 and 1850 and they were fed on home-grown food.

In summary: The death rate from infectious diseases fell because an increase in food supplies led to better nutrition. From the second half of the 19th century this advance was strongly supported by improved hygiene and safer food and water, which reduced exposure to infection. With the exception of smallpox vaccination, which played a small part in the total decline of mortality, medical procedures such as immunization and therapy had little impact on human health until the 20th century.

One other influence needs to be considered: a change in reproductive behavior, which caused the birth rate to decline. The significance of this change can hardly be exaggerated, for without it the other advances would soon have been overtaken by the increasing population. We can attribute the modern improvement in health to food, hygiene and medical intervention in that order of time and importance—but we must recognize that it is to a modification of behavior that we owe the permanence of this improvement.

But it does not follow that these influences have the same relative importance today as in the past. In technologically advanced countries, the decline of infectious diseases was followed by a vast change in health problems, and even in developing countries advances in medical science and technology may have modified the effects of nutrition, sanitation, and contraception. In order to predict the factors likely to affect our health in the future, we need to examine the nature of the problems in health that exist today.

Because today's problems are mainly with noncommunicable diseases, physicians have shifted their approach. In the case of infections, interest centers on the organisms that cause them and on the conditions under which they spread. In noninfective conditions, the engineering approach established in the 17th century remains predominant and attention is focused on how a disease develops rather than on why it begins. Perhaps the most important question now confronting medicine is whether the commonest health problems—heart disease, cancer, rheumatoid arthritis, cerebrovascular disease—are essentially different from health problems of the past or whether, like infections, they can be prevented by modifying the conditions that lead to them.

To answer this question, we must distinguish between genetic and chromosomal diseases determined at the moment of fertilization and all other diseases, which are attributable in greater or lesser degree to the influence of the environment. Most diseases, including the common noninfectious ones, appear to fall into the second category. Whether these diseases can be prevented is likely to be determined by the practicability of controlling the environmental influences that lead to them.

The change in the character of health problems that followed the decline of infections in developed countries has not invalidated the conclusion that most diseases, both physical and mental, are associated with influences that might be controlled. Among such influences, those which the individual determines by his own behavior (smoking, eating, exercise, and the like) are now more important for his health than those that depend mainly on society's actions (provision of essential food and protection from hazards). And both behavioral and environmental influences are more significant than medical care.

The role of individual medical care in preventing sickness and premature death is secondary to that of other influences; yet society's investment in health care is based on the premise that it is the major determinant. It is assumed that we are ill and are made well, but it is nearer the truth to say that we are well and are made ill. Few people think of themselves as having the major responsibility for their own health, and the enormous resources that advanced countries assign to the health field are used mainly to treat disease or, to a lesser extent, to prevent it by personal measures such as immunization.

The revised concept of human health cannot provide immediate solutions for the many complex problems facing society: limiting population growth and providing adequate food in developing countries, changing personal behavior and striking a new balance between technology and care in developed nations. Instead, the enlarged understanding of health and disease should be regarded as a conceptual base with implications for services, education, and research that will take years to develop.

The most immediate requirement in the health services is to give sufficient attention to behavioral influences that are now the main determinants of health. The public believes that health depends primarily on intervention by the doctor and that the essential requirement for health is the early discovery of disease. This concept should be replaced by recognition that disease often cannot be treated effectively, and that health is determined predominantly by the way of life individuals choose to follow. Among the important influences on health are the use of tobacco, the misuse of alcohol and drugs, excessive or unbalanced diets, and lack of exercise. With research, the list of significant behavioral influences will undoubtedly increase, particularly in relation to the prevention of mental illness.

Although the influences of personal behavior are the main determinants of health in developed countries, public action can still accomplish a great deal in the environmental field. Internationally, malnutrition probably remains the most important cause of ill health, and even in affluent societies sections of the population are inadequately, as distinct from unwisely, fed. The malnourished vary in proportion and composition from one country to another, but in the developed world they are mainly the younger children of large families and elderly people who live alone. In light of the importance of food for good health, governments might use supplements and subsidies to put essential foods within the reach of everyone, and provide inducements for people to select beneficial in place of harmful foods. Of course these aims cannot exclude other considerations such as international agreements and the solvency of farmers who have been encouraged to produce meat and dairy products rather than grains. Nevertheless, in future evaluations of agricultural and related economic policies, health implications deserve a primary place.

Perhaps the most sensitive area for consideration is the funding of health services. Although the contribution of medical intervention to prevention of sickness and premature death can be expected to remain small in relation to behavioral and environmental influences, surgery and drugs are widely regarded as the basis of health and the essence of medical care, and society invests the money it sets aside for health mainly in treatment for acute diseases and particularly in hospitals for the acutely ill. Does it follow from our appraisal that resources should be transferred from acute care to chronic care and to preventive measures?

Restricting the discussion to personal medical care, I believe that neglected areas, such as mental illness, mental retardation, and geriatric care, need greatly increased attention. But to suggest that this can be achieved merely by direct transfer of resources is an oversimplification. The designation "acute care" comprises a wide range of activities that differ profoundly in their effectiveness and efficiency. Some, like surgery for accidents and the treatment of acute emergencies, are among the most important services that medicine can offer and any reduction of their support would be disastrous. Others, however, like coronary care units and iron treatment of some anemias are not shown to be effective, while still others—most tonsillectomies and routine check-ups—are quite useless and should be abandoned. A critical appraisal of medical services for acute illnesses would result in more efficient use of available resources and would free some of them for preventive measures.

What health services need in general is an adjustment in the distribution of interest and resource between prevention of disease, care of the sick who require investigation and treatment, and care of the sick who do not need active intervention. Such an adjustment must pay considerable attention to the major determinants of health: to food and the environment, which will be mainly in the hands of specialists, and to personal behavior, which should be the concern of every practicing doctor.

Health signifies that one's life force is intact, and that one is sufficiently in harmony with the social, physical, and supernatural environment to enjoy what is positively valued in life, and to ward off misfortunes and evils.

Bantu African Medical Theory

Lois M. Verbrugge

Longer Life but Worsening Health? Trends in Health and Mortality of Middle-aged and Older Persons

Over the past decade, the United States population has enjoyed rapidly declining mortality rates at all ages and for both sexes. This was an unanticipated phenomenon; it followed two decades (the 1950s and 1960s) of virtually stationary rates for males and slowly declining ones for females. Reasons for the new decline are not known with certainty, but scientists believe that early diagnosis and treatment of life-threatening chronic diseases has been a major factor.

If people's chances of survival improve, especially at middle and older ages, what happens to the health profile of the population? Does it worsen because the people "rescued" from death are ill, and their retention in the living population boosts prevalence rates of chronic conditions?

This article discusses trends in health for middle-aged (45–64) and older (65 +) persons in the United States since 1957. The principal data source is the National Health Interview Survey, which covers the noninstitutional population of the United States. Initiated in 1957, the survey now has time series of 20–25 years for indicators of acute and chronic morbidity, restricted activity and bed disability, and long-term limitations from chronic conditions.

The article is organized as follows. First we examine the data and note a worsening health profile for middle-aged and older people, for both the leading fatal diseases and the leading nonfatal conditions. We then state possible reasons for the morbidity trends — namely, increased incidence of chronic diseases, increased awareness by individuals of their health problems, earlier accommodations in activities for health problems, longer duration and greater severity of diseases due to improved survival, increased chances of developing new diseases because of improved survival, changes in institutionalization rates, and changes in survey questions. We evaluate these reasons, especially the possible effects of lower mortality

Lois M. Verbrugge, Ph.D., is a research scientist at the Institute of Gerontology, University of Michigan, Ann Arbor, Michigan.

rates on health. Finally, we speculate about the health of middle-aged and older persons in the future and how this will be reflected in health and mortality statistics.

DATA SOURCE

The National Health Interview Survey (NHIS) provides a continuous series of information about the United States population's health since 1957. Annual reports contain rates for acute condition incidence; restricted activity, bed disability, and work loss for acute conditions; restricted activity, bed disability, and work loss for all conditions (acute and chronic combined); and limitations in major or secondary activities due to chronic conditions. Limitation rates for specific chronic conditions are not published annually, but are available for selected years. Since the late 1960s, questions about the presence of specific chronic conditions have been included each year; this permits computation of prevalence rates. In the early 1970s, an item on self-rated health status was also added to the core questionnaire.

In this analysis, we review the following NHIS indicators: self-rated health status, incidence of acute conditions and disability for them, total short-term disability (for acute and chronic conditions combined), limitations due to chronic conditions (in general), and prevalence and limitations for specific chronic conditions.

SELF-RATED HEALTH STATUS

Middle-aged people rated their health about the same throughout the 1970s. In 1972, 21.5 percent reported "fair" or "poor" health status; in 1979, 21.9 percent. Older people also showed no trend; 31.0 percent reported "fair" or "poor" health in 1972; 31.4 percent in 1979. Percentages for the intervening years were similar to the 1972 and 1979 rates, for both age groups. Thus, there has not been a rapid change in people's evaluation of their health during the 1970s. Because the series is short, we cannot know if self-rated health has changed in the past 25 years. All of the other NHIS indicators we shall review have longer series and virtually all do show trends since the late 1950s.

ACUTE CONDITIONS AND ASSOCIATED DISABILITY

Compared to children and young adults, people aged 45 and older experience fewer acute conditions. Incidence rates for men aged 45 and older are now about 110 conditions per 100 persons per year, and for women aged 45 and older they are 150 per 100 persons. More than half of the conditions are respiratory; injuries and "other acute conditions" (such as headache, acute skin and musculoskeletal problems, genitourinary problems) rank next; infective/parasitic diseases and digestive conditions are infrequent.

Since the late 1950s, incidence rates for all acute conditions have declined for men and women aged 45 and older (figure 1). Lower incidence of respiratory conditions largely accounts for this decline. Injury rates have remained constant for men but increased for women.

We would expect short-term disability to reflect the incidence trends and thus to decline over time. Restricted-activity rates for acute problems did drop for about 15 years but they then increased notably during the 1970s (figure 2). Bed-disability rates increased slightly over the whole period. These disability

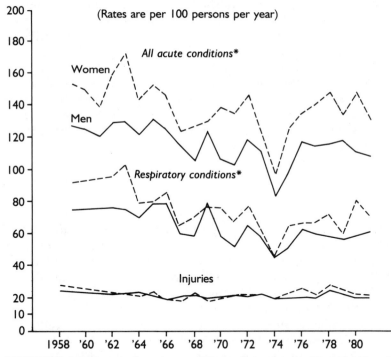

FIGURE 1 Incidence of acute conditions, for persons 45 and older, United States, 1957–1981 (per 100 persons per year).

Sources: National Center for Health Statistics, *Health Statistics.* Series B, Nos. 6, 18, 33; *Vital and Health Statistics*, Series 10, Nos. 1, 10, 15, 26, 38, 44, 54, 69, 77, 82, 88, 98, 102, 114, 120, 125, 132, 136, 139, 141 (Washington).

*Rates for 1957–58 are unusually high because of a flu epidemic, and they are often disregarded in analyses of NHIS trends.

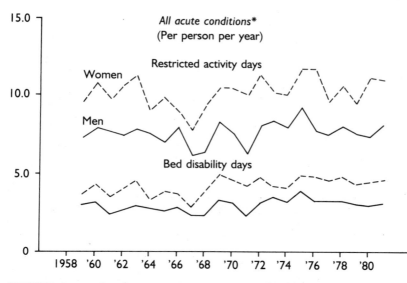

FIGURE 2 Restricted activity days and bed disability days for acute conditions, for persons 45 and older, United States, 1957–1981 (per person per year).

Sources: Same as for figure 1.

*Rates for 1957–58 are unusually high because of a flu epidemic, and they are often disregarded in analyses of NHIS trends.

trends appear for respiratory conditions and injuries separately, as well as for all acute conditions. Women show sharper increases in short-term disability than men do.

The combination of lower incidence but higher disability rates means that middle-aged and older people spend more days caring for an acute condition now than in the 1950s. In figure 3, note how the numbers of reduced activity days and bed days *per condition* have increased over time, especially for women's injuries. This phenomenon also appears for younger adults (ages 17 to 44) but is less pronounced (not shown).

In sum, men and women aged 45 and older are experiencing fewer acute conditions than before (with the exception of injuries for women), bur they are reducing activities for each acute condition more now.

DISABILITY DAYS FOR ALL CONDITIONS

Short-term disability for health problems (acute and chronic combined) increases with age. Currently, adults aged 65 and older have three times more restricted-activity days per year than children under 17, and three times more

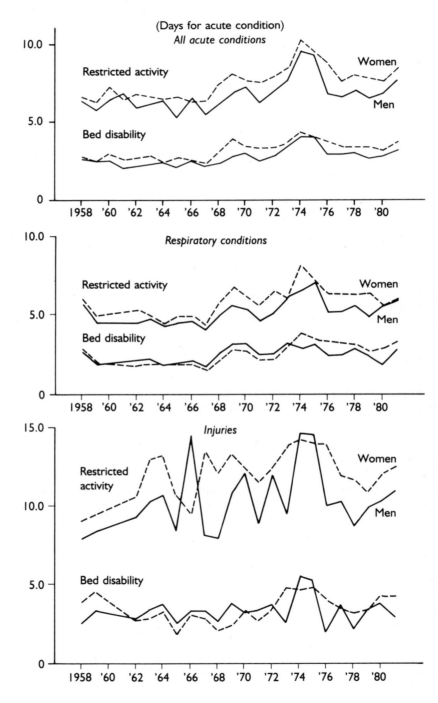

bed-disability days. The rise with age reflects rapidly increasing prevalence of chronic conditions, offset only a little by decreasing incidence of acute conditions. Men aged 45 to 64 report an average of 25 restricted-activity days per year for health problems, and women those ages report 28 days. Older men report about 35 days per year and older women 43 days. For all four groups, about one-third of the days are spent in bed. Employed people aged 45 to 64 and 65 and older report about 3 to 5 work-loss days per year.

Since the 1950s, total restricted-activity days have increased notably for middle-aged and older people (figure 4). This occurred mostly in the 1970s and it has been larger for women than for men. Nonbed days—days a person reduces usual activities but does not stay in bed—are mostly responsible for the increase. (In figure 4, bed-disability rates show no trend for older people and only a small increase for middle-aged people.) Work-loss rates have dropped for middle-aged and older working men, and they have stayed constant for working women those ages. Younger adults (25 to 44) also show increases in short-term disability over the past 25 years, but the trends (not shown) are more modest than for middle-aged and older people.

The increase in *total* restricted activity is sharper than we found for acute conditions. This suggests a substantial increase in short-term disability for chronic conditions. Is this due to more chronic morbidity especially among older adults? Or does it reflect changed health attitudes, so people are more willing to cut down their activities for bothersome chronic conditions and acute ones? We shall evaluate these and other explanations shortly.

LIMITATIONS DUE TO CHRONIC CONDITIONS

In the National Health Interview Survey, respondents are asked what their major activity was in the past year (working, keeping house, retired, school, other). Men and working women are then asked if health problems now limit them in a job, and nonworking women are asked about housework limitations. People without major-activity limitation are asked about any limitations in their secondary activities, such as church, clubs, or shopping, due to health. The questions provide indicators of long-term disability due to chronic diseases and impairments.

◀ FIGURE 3 Restricted activity days and bed disability days per acute condition, for persons 45 and older, United States, 1957–1981 (days per acute condition).

Sources: Calculated from sources of figure 1.

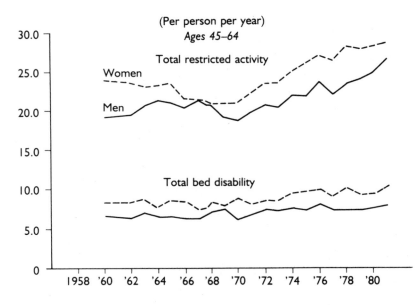

FIGURE 4 Restricted activity days and bed disability days for all conditions, for persons 45 to 64 and 65 and older, Unites States, 1957–1981 (per person per year).

Sources: National Center for Health Statistics. *Health Statistics,* Series B, Nos. 10, 29; *Vital and Health Statistics,* Series 10, Nos. 4, 5, 13, 25, 37, 43, 52, 60, 63, 72, 79, 85, 95, 100, 115, 119, 126, 130, 136, 139, 141 (Washington).

*Rates for 1957–1958 are unusually high because of a flu epidemic, and they are often disregarded in analyses of NHIS trends.

The percentage of people with major-activity limitations rises sharply with age — from 2 percent for children, to 19 percent for middle-aged adults, and 39 percent for older adults in 1981. The percentages with secondary-activity-only limitations rise from 2 percent to 5 percent and 6 percent, respectively.

Since the late 1950s, major-activity limitations have risen steadily among middle-aged people, and secondary-activity-only limitations have increased for them in the 1970s (figure 5). For older people, trends across the whole period are not clear because of highly variable rates in the earlier years. Looking just at the 1970s, we see increases in major-activity and secondary-activity limitations for older people. For young adults (17 to 44), the data suggest slowly rising limitations for both sexes (not shown).

Again, the trends could reflect rising chronic morbidity for adults. Or they could reflect more opportunities and willingness to make role accommodations for chronic health problems.

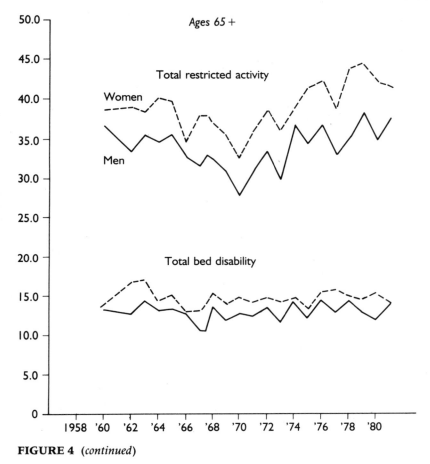

FIGURE 4 (*continued*)

PREVALENCE AND LIMITATIONS
FOR SPECIFIC CHRONIC CONDITIONS

The leading chronic conditions for middle-aged men are hypertension (20 percent), arthritis (18 percent), chronic sinusitis (16 percent), hearing impairments (15 percent), and heart disease (13 percent) (table 1). The same five problems head the women's list (arthritis, 31 percent; hypertension, 22 percent; chronic sinusitis, 21 percent; heart disease, 13 percent; hearing impairments, 9 percent). Less frequent problems (3 to 7 percent) for men aged 45 to 64 are visual impairments, back and lower extremity impairments, hemorrhoids, hay fever, diabetes, and several digestive system conditions. For women aged 45 to 64, additional problems (4 to 8 percent) are back impairments, varicose veins, hemorrhoids, hay fever, migraine, diabetes, and several

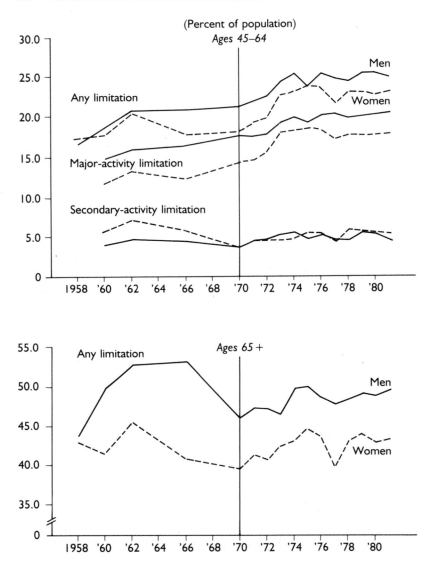

FIGURE 5 Limitations in major activities and secondary activities due to chronic conditions, for persons 45 to 64 and 65 and older, United States, 1957–1981 (percent of population).

Sources: National Center for Health Statistics. *Health Statistics*, Series B, Nos. 11, 36; *Vital and Health Statistics*, Series 10, Nos. 17, 51, 61, 79, 80, 95, 96, 100, 115, 119, 126, 130, 136, 139, 141 (Washington).

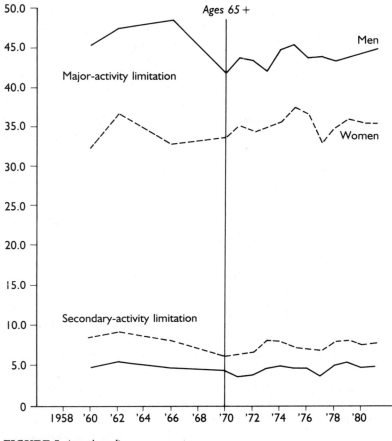

FIGURE 5 (*continued*)

skin and musculoskeletal conditions. For most chronic diseases, women aged 45 to 64 have higher prevalence rates than men do. The key exceptions are heart disease and some digestive diseases. Impairments tend to be more common for men, especially visual and hearing problems.

Limitations from chronic conditions are not common during middle age. Those which occur are mainly from heart disease (6 percent of men, 4 percent of women), arthritis (3 percent, 5 percent), various impairments (1 to 2 percent), other musculoskeletal conditions (2 percent, 2 percent), and hypertension (1 percent, 3 percent).

At older ages, prevalence rates for virtually all chronic diseases and impairments increase, but there is little change in the leading problems. The leading health problems for both sexes are arthritis (36 percent of men, 50 percent of women), hearing impairments (33 percent, 25 percent), hypertension (32 percent, 43 percent), heart disease (26 percent, 28 percent), and chronic sinusitis (14 percent, 17 percent).

Several conditions which were not important at ages 45 to 64 now become so; they are arteriosclerosis, emphysema, and prostate disease among men, and visual impairments among women. Women aged 65 and older have higher prevalence rates than men do for most chronic diseases. Important exceptions are emphysema and hernia. Compared to middle-aged people, older men and women are more similar in impairment rates; older women sometimes have higher rates than older men.

Limitations are also much more common at ages 65 and older. The principal causes of limitation are heart disease (12 percent of men, 10 percent of women) and arthritis (8 percent, 13 percent). Among men, lesser causes (3 to 4 percent) are visual impairments, emphysema, hypertension, cerebrovascular disease, and diabetes. Among women, lesser causes (3 to 5 percent) are hypertension, visual impairments, and diabetes.

The rankings for prevalence rates and limitations on rates are similar; in other words, the most common conditions also cause the most limitations in the population. This is *less* true for middle-aged people than for older ones. The reason is that, for people 45 to 64, chronic diseases are often not serious enough to force limitations, so they do not figure prominently in the list of limiting conditions. In their "absence," impairments and assorted musculoskeletal symptoms take high ranks. But for older people, chronic diseases are more severe and often require accommodations. Diseases, therefore, become prominent in the limiting conditions list, and impairments (except visual) and musculoskeletal symptoms become relatively less so.

We shall consider morbidity trends for two kinds of chronic conditions — those which are the leading causes of death and those which seldom cause death. We label them "killers" and "nonkillers" respectively.

Killer Conditions

Most of the leading causes of death for middle-aged and older people (11 titles) are chronic diseases; only a few are acute diseases (influenza/pneumonia) or external causes (accidents, suicide, homicide). Our attention centers on the chronic diseases. Choosing the same or most similar title in NHIS, what trends appear for these diseases as causes of morbidity? Do the morbidity trends mirror mortality trends for the diseases?

For middle-aged people, morbidity has risen for all but one of the diseases in the past 20 years. Cancer, diabetes, heart disease, and hypertension show especially large increases in prevalence and limitations. (The sole title with declining morbidity is kidney/ureter diseases, which includes nephritis/nephrosis.) By contrast, mortality has declined for most (8) of the diseases over the same period.

The situation is similar for older people. Morbidity has risen for most titles, especially for cancer, diabetes, heart disease, hypertension, and arteriosclerosis. At the same time, mortality rates have dropped for most (7) of the diseases.

Four patterns of change are possible: (1) rising morbidity and declining mortality, (2) rising morbidity and mortality, (3) declining morbidity and mortality, and (4) declining morbidity but rising mortality.

Nonkiller Conditions

We now examine morbidity trends for chronic conditions which seldom cause death; some are diseases, others are chronic symptoms not associated with diseases.

In the past 20 years, the following changes have occurred.

1. Varicose veins and hemorrhoids are bothersome circulatory problems. Prevalence and limitation rates for both have declined in the past two decades. This trend is opposite to those we found for life-threatening circulatory diseases.
2. Respiratory problems such as chronic sinusitis and hay fever without asthma have increased for middle-aged and older persons. This parallels the rises in bronchitis/emphysema/asthma which we noted.
3. Peptic ulcers are much less common for middle-aged men now; ulcer trends for the other age-sex groups are not clear. Most other digestive problems have decreased for all four groups, especially gallbladder conditions, frequent constipation, and chronic enteritis/ulcerative colitis.
4. Some skin problems have increased (eczema/dermatitis/urticaria, psoriasis, other inflammatory conditions) and some have decreased (corns/callosities, other hypertrophic/atrophic conditions, diseases of nail). Troubles due to corns/callosities have declined especially sharply over the period. Bunions (classified as a musculoskeletal disorder) have also diminished.
5. Musculoskeletal problems show striking rises in prevalence and limitations. Arthritis, synovitis/bursitis/tenosynovitis, displaced disc, and other musculoskeletal disorders show sharp rises for men and women in both age groups. Gout (classified as a metabolic disease but typically manifested in joint discomfort) also shows marked increases.
6. Trends for impairments are not consistent across age-sex groups. For people 65 and over, rates have declined for most titles (visual, hearing, lower extremities/hips, multiple orthopedic impairments). And although

prevalence of back/spine impairments has increased, limitations from them have diminished or remained constant. No general statement can be made for middle-aged people; some impairments show small rises, others small declines, and others no clear trend.

In sum, the most common nonkiller diseases (now and also 25 years ago) are arthritis, other musculoskeletal disorders, and chronic sinusitis. It is these problems that show consistent, large increases in rates over the past few decades. The coincidence of rising morbidity with most common nonkillers propels statistics on chronic morbidity upward. By contrast, declines in rates are attached to less prevalent diseases and to impairments.

SUMMARY OF HEALTH AND MORTALITY TRENDS

Most of the NHIS indicators show rising morbidity for middle-aged and older people since 1957. First, although acute-condition incidence rates have dropped a little, restricted activity and bed disability for them have increased. Thus, people cut down their usual activities and stay in bed more days per acute condition now than before. Second, total restricted activity (for acute and chronic conditions combined) shows especially sharp rises over time. The rise is mostly for nonbed days (cutting down activities but not staying in bed), and the data suggest that such care has increased especially for chronic problems. Third, the percentages of people who are limited in their major activity (job or housework) or their secondary activities have increased steadily since the late 1950s for middle-aged people and in the 1970s for older people. Fourth, chronic diseases which often cause death ("killers") have risen in both prevalence and limitations; this is especially true for cancer, heart disease, hypertension, and diabetes. Chronic diseases which are common but seldom cause death ("nonkillers") have also risen in prevalence and limitations; this is especially true for arthritis, other musculoskeletal disorders, and chronic sinusitis, which are the leading nonfatal diseases for middle-aged and older adults.

Examining fewer health indicators and a shorter time period (1966–1976), Colvez and Blanchet noted similar trends. Six conditions showed increased limitation rates for middle-aged people (malignant neoplasms for women, diabetes, heart conditions for men, hypertension, other circulatory system conditions, other musculoskeletal disorders). Two conditions increased in limitations for older people (diabetes and other circulatory system conditions). Our analysis shows increases for these same conditions and for many others over the past two decades. Declining morbidity appears for relatively few indicators (incidence of acute conditions, especially respiratory diseases; prevalence and limitations for some digestive and urinary chronic conditions, varicose veins and hemorrhoids, some skin conditions, and impairments for persons aged 65 and older). Few indicators show no trend over the 20 to 25 year period. In sum, signs of increasing morbidity far exceed signs of decreasing morbidity or no change.

In the same time interval, mortality has declined for middle-aged and older people. Table 3 records mortality rates in 1960 and 1978 for all causes and for chronic diseases which are leading causes of death. (The 1960 to 1978 period is chosen to be similar to the 1957–1981 span of NHIS indicators. Most of the mortality decline occurred after 1967.) For all causes, rates have dropped 15 to 30 percent for all age groups (45–54, 55–64, 65–74, 75–84, 85 +). Declines for cardiovascular diseases (diseases of the heart, hypertension, cerebrovascular diseases, and arteriosclerosis) are especially large. Diabetes, hernia, and nephritis/nephrosis also registered declines. A few leading causes do show increased rates (cancer, mainly for men; cirrhosis, mainly for people aged 45 to 64; bronchitis/emphysema/asthma, mainly for people 65 and older). (The rise of "other diseases of arteries/arterioles/capillaries" is spurious, owing to changes in disease classification between the seventh and eighth ICD revisions.) These increases are irregular, being limited to just some age-sex groups, while the other groups show declines. In sum, the main picture is one of declining mortality from killer diseases for middle-aged and older men and women.

WHAT EXPLAINS LONGER LIFE BUT WORSENING HEALTH?

First let us consider possible reasons for the increasing prevalence of chronic diseases and limitations from them in the population, and then possible reasons for declining mortality from chronic diseases.

Worsening Health

Increasing prevalence and limitations from chronic diseases can be due to six factors:

1. Higher incidence of chronic diseases. If environmental quality or personal health habits deteriorated notably since 1957, chances of developing chronic diseases (killers and nonkillers) would rise.
2. Earlier diagnosis of chronic diseases. If people now learn that they have a disease earlier in its development than they did in the 1950s, this awareness causes more (better) disease reporting in health interviews and thereby higher prevalence rates.
3. Earlier accommodations in activities for disease. If people now change their jobs and other activities at earlier stages of a disease or they cut down their usual activities more for flareups, this boosts disability indicators such as limitation and restricted-activity rates.

4. Improved survival. As mortality rates drop, some people are " rescued" from death and remain among the living. Most of these "new survivors" are ill with chronic diseases, though not so ill as those who died. By staying alive longer, they have more years for their illnesses to advance in severity and more time to develop other chronic conditions, both killers and non-killers. The survivors may actually be more susceptible to new illnesses than their healthier age peers are; this is an intriguing question. Lower mortality, therefore, makes population health worsen in three ways: by immediate increases in prevalence rates, by more gradual increases in limitation rates and other severity measures, and by further gradual increases in prevalence rates due to new illnesses among the rescued.

5. Less institutionalization. Illness and impairment are principal reasons for entry into nursing and personal care homes. If ill people are more able to receive home and community care, this can reduce rates of institutional residence. Prevalence and limitation rates in the noninstitutional population should rise accordingly.

6. Questionnaire changes. Changes in procedures for eliciting chronic disease reports can influence morbidity rates.

How plausible are these changes over the past 25 years?

1. Risks of developing chronic diseases have probably fallen due to safer work and home settings and to better lifestyle behaviors (less smoking by adults, reduced fats and alcohol, increased aerobic activity). Health habits affect disease risks in a slow and cumulative way; so the consequences of lifestyle changes by the population emerge gradually over decades rather than by immediate effects on disease incidence and severity.

2. People are now more aware of their chronic diseases than before due to marked improvements in diagnostic techniques and to more frequent visits to physicians (the percentage with a visit in the past six months has risen steadily over 20 years).

3. It is quite likely that people are more willing and able to adopt the sick role now than in the 1950s. People now know more about how their own behaviors affect disease onset and prognosis; in particular, the belief that disability slows the progress of chronic diseases and speeds recovery from acute ones may be stronger now. Furthermore, there are now ampler social supports for disability. Employer policies about work absence are more flexible, and public assistance programs, pension plans, and health insurance make it easier and more remunerative to be ill or disabled on a long-term basis. Finally, public attitudes about disability—both about short-term reductions and about permanent disability—seem more empathic and flexible.

4. Mortality declines have principally occurred in the 1970s. Increases in chronic morbidity are most pronounced in that decade as well. This

sensitivity of morbidity trends to mortality trends is not surprising especially for older ages, since every added year of life entails high risks of having diseases worsen or developing new ones.

5. Institutionalization rates have risen sharply in the past 20 years. Residence rates in nursing and personal care homes have increased for middle-aged and older persons, especially for those aged 75 to 84 and 85 and older.
6. Changes in data collection procedures can cause sudden jumps in rates, but they are unlikely to cause secular trends. The NHIS questionnaire has changed in several important ways, but there is no evidence this underlies the observed morbidity trends.

Overall, the most plausible reasons for increased morbidity are people's greater awareness of their diseases due to earlier diagnosis, lower population mortality rates, and, possibly, earlier accommodations for disease. Trends in disease incidence and institutionalization have probably acted to decrease morbidity, and procedural changes in NHIS cannot account for the long trends.

Longer Life

Decreasing mortality from chronic diseases can be due to four factors:

1. Lower incidence of chronic diseases. If environmental quality or personal health habits have improved over time, risks of developing chronic diseases would fall. This would ultimately (but not rapidly) be reflected in lower mortality rates.
2. Earlier or better treatment of chronic diseases. If medical intervention is now applied at earlier stages of a disease because of earlier or better diagnosis, diseases advance more slowly and case fatality is lower. Similarly, if medical treatments are more efficacious now, this too slows the course of disease and lowers case fatality.
3. Earlier or better self-care for disease. When diagnosed with a chronic disease, people can change their health habits in hopes of slowing its development. If people are now more likely to change their risk factors such as smoking, alcohol consumption, and stress level than before, this will delay death from their disease.
4. More heroic medical care near death. When disease has advanced and death is near, intensive drug therapy and technical procedures may stave off death. If heroic measures are applied more now than before, death can be delayed for days, months, and occasionally years.

How plausible are these changes for the past 25 years?

As noted above, incidence rates for many chronic diseases have probably fallen. Few data are available to document trends in incidence; for cancer, incidence rates have fallen for women but have increased for men.

Early diagnosis and improved medical therapy for cardiovascular diseases are thought to be key reasons for declining mortality rates from them. Better drugs and surgical procedures for diabetes, early-stage respiratory diseases, and hernia have probably improved the prognosis for those conditions. By contrast, although some cancers are now detected earlier than in the 1950s, there have been few significant improvements in cancer therapy.

Lifestyle changes by the population have probably influenced the progression of chronic diseases. When diagnosed with a killer disease, adults are now strongly encouraged to alter their habits and many do so in hopes of prolonging life. Earlier diagnosis has improved individuals' chances to make adaptations that do, in fact, influence the disease process.

Although heroic medical care is more common now than before, it is applied to relatively few people and probably has a negligible effect on mortality rates.

Overall, the most plausible reasons for decreased mortality are earlier and better medical care of diagnosed cases, earlier and better self-care after diagnosis, and possibly lower incidence of some chronic diseases. Heroic measures have minimal effect.

The Compatibility of Longer Life and Worsening Health

The conjunction of increased morbidity and decreased mortality for American adults is not contradictory, but is instead a logical result of medical and social changes in the past 25 years. During this period, secondary prevention—the early detection of disease and subsequent intervention to slow its progress—was emphasized in medical care and personal health care. Numerous drugs to control diseases were developed and widely disseminated through medical practice. Increasingly, individuals were encouraged to take more responsibility for their long-term health—to have persistent symptoms diagnosed, to follow drug regimens for diagnosed conditions, and to view short-term restrictions and long-term disability as means to improve health and longevity. Social programs made it easier for people to be disabled for a short time or permanently. These changes led naturally to increased chronic prevalence rates and increased acute and chronic disability rates in the population. At the same time, these medical and social changes slowed the progress of diagnosed chronic conditions, leading to decreased mortality rates. The mortality declines further spurred morbidity rates upward as the "new survivors" had their conditions worsen and as they developed new illnesses during their extra years of life.

Trends for specific chronic conditions are also consistent with these medical and social changes. Recall that morbidity increased while mortality decreased for most killer diseases (diabetes, diseases of heart, hypertension, cerebrovascular diseases, arteriosclerosis, bronchitis/emphysema/asthma at ages 45 to 64, and hernia). This is a logical outcome of earlier diagnosis, better medical care, and better self-care. Several killers show rising morbidity and mortality (malignant neoplasms, bronchitis/emphysema/asthma at ages 65 and older, cirrhosis at ages 45 to 64). (The mortality rise for "other diseases of arteries, etc." is spurious.) Medical advances have been slow for these diseases especially at later stages. Also, although awareness and accommodations may have increased, lifestyle changes do nor deter their progress much. And as cohorts with heavy smoking and drinking histories entered middle and older ages, incidence may have actually risen for these diseases. (Cancer incidence rates have risen for men.) Several killer diseases show declining morbidity and mortality in some age-sex groups (hernia, nephritis/nephrosis). These conditions are more amenable to medical treatment than those just mentioned. Lower morbidity rates also suggest lower incidence for them now.

The principal nonkiller diseases have risen in prevalence and limitations. This would be a logical outcome of more awareness, more accommodations, and longer lives. For impairment trends, we must look for different causes than for disease trends. Impairments (especially orthopedic ones) are often initiated by accidents, and physical aids are often used in their treatment. The decline in impairment rates for older people may reflect improvements in prosthetic devices and rehabilitation. (Injury rates have not fallen for people aged 65 and older, so we cannot argue that risks of acquiring impairments are lower now.)

The morbidity and mortality trends are contradictory only if we adopt a limited epidemiological approach and see them as straightforward outcomes of disease incidence and duration (severity). But once we invoke medical and social changes that affect health status and health behavior in contemporary America, the contradiction evaporates and the trends are consistent and even expected.

MODELS THAT LINK MORBIDITY AND MORTALITY

In premodern society, the links between morbidity and mortality are simple, since acute conditions are the main causes of illness and death and interventions are uncommon (or at least not very effective). But in modern society, chronic conditions predominate and interventions are common. Many chronic conditions are not fatal but do bother people and induce them to change activities and seek medical care. Others are fatal and will ultimately cause death, though personal and medical interventions can delay that outcome and provide symptom relief. Health habits and medical care are aimed at slowing the progress of chronic diseases, more than toward preventing them in the first place or curing them entirely. This can change as research identifies causal factors of chronic disease or finds ways to arrest it. Overall, the causal links between morbidity and mortality become more complex, and we must look to medicine and social behavior as well as epidemiology for explanations of aggregate change (trends in morbidity and mortality rates).

Ultimately, health scientists would like to develop a model that states how changes in chronic disease incidence and prevalence affect mortality rates. The model would also allow us to specify how changes in mortality will affect the population's health profile. The model would include risk factors, showing how changes in medical practice, physical environment, and individual behavior propel changes in disease incidence, prevalence, and mortality. The model could be elaborated to include assumptions about biological limits to mortality and disease reduction or about changes in virus structure and potency. And it could be extended to study the implications of morbidity and mortality changes on health expenditures and services. To craft a model linking morbidity and mortality is difficult but not impossible.

With a model, scientists could interpret recent trends and make future forecasts about morbidity and mortality with more confidence and rigor than is now possible. Contemporary analyses are necessarily more speculative, and they can easily differ from each other by using different assumptions about medical and social changes.

THE HEALTH OF FUTURE COHORTS

In predicting how healthy or ill future cohorts of middle-aged and older persons will be, we must, therefore, keep myriad factors in mind. The chances of acquiring and dying from chronic diseases are influenced by individuals' lifestyle habits and health care practices, the safety of work and residence environments, and medical drugs and procedures. The chances of being limited by a chronic disease or impairment are further influenced by public attitudes about illness, definitions of disability used by public assistance programs, employer policies about work absence, health insurance coverage, and pension supports. Moreover, the health and mortality profile of an age group reflects not just their contemporary risks but the cumulation of lifetime risks. Cohorts who will be middle-aged and older several decades from now will have had very different inputs to their health and longevity than current cohorts of those ages. Here, we offer some thoughts about those inputs and their consequences for health and mortality.

Future cohorts of middle-aged and older people will probably have more years of healthful lifestyles than current cohorts. Work environments will probably pose fewer hazards for chronic disease development; whether community environments will improve is less certain. Medical diagnosis and treatment will be more efficacious, so that diseases are slowed and sometimes even arrested or reversed. Public attitudes and financial supports may make it easier for people to adopt the sick role temporarily or permanently. But more than ever today, ill people may wish to remain socially active, and employer policies may help them remain employed. Whether seriously ill people are more likely to remain in the community than enter institutions is uncertain, and it will depend greatly on public financing of care in both places. Summarizing this array of medical and social changes, we can anticipate (1) lower incidence of chronic diseases, (2) earlier diagnosis of chronic diseases, though the gains may be smaller than in the past 25 years, (3) earlier accommodations in activities for disease (the net results of some factors which encourage disability and some which discourage it), (4) earlier and better medical treatment of chronic diseases, and (5) earlier and better self-care for diseases.

The consequences for health and mortality statistics would be as follows. Mortality rates will continue to fall as fast or faster than in the 1970s. Prevalence rates for killer diseases could rise in the next few decades, mainly due to earlier diagnosis and to mortality reductions. In fact, further mortality declines will have a pernicious effect on population morbidity since future "new survivors" will be even more ill and susceptible than those in the 1970s. Gradually, as primary prevention succeeds and incidence rates fall, the upward trend in prevalence rates may be slowed or stopped. Prevalence rates for nonkiller diseases will probably increase further, because longer life gives people more opportunity to develop them and because advances in primary prevention are unlikely. Little is known now about the causes of nonfatal chronic conditions, and medical research will continue to focus on killer diseases in coming decades. Short-term disability rates may continue to rise, a reflection of earlier diagnoses, mortality reductions, and personal motivations to care for illness. So many factors affect long-term disability, it is difficult to make any forecasts. One possibility is that complete disability rates fall while partial disability rates rise; this can occur if medical treatments improve and if ill people choose to make minor accommodations but not relinquish social roles entirely. Overall, morbidity for middle-aged and older people will probably shift toward nonkiller conditions, less severe symptoms, and partial accommodations.

Underlying the statistics will be individuals experiencing diseases, symptoms, and disability. What will their daily lives and later years be like compared to current individuals? At a given age, they will probably have fewer chronic diseases (both killers and nonkillers). Symptoms from the diseases they do have will tend to be less severe than at present, partly because diseases are less advanced and partly because the diseases will more often be nonkillers. People will probably have fewer serious limitations in their social activities, physical functioning, and mobility. And individuals who do have severe conditions may still be more independent than now because of better special aids and public accommodations. Thus, middle-aged and older people may be more comfortable and active even when chronic diseases are present. Individuals can expect to live longer. An unfortunate consequence is that they may ultimately develop more chronic conditions in their lifetime than now, especially the nonkiller conditions. And symptoms due to natural aging processes (such as graying of hair and loss of skin elasticity) will also accumulate. The death process might be swifter than now and involve the breakdown of several body systems at once; this endpoint scenario will be more common as primary prevention of disease succeeds.

In conclusion, for the rest of this century some health statistics will continue to show increasing morbidity in the United States population. This is especially likely for statistics on prevalence and limitations for nonkiller conditions. Increasingly, individuals will choose behaviors early in life with the hope of preventing killer diseases and debilitating nonkillers such as arthritis and hearing loss. Medical research and care will continue to focus on diagnosis and control of killer diseases. But as medical advances for them slow and as nonkillers assume prominence in patients' lives, medicine will gradually shift emphasis toward musculoskeletal diseases and symptoms, sensory impairments, allergies, and skin problems of middle-aged and older persons.

Health is not a condition of matter, but of Mind; nor can the material senses bear reliable testimony on the subject of health.

MARY BAKER EDDY

James F. Fries

An Introduction to the Compression of Morbidity

The thesis of the compression of morbidity presents a paradigm for the aging process and suggests new approaches toward preventive gerontology. An allegory is that of Oliver Wendell Holmes Sr.'s "One Hoss Shay," which functioned perfectly over a long period of years until all parts simultaneously wore out and the shay collapsed into a pile of sawdust, nuts and bolts. If a human organism can lead a long and vigorous life, terminated by a sharp decline mandated by senescence, then a social and individual ideal for many might be reached.

The basic syllogism of the compression of morbidity is that since the age of first infirmity can be postponed but the lifespan itself is genetically fixed, the period of infirmity can be shortened. In more general formulation, the theorem holds that for the average person a) if morbidity may be defined as that period from the onset of the first irreversible chronic disease or aging marker until death, and b) if the date of occurrence of that marker can be postponed until later in life, and if c) the rate of such postponement can be greater than the rate of increase in adult life expectancy, then d) morbidity for the average person can be compressed into a shorter period of time.

Interest in this paradigm has been high, in part because the implications of the compression of morbidity both for health policy and for demographic predictions are substantially different from those previously suggested. Further, the concept puts emphasis on prevention rather than on cure, postponement rather than palliation, and personal autonomy rather than paternalistic care. This paradigm is more pessimistic than some previous forecasts with regard to the capacity to infinitely extend life, but more optimistic with regard to the ability to improve the quality of the later years of life.

On the other hand, in the first three-quarters of the 20th century there seems little doubt that morbidity for the average person increased. Health advances over this period were characterized by sharp reductions in infant

---

James F. Fries, M.D., is professor of medicine at Stanford University, Stanford, California.

mortality, major increases in life expectancy from birth (from 47 years to 74), decline and virtual elimination of most of the acute infectious causes of death prominent early in the century, and a concomitant major increase in chronic and morbid diseases such as atherosclerosis, neoplasia, and osteoarthritis.

However, a dramatic reversal both in the incidence and prevalence of chronic illness (figure 1) began in the mid-1970's, defying previous predictions. The implications of this impressive decline with regard to mortality are now slowly being worked into predictive models, but the implications for morbidity (figure 2) remain far from fully appreciated.

A number of semantic contradictions have become imbedded in the models with which we traditionally view illness and in which we contemplate the health problems of the future. Several corollaries to the thesis of the compression of morbidity are of importance in understanding the biology which underlies the statistical record. These may be discussed under seven headings.

The Lifespan is Finite

Statistical (and medical) models have contained the implicit assumption that if all diseases and all accidents were eliminated, there could be no death. Such assumptions have been maintained despite abundant evidence to the contrary.

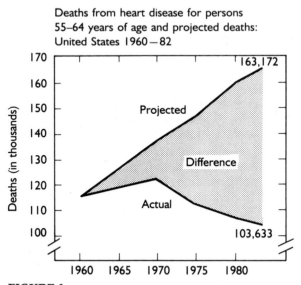

Deaths from heart disease for persons
55–64 years of age and projected deaths:
United States 1960 – 82

FIGURE 1
Reprinted with permission from the National Center for Health Statistics, P.M. Golden: *Charting the Nation's Health, Trends since 1960.* DHHS Pub. No. (PHS) 85-1251. Public Health Service, Washington, D.C., U.S. Government Printing Office, Aug. 1985.

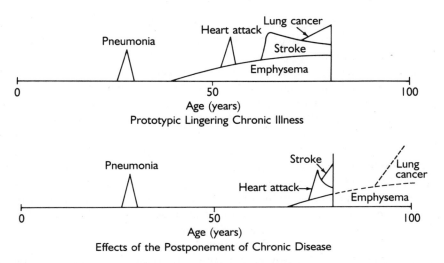

Prototypic Lingering Chronic Illness

Effects of the Postponement of Chronic Disease

FIGURE 2 The Compression of Morbidity. Two health-lives are diagrammed, the upper with poor health habits and the lower with better health habits. The period of adult vigor prior to infirmity is reduced in the lower example.
Reprinted with permission from Fries, JF and Crapo, LM, *Vitality and Aging*, W.H. Freeman, San Francisco, 1981.

At least ten general lines of evidence indicate the finitude of the human lifespan, and have been discussed more fully elsewhere. First, there have been no fortunate individuals who have outlived the natural laws. In the United States, for example, the oldest individual has lived to 113 years, 274 days. Sporadic claims of extreme longevity, in individuals or in populations, have been disproven and are now seldom advanced. Second, the steadily rectangularizing mortality curves frequently shown to demonstrate the major advances of health in this century point clearly toward an upper bound. Third, Gompertz's law, first formulated in 1825, notes exponential increase in mortality with age in all populations. Fourth, different animal species clearly have different lifespans, ranging from minutes or days to nearly 200 years, and it seems unlikely that the human species should be different. Fifth, anthropological estimates of lifespan based upon brain size/body weight ratios imply little change in human lifespan over the past 100,000 years. Sixth, no reasons why important genetic change in the longevity characteristics of the species over recent time periods might have occurred have been advanced. Seventh, in the laboratory, the Hayflick phenomenon suggests a finite number of doubling cycles for somatic cells in tissue culture. Eighth, physiologic studies of organ reserve show a decline in maximum functional capacity of the average organism approximating 1½% per year which mandate eventual function insufficient to maintain life. Ninth, data since 1932 on longevity in the developed nations are marked by approximate constancy, with changes statistically consistent with the larger number of individuals at risk in successive cohorts and the larger number of individuals escaping early death. Finally, the phenomenon of increasing frailty with age, although poorly documented in available national statistics, is a matter of daily observation.

We have estimated the average human lifespan at approximately 85 years, with a standard deviation of four to five years, based on projection of life expectancy changes from different age points, observed declines in physiologic reserve, estimation of a normal curve from a known "tail" and other types of convergence extrapolations. Such estimates are obviously "soft" but are surprisingly insensitive to major changes in assumptions. Moreover, even competing projections which ignore senescence as a factor for mortality project only an eleven month increase in life expectancy after age 100 over the coming 40 years. The markedly higher estimates of average maximal life potential occasionally advanced are based either on a confusion of the concepts of the maximal individual lifespan with the maximal species lifespan (i.e., because one person has lived to 113, everyone has the potential to live to age 113) or to the belief that a particular intervention (e.g. gerovital, under-nutrition, vitamin C) will remove the limits.

We Reduce Premature Death, We Do Not Save Lives

Reduction in infant mortality, passage of seat belt laws, and elimination of smallpox improve statistical "life expectancy," which is a pejorative and somewhat misleading term. Lives, however, are not thereby saved; rather, deaths are postponed. An early life death from an acute cause prevented becomes a death from chronic illness later in life. Postponement of a death from chronic illness takes one toward old age.

Natural Death Must Exist if There Is a Natural Force of Senescence

The semantics of recording of death require specification of cause. In this regard, the concept of cause implies the striking down of a healthy individual. The frailty of the host is not considered. A major confusion develops between "underlying" and "proximate" cause. The certifying physician records "bronchopneumonia," "influenza," or "heart failure" when a terminally frail individual meets one of the unavoidable perturbations to homeostasis which are part of daily life. The effects of such recording are insidious, perpetuating myths that only the lack of perfectly effective treatment for the proximate "cause" prevents immortality, and encouraging heroic attempts to save the life of the terminally ill patient. The nomenclature of senescence becomes thus confounded with that of disease. Arteriosclerosis, cataract, hearing loss, slowed reflexes, diminished muscle power, or depressed maximum cardiac output are for many individuals a part of their biology over time rather than the result of disease processes as generally conceived.

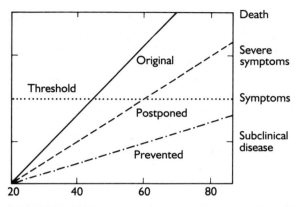

FIGURE 3 An incremental model of chronic disease. The model is characterized by early age of onset, progression of various rates in different individuals, and passage of symptomatic threshold at which time a clinical diagnosis may be made. Reprinted with permission from Fries, JF and Crapo, LM, *Vitality and Aging*, W.H. Freeman, San Francisco, 1981.

The Major Chronic Diseases, Like Aging, Are Universal, Progressive, Presymptomatic Usually for Decades, and Relatively Resistant to Treatment

Atherosclerosis, emphysema, osteoarthritis, the statistical likelihood of malignant change, and the other major disease processes making up most of current mortality and morbidity are increasingly recognized as having antecedent presymptomatic findings identifiable early in life, increasing to universal prevalence with age, and marked by rates of disease accumulation which are remarkably different between individuals, some persons exhibiting rapid progression to severe disability or death while others remain presymptomatic throughout their entire lives (figure 3). Emphasis on the universality of these disease phenomena and upon the long pre-symptomatic period is important, since it focuses attention upon factors (and possible interventions) which alter the rate of accumulation of the chronic disease pathology and which very well may need to be undertaken at periods of life long before emergence of the first irreversible symptom.

Chronic Diseases Are Characterized by Risk Factors which Accelerate or Decelerate Progression

A large and growing literature has identified many factors (such as cigarette smoking, lack of exercise, obesity, hypertension, saturated fat intake, alcohol intake, fiber intake, occupational toxins, and environmental toxins), which are strongly associated with chronic disease and for which mechanisms have been identified by which the risk factor might be expected to accelerate disease progression. Conclusive evidence of causality, and in some instances proof of effective intervention, is now available for a number of these factors, such as cigarette smoking, dietary fat intake, control of hypertension, asbestos and silica exposure, and exercise, and strong circumstantial evidence exists for others. Most authorities conclude that the major recent improvement in the most important disease category, cardiovascular disease, is largely a result of improvement in a combination of these factors.

Aging, Like Chronic Disease, Is Universal, Progressive, Presymptomatic Usually for Decades, and Relatively Resistant to Treatment

No formal justification for such an assertion should be required; indeed, it might be considered a summary statement of the physiological, pathological, functional, and observational studies of gerontologists.

Aging is Characterized by Risk Factors which Accelerate or Decelerate Progression and which Prevent the Organism from Expression of Its Full Biologic Potential at a Given Age

An emergent and fascinating literature documents the increasing variability in various markers of aging between individuals as they grow older. Unlike an intuitive assumption that individuals might differ most in their various abilities at the time when their powers were greatest, the differences between individuals increase with age. This increasing variability holds for physiologic processes, functional abilities, cognitive processes, and social variables.

Moreover, intervention studies have documented the ability to improve performance in a great many areas despite advancing age. The ability to improve performance at cognitive tasks, at athletic achievements, and in personal autonomy have been repeatedly demonstrated. Interventions have generally been directed at countering what might be generally termed "detraining," in which lack of sufficient use of a particular faculty had resulted in its relative atrophy.

Clearly, these studies imply that a considerable part of the increasing variability with age and the decreasing functional capacity with age are a consequence of the failure of average individuals to express their full biologic potential at a given age (figure 4). The magnitude of these effects suggests the ability to effect major decreases in the morbid burdens associated with aging by decreasing the risk factors of disuse, in a manner analogous to those which are successfully helping to reduce the morbid burdens of chronic disease. Despite biologic limits therefore, there are potential initiatives for significantly compressing the terminal morbidity associated with senescent decrements as well as those elements of morbidity associated with well-known

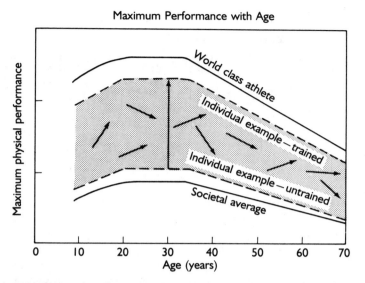

FIGURE 4 The plasticity of aging. Within the biological potential of the organism are multiple possible pathways to improvement of performance despite age, bounded by present performance and maximum potential performance. Reprinted with permission from Fries, JF and Crapo, LM, *Vitality and Aging*, W.H. Freeman, San Francisco, 1981.

disease processes. To effect such reductions, however, requires a change in our traditional views of disease and senescence. These considerations suggest that the numerically most important health advances over the next decades may occur in the area of preventive gerontology, practiced throughout the adult life cycle.

In America the passion for physical well-being . . . is general.

ALEXIS DE TOCQUEVILLE

Jack M. Guralnik/Edward L. Schneider

The Compression of Morbidity: A Dream Which May Come True, Someday!

Trends in mortality and morbidity are of great interest and importance to a variety of disciplines. They have been employed by groups ranging from insurance actuaries in determining premiums for life insurance and annuities to Congressional committees planning social security programs. They are currently of interest to Federal, state, and local governments as well as the private health care industry in planning for acute and long-term care provision. In the future they will probably be employed for numerous additional unanticipated uses.

Because of the enormous policy and planning implications of changes in mortality and morbidity rates, it is important that the issues be presented in an accurate, yet uncomplicated manner. In an eloquent article, Fries proposed the very seductive concept of an ongoing and continuous compression of morbidity. He made four predictions: the number of very old persons will not increase, the average period of diminished physical vigor will decrease, chronic diseases will occupy a smaller proportion of the lifespan, and the need for medical care in later life will decrease. Recognizing the enormous policy implications of these predictions, a number of individuals analyzed the data and logic upon which these hypotheses were based and arrived at very different conclusions.

The compression of morbidity should be the highest goal of gerontology. It would be wonderful to have disease, illness, disability, and dependency compressed into a few short years or even months! It is a goal we all share with Dr. Fries. We also concur with Dr. Fries that, with increased understanding and effective treatment and prevention of the diseases and disorders of aging, this goal will *eventually* come true. However, our disagreement with Dr. Fries is in the timing of this compression of morbidity. He believes that it is occurring now and will continue to occur, while we find no evidence that a

Jack M. Guralnik, M.D., is an epidemiologist with the Epidemiology, Demography, and Biometry Program, National Institute on Aging, National Institutes of Health, Bethesda, Maryland.

Edward L. Schneider, M.D., is executive director of the Ethel Percy Andrus Gerontology Center, University of Southern California, Los Angeles.

compression of morbidity is occurring now or will occur in the near future without significant breakthroughs in the prevention and treatment of the diseases and disorders of aging.

Assessing Compression of Morbidity

Compression of morbidity is dependent on two independent factors: the time of onset of morbidity and the life expectancy of the population. This is a dynamic process which can only be assessed by documenting, at two points in time, both average life expectancy and average age of onset of some measure of significant morbidity.

In order to facilitate discussion of trends in the compression of morbidity, we present a simple model (figure 1) which illustrates the change in population morbidity level as a function of changes in life expectancy and disability-free life expectancy, a measure of the time of onset of significant morbidity. Life expectancy is defined here as the average number of years of life expected by a given population at a specific age. Disability-free life expectancy is the average number of remaining years of life free of significant morbidity, defined in terms of severe disability. We prefer to use disability since it provides a meaningful measure of the burden of morbidity in an older population. If, from time 1 to time 2, life expectancy increases by a certain number of years (x axis) and disability-free life expectancy increases by that same number of years (y axis), then the average burden of morbidity of the population will be unchanged (this is represented by the line drawn at 45 degrees in figure 1A). If life expectancy is increasing at a rate in excess of disability-free life expectancy, then the average burden of morbidity in the population will be expanding (area below diagonal line in figure 1B). If, on the other hand, there is an ongoing increase in disability-free life expectancy which exceeds increases in life expectancy, then a compression in the average burden of morbidity in the population will be occurring (area above diagonal line in figure 1C).

IS THERE AN ONGOING COMPRESSION OF MORBIDITY?

To assess if an ongoing compression of morbidity is occurring, we must examine recent changes both in life expectancy and in disability-free life expectancy. Fries argued that the rates of increase in life expectancy are slowing down and that the age of death is being compressed into a smaller range of years. We certainly do not question the impressive compression of mortality that occurred in the first part of this century. The dramatic reduction in deaths in infancy and early adulthood in the first forty years of this century led to a trend toward rectangularization of survival curves from 1900 to 1940 (figure 2). However, this trend is related almost entirely to improved survival in

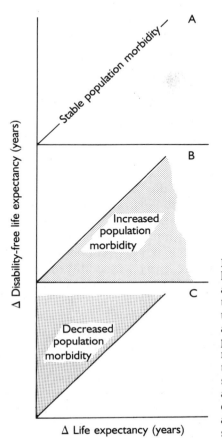

FIGURE 1 Change in population morbidity level as a function of changes in life expectancy and disability-free life expectancy. In figure 1A, the diagonal line represents no increase in population morbidity when increases in life expectancy equal increases in disability-free life expectancy. In figure 1B, the shaded area represents an increased burden of morbidity in the population as increases in life expectancy surpass increases in disability-free life expectancy. In figure 1C, the shaded area represents a decreased burden of morbidity in the population as increases in disability-free life expectancy surpass increases in life expectancy.

the early years of life. If we look at survival curves from 1900 to 1980 for females who survive to age 60, there has been no trend toward rectangularization (figure 3). These curves remove the effects of mortality at early ages and more clearly reveal the ongoing progress in increasing life expectancy in the last decades of life.

Another way of examining ongoing trends in mortality is by examining death rates during the twentieth century (table 1). From 1954 to 1968 there was a deceleration in the increases in survival that had been occurring during the preceding two decades. This may have led Fries to his conclusion that life expectancy was beginning to approach its upper limit and mortality was being compressed into a narrow ranges of years. However, the annual changes in mortality rates since 1968 have resumed the same pattern of increases in survival that was present from 1936 to 1954. Survival curves in 1960 and 1980 (figures 2 and 3) reflect this change and show no compression of mortality. Examination of the survival curves in figures 2 and 3, and an understanding

TABLE 1 Annual changes in mortality rates,* 1900–1982.

Year	Males	Females
1900–1936	−0.9	−1.0
1936–1954	−1.7	−2.6
1954–1968	+0.1	−0.8
1968–1982	−1.8	−2.1

*Rates are percent changes in central death rates, adjusted to take into account the age distribution of the population.

Source: Social Security Administration. Office of the Actuary. 1983. *Life Tables for the United States: 1900–2050.* Actuarial Study No. 89. SSA Pub. No. 11-11536.

of the factors that led to the trend toward rectangularization of these curves in the first part of this century lead us to conclude that the trend toward rectangularization has slowed or stopped.

EVALUATION OF CHANGES IN DISABILITY-FREE LIFE EXPECTANCY IN THE ELDERLY

It is difficult to accurately assess long-term changes in morbidity in older persons. Changes in reporting of diseases may simply result from increased access to medical care or changes in medical practice in the community. Measures of health care utilization may also offer a distorted picture of morbidity over time, as rates of doctors' visits, hospitalizations, and nursing home admissions may reflect changes in health care availability and financing rather than changes in population morbidity. Since measures of disability status probably offer the best tool to evaluate morbidity, we have examined a number of studies of trends in disability over the last few decades.

Several investigators have used the U.S. National Health Interview Survey (NHIS) to evaluate changes in disability in the population (see table 2). The advantage in using these data is that information on activity limitation has been collected for a representative sample of the U.S. population for the past 20 years. Activity limitation is assessed in older people in the NHIS by ascertaining whether they are retired and whether their retirement was due to poor health. If they ever worked, respondents are asked whether their health currently limits the kind or amount of work they *could* do and whether they are limited in the kind or amount of other activities. Those keeping house are also asked about limitations in the kind and amount of housework and other activities. As indicated in table 2, studies of activity limitation over various time intervals have shown either an increase in limitation or no change. Kovar

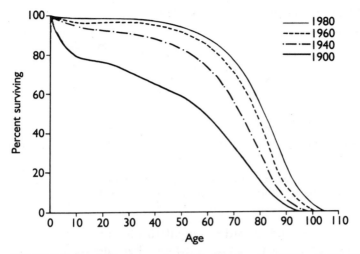

FIGURE 2 Survival curves for U.S. females for 1900, 1940, 1960, and 1980, from Social Security Administration, DHHS Publication #11-11536, *Life Tables for the United States, 1900–2050,* 1983.

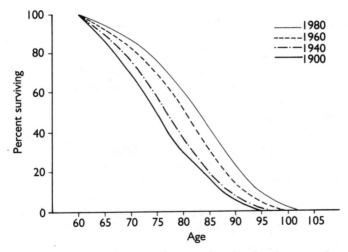

FIGURE 3 Survival curves for U.S. females for those reaching age 60 in 1900, 1940, 1960, and 1980. Social Security Administration, DHHS Publication #11-11536, *Life Tables for the United States, 1900–2050,* 1983.

attributed the increase she found between 1965 and 1975 for the population aged 65 and older to be due entirely to the change in the age distribution (increased percent over age 75, 85, etc.) of that population.

An important problem in using activity limitation as a measure of morbidity in older persons is that those who are retired are asked to estimate how

TABLE 2 Changes over time in selected measures of morbidity in the elderly.

Reference	Data Source	Years Evaluated	Age Group	Parameter Measured	Outcome
Kovar 1977	National Health Interview Survey	1965–1975	65+	Limitation in Activity	Increase
Colvez and Blanchet 1981	National Health Interview Survey	1966–1974	65+	Main activity impossible Main activity restricted	Increase men and women Decrease men Increase women
Crimmins 1986	National Health Interview Survey	1970–1980	65–79 80+ 65–74 75–80, 85+ 80–84 75+	Limitation in activity	Increase women NC* or Decrease women Increase men Increase black men Decrease black men NC white men
Verbrugge 1984	National Health Interview Survey	1958–1980 1972–1979 1970–1980	65+	Days of restricted activity Days of bed disability Self-reported health Limitation in activity	Increase NC NC Increase
Palmore 1985	National Health Interview Survey	1961/65–1976/81	65+	Days of restricted activity Days of bed disability	NC Decrease
Wilkins and Adams 1983	Canada Health Survey	1951–1978	65+	Bed days Total short-term disability days Long-term disability (%)	NC NC Increase
Shanas 1982	National Survey of the Aged	1962–1975	65+	Bedfast Housebound Difficulty: Walking stairs Getting about house Washing, bathing Dressing, putting on shoes Cutting toenails	NC NC Decrease NC NC NC NC

* NC = No change

their health might limit the work they could do. This forces respondents to evaluate their current health in terms of their past work. The problems in evaluating function by relating it to work are particularly apparent when comparing men and women. Using NHIS activity limitation measures, men appear to be more disabled than women. However, virtually all studies which have used measures of current performance, for example, activities of daily living, have shown women to have more disability than men for all age groups.

Other measures of morbidity from the NHIS, including days of restricted activity, days of disability confined to bed, and self-reported health status have been evaluated (table 2). These also show no consistent pattern over time. One of these studies has been used as an example of evidence for an ongoing decline in morbidity. This study found a slight increase in days of restricted activity and a small decrease in days of bed disability on examination of NHIS data. However, consistent declines in these measurements were only found after adjusting NHIS data for national trends in reporting of disability by calculating the ratio of disability in those 65 and older to the entire population.

In another large study, the Canada Health Survey, no change was seen in days spent in bed or short-term disability days between 1951 and 1978 (table 2). During this same period, long-term disability based on activity limitation and permanent physical disabilities increased in those aged 65 and older. The two National Surveys of the Aged conducted by Shanas in 1962 and 1975 offer perhaps the best available means to evaluate changes in morbidity as reflected by functioning. The ability to perform specific activities was queried in the same way in both studies. As demonstrated in table 2, there was no substantial change in any parameter measured except for a decline in disability related to stair climbing. In summary, examination of selected measures of morbidity in the elderly in a variety of surveys does not show any distinct trends toward either increasing or decreasing disability.

By using data from the Canada Health Survey it is possible to examine the change in overall population morbidity as applied to the model presented in figure 1 (figure 4). Over the 26-year period from 1952 to 1978, disability was postponed 1.3 years for men and 1.4 years for women while life expectancy was increasing by 4.5 and 7.5 years, respectively.

These changes clearly fall into the range of an increased burden of population morbidity. It is unfortunate that data from other studies spanning comparable time periods are not available for application to this model.

Will There Be a Future Compression of Morbidity?

A future compression of morbidity will require that increases in disability-free life expectancy surpass increases in life expectancy. Obviously, one can only speculate about future changes in these parameters. It is particularly difficult to predict future trends in disability-free life expectancy. As previously discussed, there is no strong evidence that morbidity or disability has declined in

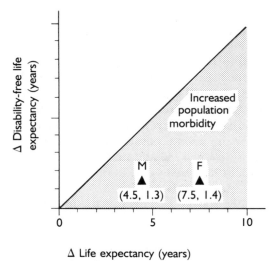

FIGURE 4 The results of the Canada Health Survey plotted on to the model presented in figure 1. Change in life expectancy vs. change in disability-free life expectancy, 1952 to 1978, in males (M) and females (F).

recent years even in the face of substantial improvements in life expectancy. The thrust of this section will therefore be to discuss future trends in life expectancy, for which better predictions are available than for morbidity. As long as life expectancy is increasing, then compression of morbidity will take place only if disability-free life expectancy increases at an even greater pace.

Considerable discussion about future mortality has centered around the debate on rectangularization. The two necessary conditions under which rectangularization will occur are: 1) a fixed life span and 2) increasing life expectancy. Life expectancy is certainly increasing and while there is debate about just what the maximum human life span might be, there likely is some upper limit on life span. It is therefore probable that at some time in the future there will be a full rectangularization of the survival curve. If rectangularization is considered a process rather than an endpoint, then it is likely that we are at some stage in this process. But the reality is that while the promise of rectangularization is enticing, it is a very long way away.

Fries offers the appealing view that "ideal average life span," which we interpret as maximum human life expectancy, is fixed at a specific age and that as we approach that age, gains in life expectancy will decrease and then cease entirely, resulting in almost complete rectangularization of the human survival curve.

Fries, presenting his view that complete compression of mortality (rectangularization of the suvival curve) will occur before the middle of the next century, defined the characteristics of his "ideal" rectangular survival curve. In listing the parameters for this curve, Fries proposed that the age of death will be distributed around his proposed average life expectancy of 85 years, with a standard deviation of age at death of 4 years. In presenting his "ideal" survival curve, he also assumed that a small percentage of deaths will occur at all ages from trauma. We present in figure 5 the "ideal" rectangularized curve as defined by Fries together with the actual U.S. survival curves for women from 1900 to 1980. There are important differences between the "ideal" and 1980 survival curves presented in figure 5 and those originally presented by Fries. In Fries' original figure, the 1980 survival curve approaches but does not overlap his "ideal" survival curve. In figure 5, the 1960 survival curve overlaps and the 1980 survival curve clearly exceeds the "ideal" survival curve at older ages. There are several possible explanations for these differences: Fries published his article in 1980 and he may have used estimates since he did not have the actual 1980 census data at that time. Furthermore, the sex of the group was not indicated in this article; thus, he may have used data for men or men and women together. However, the important issue is that in the year 1980, the 30% of American women surviving the longest have already surpassed the "barrier," the "ideal" survival curve! Another important point is that the survival curves in 1980 and 1960 are relatively parallel to each other and there is no trend between 1960 and 1980 toward the shape of the ideal survival curve presented by Fries.

There are many possible scenarios for future trends in life expectancy. We would like to discuss two that particulary bear on the issue of the limits of human life span: 1) that life span is fixed and that eventually, increases in life expectancy will halt, or 2) life span is not fixed and that increases in life expectancy may continue indefinitely.

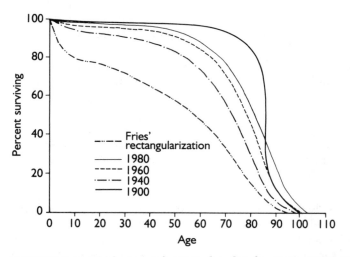

FIGURE 5 Survival curves for U.S. females for 1900, 1940, 1960, and 1980 (as per figure 2) and the "ideal" survival curve hypothesized by Fries of an average life expectancy of age 85 with a standard deviation of age of death of 4 years.

Consequences of a Fixed Life Span

In the first scenario, the key issue is how long it will take before increases in life expectancy stop as life expectancy approaches the fixed limit to human life span. Fries has implied that we are close to maximum life expectancy, which he predicts will be reached by the middle of the next century, his predicted time of complete rectangularization. We have demonstrated that the rectangularized survival curve proposed by Fries has already been surpassed by 30% of women alive in 1980. Furthermore, there would have to be a dramatic change in the shape of the survival curve in order to approach Fries' "ideal" survival curve.

According to the first scenario, rectangularization of survival curves will occur eventually; the key question is when it will occur. Figure 6 shows survival curves for those surviving to age 60 and older for years 1980 through 2050. Future survival curves are derived from projections from the Social Security Administration. These curves are drawn with maximum survival fixed at just over 100 years. It is clear that in 1980 the shape of the curve is not rectangularized and that even for the projected curve for 2050, rectangularization is still quite far away. The implication of this argument is that even with the right tail of the survival curve fixed, life expectancy can continue its rise for a very long time before theoretical rectangularization is reached. The theory of rectangularization, as provocative and optimistic as it might be, will therefore play no role in the dynamics of population survival at any time in the foreseeable future.

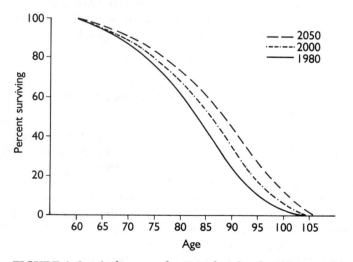

FIGURE 6 Survival curves for U.S. females for those reaching age 60 in 1980 and projected curves for 2000 and 2050, from Social Security Administration, DHHS Publication #11-11536, *Life Tables for the United States, 1900–2050*, 1983.

Consequences of an Increasing Life Span

In the second scenario, let's start by questioning Fries's assumption that the maximum human life span will remain at 114. While we agree with Fries that human life span is genetically defined, we are not sure that the 114 years that Fries derived from the Guiness Book of Records can be definitively called the limit to human life span. Certainly, few scientists would draw conclusions from one or two data points. With centenarians reported to be the fastest growing age group, we would not be surprised to see individuals living past 114 years by the end of this century.

In assessing how long life expectancy can continue to increase before reaching an upper limit, the argument above assumed that life span is now fixed and that the tail of the survival curve cannot continue to move to the right. If the tail does move to the right, then the entire survival curve has room to shift to the right and the upper limit on how far life expectancy can be extended will be even higher.

There has been much debate over whether the tail of the survival curve represents a Gompertz function (reflecting exponential increases in death rates with age) or some other function which would result in a normal or a flattened distribution of ages at death for the very old. However, these debates concern the shape of the tail of the survival curve and do not definitively answer the question of whether the tail is stationary or moving to the right. Empirically evaluating the upper tail of the survival curve is quite difficult due to the sparse data available. There is some evidence, though, that the tail is slowly moving to the right. Life tables from the past 30 years indicate that remaining life expectancy for the very oldest people has increased. Between 1950 and 1980, life expectancy for those reaching 90 years of age increased by nearly one year while life expectancy for those reaching 100 years increased by about a half-year.

Implications of the Continued and Long-Term Increases in Life Expectancy for the Compression of Morbidity

In a sense, compression of morbidity is easy to achieve in a population which has a stable life expectancy. Any postponement in morbidity in this population means that morbidity will be compressed. This explains why Fries promotes an early occurrence of rectangularization when making his case for compression of morbidity. Rectangularization is a special case when life expectancy can no longer increase. In this setting, total population morbidity will decline if there is even the smallest postponement of morbidity onset.

Compression of morbidity is much harder to achieve in a population in which life expectancy is still increasing. For this to occur, between time 1 and time 2 the onset of morbidity must be postponed for a greater number of years than the average age of death is postponed, as demonstrated in figure 1. The data from the Canada Health Survey plotted on figure 4 clearly exemplify a situation of expanding population morbidity.

Conclusion

In summary, while the concept of a compression of morbidity is a noble goal for society, it is not occurring now and there is little evidence that it will occur in the near future. It is hoped that through basic and applied research and through education and preventive medicine, we will prevent and/or effectively treat those diseases and disorders which have their onset late in life and which cause long-term disability. It is important to emphasize that the major causes of disability today are these diseases and disorders of aging: arthritis, dementia, peripheral vascular disease, stroke, and hip fractures. These disorders cause more disability in the elderly, in terms of limitation of activity, than the two commonest killers, ischemic heart disease and cancer. While there has been a significant drop in deaths from the number one killer, ischemic heart disease, there have been no comparable inroads into many of the major causes of disability. Thus, individuals escape death from heart attacks in their earlier decades only to live longer into the later decades where the chronic diseases and disorders which cause disability take their toll. As gerontologists, we strive to achieve a compression of morbidity. However, it will not come spontaneously or as a result of rectangularization in the near future. It will not come solely through application of current knowledge in prevention. It will only come through intensive research on the nature of aging and age-related diseases.

Health is a very large term indeed. It goes beyond the condition of the flesh. It's also a condition of the spirit. Everything we do is reflected in the physical. Over a period of years, the strains and stresses residing in the body often manifest themselves as diseases. The opposite can also be true. And ultimately health doesn't just involve isolated parts of the body. It also involves the whole way we live, the way we think, our social responsibility, our attitude toward the world, our enthusiasm for life.

GEORGE LEONARD

S. M. Miller

Race in the Health of America

At the beginning of this century W.E.B. DuBois prophetically declared that "the problem of the twentieth century is the problem of the color line — the relation of the darker to the lighter races of men in Asia and Africa, in America and the islands of the sea." Much has happened since DuBois first published his stirring, brilliant essays but the color line continues to be a disturbing force in the United States as well as in South Africa. Certainly, the issue of race is different today in America from what it is in South Africa, but progress in the United States has not erased racial divisiveness.

PATTERNS

Health cannot be understood simply as a biological phenomenon. Consequently, the health of black America is first discussed in terms of economic and social conditions and racial attitudes, and, then, in terms of the differential data between blacks and whites.

Economic Conditions

Poverty, as it is now understood in the United States, is defined by a simple measurement: a poverty line is determined by 30-year-old food expenditure data; those with incomes below that line are officially designated as poor. The result is that the poor are probably worse off relative to the rest of society today than they were in 1960.

Racial inequality is measured by comparing blacks and whites on a variety of conditions. Some view the last 20 years as a movement toward a "melting pot" that has narrowed economic and social differences between the races, so that blacks are now experiencing the pattern of various ethnic groups who began as poor immigrants and achieved sizable economic gains over time. In this view, race is becoming less important; class-linked factors like schooling are pointed to to explain income differences among blacks. Others see increasing "polarization"; for them, the differences between blacks and whites are

Seymour M. Miller, Ph.D., is a professor of sociology at Boston University, Boston, Massachusetts.

widening rather than declining. Farley sees both of these perspectives as misleading. My own view is that evolving and revolving sets of relationships form "jagged changes," with some reductions in inequalities, small changes, and some widening inequalities all occurring at the same time.

Poverty and unemployment are two economic areas in which wide racial differences are disturbingly apparent. The white poverty rate in 1986 was 11 percent while the black rate was 31 percent. Between 1985 and 1986, the poverty rate declined slightly for both blacks and whites but was higher than it was in 1978. The percentage of the black population below the poverty line was higher in 1986 than in 1969. The most dismal statistic is that 45.6 percent of black children were living in households with incomes below the poverty line in 1986; this compares with a figure of 17.7 percent for white children. A broader measure of the poor is the near-poverty line, which refers to all those whose household incomes are below 125 percent of the poverty line; in 1984, more than two-fifths of blacks lived below this standard compared to somewhat more than one of six whites. While black and white rates are closer than they were in 1959, the percentage of blacks living in poverty or near poverty today does not support a melting-pot interpretation.

The median family income of black households is a smaller percentage of white household income today than it was in 1969, 1974, or 1979. The continuing difference is partially due to the growth of single-parent households among blacks but, controlling for this factor, black household incomes are still only 80 percent of those of whites.

The greatest relative gain for blacks is in the occupational earnings distribution for women. The differences have declined to close to zero; in some comparisons, employed black women do better than employed white women. Two limitations should be noted, however. Women, both black and white, still substantially lag behind white men who have a big income advantage even when differences in education are controlled. When attention shifts to one-parent families, black female heads of households have smaller incomes than do their white counterparts.

Unemployment continues to plague black communities. The black unemployment rate is twice that of whites and has remained at that multiple for 30 years. The unemployment rate among young black males is staggering: over 30 percent of those in the labor force. Perhaps of greater damage is the high percentage of young black males who are not considered to be looking for employment, those "out of the labor force." "Indeed, all indicators report," according to R. Farley, "that the employment situation of young blacks vis-a-vis that of whites has deteriorated since 1960".

Social Conditions

Black fertility rates have declined very dramatically and are much closer to those of whites than in 1960. While the number of black teenage births has not increased, they are a larger percentage of all black births. In part, the importance of these teenage births is due to what sociologist Cheryl Townsend Gilkes terms the "constrained fertility" of older and/or middle-class black women who do not have children or have only one. The concern about black teenaged mothers is not misplaced but has narrowed the analysis of what is occurring. Some analysts partially attribute the large number of unmarried black mothers to a shortage of suitable males — men who are not in jail and are employed at a decent wage.

Housing has decidedly improved, partly because fewer blacks live in the rural South, but even there black housing has advanced. This overall gain may mask the deterioration of housing in many centercity areas and ignores the fact that blacks spend a higher proportion of their incomes for housing than whites. The general housing gain has been accompanied by continuing and perhaps increasing residential segregation.

Differences between blacks and whites in years of schooling have decreased markedly, especially for women. A warning sign is that the percentage of blacks in colleges and universities has declined in recent years, possibly due to the contraction of funds available to minority students. The overall improvement in years of schooling of blacks is not as positive as it appears, for the gap between blacks and whites in school skills has not diminished and may have increased. School segregation has been reduced in the South but not in the North.

What is to be made of these changes in economic and social conditions? A sizable slice of the black population has improved its economic position, but a large, perhaps larger, group of blacks is living under very inadequate conditions. American society is less occupationally segregated than in the past, but it is still residentially and (especially in the North) school segregated.

Health Differences

Health is a key indicator of well-being, and health statistics a measure of both progress and continuing inequalities. The health of blacks has improved considerably but inequalities between blacks and whites are still significant.

Mortality Differences   Black longevity has certainly increased, but a 50 percent difference remains in adjusted death rates for blacks and whites. If blacks had the same death rates as whites, 59,000 black deaths a year would not occur. Infant mortality in 1984 was almost twice as frequent among blacks as whites; this difference is not completely attributable to more young black mothers. Except for stomach cancer, the cancer survival rate of blacks is lower than that of whites.

That considerable progress has been made (and presumably could be made) is revealed in the relative change in mortality rates in the Carolinas between 1900 and 1940. In the earlier year, black mortality rates were 40 percent higher in the more urban northern state; by 1940, the New York State black mortality rate was at least 25 percent lower than that of the more rural Carolinas. Various influences were involved, but improved housing, water supply, and other public measures in New York undoubtedly contributed to the absolute and relative decline in mortality races.

Morbidity Differences   Blacks have more undetected diseases than whites, and black children may be in worse health than white children. The incidence of low-weight births (and their attendant difficulties) is almost twice as frequent among blacks as whites. This difference, as with infant mortality, is not completely attributable to more young black mothers. Older blacks suffer from more functional limitations than older whites, a situation of "accelerated" or "unequal" aging, which is associated with poverty, low education, and low-level occupations. At the young end of the age ladder, black children seem in worse health than whites.

Self-report data indicate that 50 percent more blacks than whites are likely to regard themselves as only in fair or poor health. Blacks report more frequently that they feel "little" satisfaction with their health and physical conditions. Yet, there is more undetected disease among blacks than whites. While whites report more acute conditions, blacks report more chronic conditions. The statement by Manton et al. that "differentials in health between blacks and whites are pervasive and long-standing, despite recent advances in black life expectancy" summarizes what the morbidity and mortality data record.

To be poor *and* black is to run the risk of ill health; those who are black alone share the same health risks.

Use of Facilities   Medicaid has made a difference in access to and use of physicians and hospitals. Differences in utilization (as measured by visits to physicians) between blacks and whites have been eliminated. A further indication of the importance of financing mechanisms to provide access to and use of medical care is that poor blacks with health coverage make twice as many visits to physicians as do poor uncovered blacks.

Nonetheless, some important differences persist. Whites receive more skilled nursing home care than blacks, although the differences are decreasing. Blacks have a lower cancer survival rate than whites, except for stomach cancer.

Despite Medicaid, 22 percent of blacks are without any medical insurance coverage, compared to 15 percent of whites. Furthermore, in terms of physician contact, the factors of emergency room and hospital treatment are almost twice as important among blacks as whites.

While the number of black physicians has increased, the rate of increase is diminishing. The fear is that the number of black physicians will not expand as a percentage of all physicians as market pressures become more significant and financial aid to black student physicians does not expand. Since black physicians are more likely to serve black patients than do white physicians, this limitation could prove important.

The utilization issue has three important components: (1) Does medical care make a difference? An influential survey by Levine and associates argues the importance of medical attention. The improvement in the survival rates of low-weight babies is attributed to advances in hospital care, not to other conditions. (2) Will blacks, and especially the black poor, take advantage of opportunities for care? Again, surveys show that when poor individuals are provided services that are accessible and appear to them to be useful they will be used, undermining the notion of under-utilization of services by the uneducated or resistant poor. (3) Do finance and delivery systems affect utilization? A strong conclusion is that they "have played a critical role in improvements in health and access to care."

The clear inference is that health conditions of blacks and the poor can be influenced by governmental actions. The distribution of medical resources relative to need affects causality and successful treatment. General economic gains, the reduction of barriers to blacks, and governmental programs including occupational health regulations have improved the health situation of blacks. Some important differences still persist. Black mortality and morbidity could be reduced by further government-sponsored economic and health programs.

INTERPRETATIONS

Studies show that racial differences in health exist; numerous investigations report that class or income level influence health conditions. Surprisingly few analyses try to discern whether race is related to health conditions when differences in income levels are controlled. Studies that have made this type of cross-tabulation point to the significance for health of being black, even at higher income levels.

In Oakland, California, a comparison by Haan et al. of age-specific mortality rates in poverty and nonpoverty areas shows that differences between blacks are much less than between whites. Improved housing, a lower concentration of poor people, and more income seem to have less effect on blacks than on whites.

A study of stress found its severity highest in lower-class blacks and lowest in middle-class whites. This result would confirm the importance of class factors, but an additional comparison by Dohrenwend and Dohrenwend points to the significance of racial experience: middle-class blacks and lower-class whites had similar levels of stress.

We turn from the limited data on the important question of whether race as well as class is important in health conditions to interpretations of why black and white health differences persist despite distinct improvements in black health. Five sets of explanations are examined: biological, cultural, economic, social, and service.

Biology

Sickle cell anemia is often cited as a genetic factor among blacks. But such genetic influences would by themselves not explain higher mortality and morbidity rates for particular disease conditions. A somewhat more compelling argument is that certain black genetic characteristics conduce toward disease. But if such biological influences were important, they would interact with economic, social, or psychological situations to produce effects.

It is difficult to explain black women's pronounced gains in health without introducing nonbiological influences. Nor would it be easy to contend that black health could not be further improved because it has met the limits placed by genetic factors. For example, "there does not appear to be any inherent biological reason for the differences in cervical cancer rates between blacks and whites" (Baquet and Ringer, 1987). Extending this point to other diseases and afflictions, we need to rethink health policy in broader than strictly medical terms. The cloudiness of the concept of race and the many genetic strains among American blacks make purely biological explanations questionable.

Culture

Cultural explanations of health problems have even reached the extreme concept of "health criminals." Blacks and others, because they do not take proper care of themselves (e.g., poor diet, lack of exercise, homicide) are indicted as the producers of their sad fate, driving up medical expenditures and exacting tribute from the careful healthy. Certainly, a healthy life is in large measure produced by what people do for themselves, but not completely. It is too easy to blame a group's behavior rather than to look for broader or deeper causes and outcomes.

Where cultural influences might be significant, the questions become: Why the pattern? What maintains it? Since not all practices of one generation are exhibited in the next, continuity has to be explained rather than taken for granted. In the case of black and white health differences, the implication is that blacks do not behave in ways that are as conducive to health as do whites. The further implication is that conditions for blacks and whites are the same and that health differences are due to malperformance on the part of blacks.

A cultural explanation does not adequately reveal the dynamics of at least one health hazard, particularly important for blacks, which seems particularly suited for such an explanation—the high incidence of obesity. The continuation of eating habits of a poor childhood that relied on cheap, fattening food; work and family tensions that make planned, diet-conscious eating difficult; inadequate incomes that reduce possibilities and choices; a low sense of destiny control; and limited knowledge are all implicated in obesity. Even in this most personal of behavior, simply relying on an explanation in terms of habit and attitudes may be inadequate. Nor does the cultural approach lead to a comprehensive strategy for dealing with the issue.

Economic Factors

"To be a poor man is hard, but to be a poor race in a land of dollars is the very bottom of hardships," according to W.E.B. DuBois. Black and white disparities in economic conditions contribute to health differentials despite black gains. Since a much larger and very sizable slice of blacks is poor, economic conditions and their ramifications undoubtedly adversely affect black health. Inadequate incomes affect many aspects of daily life that impinge on health. These range from housing problems (e.g., rat-infested neighborhoods and overcrowding, which quicken the spread of communicable diseases), malnutrition, the stress of struggling to make ends meet, and dangerous jobs. Job and housing conditions may expose blacks to certain cancers to a much greater extent than whites.

The emphasis on improvements in economic gains for blacks ignores the possibility that early deprivation can affect later health states. Nutritional deprivation of children during World War I affected their health, especially of women, in later life. Recent advances in material circumstances of blacks may not overcome the effect of earlier life experiences. With perhaps one-half of black children under the age of 6 living in poverty, this current deprivation may maintain later health differences, even if many of these children later improve their economic conditions.

Social Explanations

The problem is not only that of poverty but of economic and social inequalities associated with race. A British study provides a suggestive line of thought: A pronounced difference in mortality risk exists between high- and low-level members of the white-collar civil service. Both groups had secure tenure, relatively good pay, and fringe benefits. The author's point is that hierarchy produces tensions and stresses even where individuals seem somewhat similarly situated. For blacks in the United States the sense of economic inequality, social distance, discrimination and hierarchy—of not being accorded full equality—is undoubtedly strong and persisting. In the words of H. W. Neighbors, racial discrimination probably "exacerbates the mental health-damaging effects of poverty status among blacks."

In the health area, then, the call for individuals to change to more positive health practices may not be effective among blacks because the shift requires exploration of new roles, norms, and practices, as well as access to facilities, information, and support: "Maladaptive patterns of coping . . . and hazardous forms of consumption . . . can be seen to reflect the molding of social and cultural life by contemporary economic (and race) relations," according to M. Susser and associates.

A more specific influence on blacks may be widespread and disturbing uprooting and resettlement. Although the black population of center city areas is declining, it may be that new blacks are moving in as long-time residents move out. The data on this point are uncertain. The new residents may experience heavy pressures in accommodating to a difficult set of center city circumstances and lack the social supports that would be helpful.

What is clear is that black neighborhoods suffer disruption resulting from urban renewal, abandonment, and arson. People are forced to move, severing networks of relationships, which are important for social well-being and which impinge on health, especially of the aged.

Some investigators believe that racial discrimination is almost inevitable in a market economy and infer that the stress resulting from discrimination continues to affect health. Many successful blacks point not only to limitations on their occupational progress but to stressful encounters around the job.

Medical Services

Despite noticeable improvements in health care for the poor and blacks resulting from Medicare and Medicaid, there is still less adequate medical attention for blacks than whites. The quality of health care is likely to be better in white areas, especially in access to physicians and hospitals. At every income level, blacks have substantially higher reliance on emergency room and outpatient departments for contacts with physicians than do whites. Indeed, racial differences are greater above the $10,000 annual income level than below it. Since 1980 blacks have experienced decreased medical attention as a result of federal cutbacks. If such patterns continue, black and white differences in health services will not be reduced.

POLICY

The burdens of knowledge are heavy. Knowing that health care can be improved and health inequalities reduced, it is immoral as well as economically wasteful to refuse to pursue these goals. For in the realm of health, rights to equal consideration and conditions are much less controversial than in the realm of employment. In the 1960s a president of the American Medical Association declared that health care was a privilege, not a right. Today, few would agree. There is now a consensus that blacks should have mortality and morbidity rates much closer to those of whites. Much less agreement exists about what to do to close the gaps.

Policy Criteria

In this section, we deal with three policy issues: creaming; universality vs. targeting; and poverty or inequality reduction.

Creaming   The jagged progress characteristic of blacks can be partly considered a result of creaming. Creaming is a policy, intentional or unintended, of concentrating on the "easiest cases." Where the poor or disadvantaged are involved, it improves the situation of the better-off of the badly-off population—those least disadvantaged of a disadvantaged group. The expectation is that as each layer moves up, those worse off gradually become the recipients of attention and will then improve their situation.

The methods which led to the improvement among the better-off of the badly-off will be equally useful for the worse-off who were left behind; the departure of the better-off will not adversely affect the worst-off who remain. Both assumptions are frequently, perhaps usually, wrong.

Poverty Reduction or Equality   Is the objective only to reduce poverty or unemployment among blacks because of the damage inflicted by that economic condition? Or is it to reduce economic inequalities between blacks and whites? In the latter case it would be unsatisfactory if black poverty rates were reduced while white household income increased and widened the gap between blacks and whites. Despite strong disagreements about the goal of economic equality, the dismay when economic inequality between blacks and whites is increasing indicates widespread agreement that these inequalities should be decreasing, even if complete equality is not the objective.

The consensus seems to be that poverty and inequality should not be disproportionately concentrated in an ascriptive group (i.e., one characterized by unchangeable characteristics like race, ethnicity, or gender), and should be dwindling rather than expanding. While this outlook is not as demanding as the right to equal health and health care, it demands reductions in inequalities as well as in poverty.

The underlying issue from the perspective of health policy is the strong likelihood that the persistence of economic, social, and political inequalities, even if black poverty is reduced, is injurious to the health of black Americans. This outlook treats equality as instrumental to health; the deeper question is, of course, the moral one of the nature of our obligations to one another.

Black and white equality may be insufficient in some health respects. The concept of "excess deaths" points to American morality rates for certain diseases that exceed those of other nations. More effective interventions would be likely to lower American rates. If black rates were the same as white rates, that achievement would be unsatisfactory. The case of "excess deaths" illustrates a general point about equality: incorporating the excluded or disadvantaged into existing structures and improving their situation may be inadequate; the general situation for all may have to be improved. American medical care may have to face that challenge.

Universality or Targeting   The specific policy questions of how to improve the situation of blacks is part of the general policy debate about the competing principles of, on one hand, universality or comprehensiveness and, on the other, targeting, selectivity, or means-testing. The first set of terms refers to programs available to (almost) all; by virtue of being a citizen, resident, or wage earner, one receives benefits from a program. In practice, no program is available to everybody, but Social Security and Medicare come closest to it. Age and past contributions of the former and age alone for the latter make one eligible for benefits. The targeted principle sets out conditions, usually of income inadequacy, that must be met in order to receive benefits. Eligibility is not on the basis of a noneconomic characteristic like age or sickness alone; rather, one must show need, the inability to provide for one's household, or to seek the needed service in the marketplace. Targeted programs like Medicaid are aimed at "needy" persons; untargeted or universal programs do not require that the individual or household demonstrate a lack of means to cover needs.

The advantage of a universal-type program available to (almost) all is that it builds support because so many, especially politically potent nonpoor persons, benefit from it. Other gains are that it avoids stigmatization of beneficiaries, may promote social solidarity by establishing institutions and activities in which all are involved (at least at some point in their lives), and is likely to promote higher quality service because of the threat of widespread political discontent if quality is low or deteriorating.

The negative side, emphasized by economists in their benefit-cost calculations, is "leakage," diffusion of program resources, which reduces the "target efficiency" of a program because it aids those not in need. By providing to all rather than to only those with insufficient resources, less is available to low-income people who need more substantial aid. Public resources are "wasted" or "leaked" to those who could handle the burden of the costs that they face. By eliminating this diffusion and concentrating the public program on those with real resource needs, more funds would be available to those who need them.

The assumption is that cost savings resulting from targeting and removal of benefits from those who do not lack resources would lead to a practice where greater resources are expended on those who lack means. No iron law of policy or politics dictates that result.

Indeed, the argument against selectivity or targeting goes further and contends that participants in means-tested programs tend to be or feel stigmatized, so that some of the benefits to them of the program may be lost because of the burden of the disgrace.

Programs that are seen as for the poor, the underclass, welfare cheats, and blacks in general face political, financial, and operational obstacles. The contrast between a universal program like Social Security and a targeted program like Aid to Families with Dependent Children (AFDC) is instructive: in the 1970s and 1980s Social Security payments more than kept up with inflation while AFDC suffered real income losses as many states did not increase benefits at all despite the high rise in prices.

The Reagan administration's objectives of drastic reductions in the levels of and eligibility for means-tested programs were largely unsuccessful. That is not to say that they achieved no significant reductions but they could not institute the depth of cuts that were initially predicted. Considerable public and political pressure for maintenance of these programs blocked many Reagan efforts. While many people are critical of something called "the welfare state," they often recognize the usefulness of specific programs.

The first line of defense or improvement should be universal programs; they are likely to be better programs and to have strong political constituencies. The general principle is to make the needs of the black low-income population part of efforts to improve the situation of all or most Americans. Where that principle is inadequate, then targeting within the universal program can be a desirable and effective instrument. The outstanding example of the merger of these approaches is the Social Security program, which favors low-income participants. Their benefits are greater relative to their contributions than are those with higher income. Differences in preretirement wage incomes are narrowed in postretirement Social Security benefits. Elderly blacks who suffered from low wages during their working lives are somewhat improved relative to those who were in a better situation in the preretirement period. Yet, elderly blacks are not singled out for this gain, a situation which makes that advance more politically secure.

In practice, both universality and targeting have to be utilized. When and how are the issues. Universality is the policy of first resort, but such programs often cream, are more effectively utilized by those with more education and resources, provide inadequate resources for those in greatest need, and have only a limited effect on reducing economic inequalities. Universality reduces the likelihood of two Americas or two sets of institutions—one for the "disadvantaged," the other for those who are better off. It improves the political chances of maintaining and improving funding for programs and enhancing their quality. Nonetheless, universality has to be supplemented and sometimes supplanted by targeting on those who are disadvantaged and discriminated against.

Economic and Social Policies

Employment is a prime area for improvement of the situation of blacks—more and better jobs and a more effective upgrading of existing jobs are all needed.

Following the approach just discussed, the first step is an expanding economy that produces more jobs and good jobs at that. Blacks do better in an expanding than in a contracting economy. An effective macroeconomic policy that stimulates the economy is an important first step. At issue within job growth is the quality of jobs produced. Many of the new jobs of the 1970s and 1980s have been low-paying, part-time, and devoid of fringe benefits; many of the good blue-collar jobs in mass-production industries have disappeared.

An increase in jobs, especially good jobs, does not assure that blacks will get them. Affirmative action, to which we shall return, is one route. Encouraging black entrepreneurship is another. But education, training, improved transportation, and child care are of greater importance in helping blacks to move into good jobs in greater numbers.

The current emphasis on higher standards in public education may worsen the schooling of many poor and black children if particular effort is not put into improving their learning. Federal aid to education has diminished; the downward cycle should be reversed. The Elementary and Secondary Education Act, which provides funding to school districts with many low-income children, should be better funded and strengthened to insure that the funds are spent in ways that benefit low-income students.

A difficulty within the dual pressures on schools today—pressures toward "excellence" as well as on general learning and vocational preparation—is that schools for the poor, especially the black poor, may become so heavily vocationalized that students learn little of the world around them. If the vocational training does not lead to a good job and provides few adaptable skills, then poor blacks will be doubly handicapped—ill-prepared for employment and uninformed about significant matters. And, if they fail to measure up to "excellence," they will drop out or be pushed out of school.

The United States lacks a comprehensive, accessible, well-funded system of worker training and development like the permanent or recurrent education schemes of France and Sweden. We have community colleges, adult education programs, and nationally funded and state and locally operated job training programs. They do not add up to a national program with priorities and direction. A comprehensive national program is needed with specific targeting to improve the employment prospects of those who are more difficult to place. At the same time, access to higher education should be facilitated by expanding aid and loan programs for low-income students. Where higher education is concerned, targeted financial help is not stigmatizing nor politically unattractive.

Affirmative action has a definite role to play, but it is certainly not the most important item on the economic agenda for blacks. Without affirmative action, many educated and trained blacks would not have attained middle-class positions. Indeed, they might not have been willing to seek further education and training if they did not believe that affirmative action would open up positions that had been closed to their parents.

A charge against it is that it has not improved the situation much for those blacks with limited schooling and training and low initial job motivation and capacity. To benefit the black poor, not only does affirmative action need to be strengthened but programs going beyond it need to be devised.

Even with a successful welfare-type program, direct aid or transfers to low-income people would still be necessary. Again, if universal programs reduced the need for targeted transfers, the poor would benefit. Improving Social Security benefits for low-wage earners would benefit the aged black poor without invoking a special system for them. If unemployment insurance payments were weighted so that not only previous wage income but the number of members in the household influenced the benefit, some large unemployed white and black families would gain.

Health Services

Unfortunately, only two approaches to extend medical insurance coverage are on the current congressional agenda. Both are limited. One would nationally mandate that employers provide a minimum package of medical insurance for their employees. A difficulty with this approach is that those who are unemployed or out of the labor force would not benefit nor would those sporadically employed if mandatory coverage applied only to those who have been with an employer for some period. A second consideration is whether all firms would be covered or only those with a minimum number of employees. It is quite likely that poorer blacks work in very small enterprises and would not be covered by the minimum-worker requirement. A third issue is the content of that mandated package and to what extent it meets the needs of blacks. A fourth point is that larger, better-off firms that are likely to be unionized have sizable medical benefits. While a mandatory program will reduce the gaps in medical coverage resulting from employment in differently situated firms, inequalities in access to health care will continue.

The alternative proposal is to extend Medicaid to more people by raising income eligibility limits (and continuing for some time Medicaid coverage for those who were on AFDC and left the rolls for a job). This approach makes sense because Medicaid in the 1980s has been serving a smaller percentage of the poor than in the early 1970s. The negative side is that by extending Medicaid we maintain a dual system of medical insurance coverage, which provides lower quality service for the non-aged poor compared to older persons covered by Medicare and those at all ages with private insurance. Further, state variations in Medicaid provisioning would continue, so that access to health care by the poor would still depend on where they lived. Expenditure patterns are important as well. Two-thirds of Medicaid spending goes for the medical needs of the aged and disabled; the more ordinary medical needs of lower-income people, especially blacks, may not be met by extension of Medicaid, particularly if the extension of coverage to more people leads to limits on the services available.

Each proposal does take an important step toward increasing medical access for lower-income citizens. Neither meets the objective of a universally based system especially targeted to aid the poor. Neither assures that hospitals and physicians would be easily available to blacks in center-city areas. Neither deals with primary and preventive health care.

Since national health insurance appears remote, the highest, somewhat realistic, hope in the next years would be to move to mandatory employer provision of a medical insurance package, to extended Medicaid eligibility, and to expanded Medicaid services. In addition, the accessibility issue could be partially met by increasing the number of black physicians through scholarships and start-up loans and by expanding incentives for physicians to locate in low-income areas.

The attention to improving financial access to medical personnel and hospital care draws concern away from the advancement of public health measures (e.g., reduction of air and water pollution, improved regulation of food and drugs, reduction of work injuries and diseases, elimination of dangerous dumps). Public health measures are particularly important for lower-income citizens. Good health is not only a result of what physicians and hospitals do for us, or what we do for ourselves; our environments, broadly viewed, are implicated in our health status.

A final, difficult-to-resolve issue is how much should be spent on health measures to improve health and how much on improving economic and social conditions that affect health. Class and race data point inevitably to the conclusion that improving incomes and social conditions would enhance the health of blacks, especially low-income blacks. Even those who espouse the importance of personal health practices (e.g., quitting smoking, good nutrition, exercise) have to question whether improved incomes or social conditions will do more for health outcomes than medical interventions or health education. It is difficult to change practices without changing circumstances. Is the way to improve the health of blacks through the economy and society rather than through the clinic, hospital, or health maintenance organization? Reducing economic and social inequalities may be the road to the achievement of individual health and a healthy society.

Every doctor believes that he should have legal powers to compel his patients to swallow drugs, to have their limbs and breasts cut off, their internal organs extirpated, and their blood provided with exceedingly unpleasant stimulants for the phagocytes (opsonins, resulting from immunization), besides dictating whether they shall stay at home or go out or go to bed.

GEORGE BERNARD SHAW

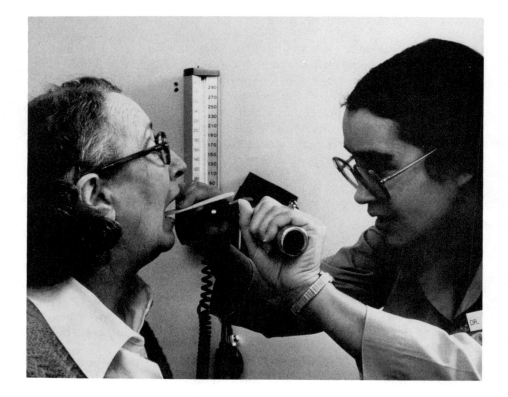

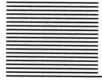

2

Shaping the Health Care System

I N THIS CHAPTER, we shift our perspective from disease, disability, and death, in order to look at the health care system. As we have seen, the causes for sickness and death have changed dramatically in the last one hundred years; so have medical treatment, health professions education, the organization and provision of health care, the costs and methods of payment for health care, the role of government in health care, and the attitudes and values of the American people about health care.

A look at the history of American medicine reveals the societal forces that have shaped modern medical care. We began with a system of faith and superstition subscribed to by the colonists, and we progressed to a system based on a strong belief in science and the germ theory of disease, a highly developed technology, and deeply held values about individualism, free enterprise, and competition. We can trace two major influences on the evolution of medicine: (1) the free enterprise system with its emphasis on competition and fee-for-service payment, as well as the predominance of the private sector, including private practicing physicians, dentists and pharmacists, nonprofit and proprietary hospitals, drug companies, and nursing homes; and (2) the science-based, disease-oriented system of medical research and education.

Intractable increases in the costs of health care have resulted in various interventions in the traditional system in recent years, and a major revolution is underway in the delivery of health care services because of resultant changes in payment systems. The results of these forces are manifest in a complex structure involving over seven million health care workers, many of them highly specialized, 7100 hospitals that range in size and complexity from small rural hospitals to major urban tertiary care centers that are equipped with streamlined medical electronics systems and technologies for diagnosis and treatment; giant private health insurance companies that serve in some capacity over 80 percent of the population; and federal, state, and local government programs that provide direct care for millions and finance care for the aged and the poor to the tune of billions of dollars a year. The dramatic increase in the size and scope of health care has transformed the medical care of only fifty years ago, when physicians practiced more art than science and prospects for cure were severely limited.

Increasing industrialization, urbanization, and modernization have created a host of new disease problems that have largely replaced those that responded earlier to advances in medicine and public health. Many of these problems are as much social as they are medical, and they offer new challenges to health care workers as well as to policymakers. Improvements in lifestyles and advances in medical science have resulted in a vast increase in the number of older Americans, and the aging population places a greater burden on the health care system.

In her article, "The Medical Care System: Past Trends and Future Projections," Dorothy P. Rice, a former Director of the National Center for Health Statistics, discusses the implications of current demographic trends as well as changes underway in medical care services, financing, and insurance benefits. Ms. Rice provides a masterly condensation of the state of the nation's health care system, including evolving reimbursement policies, access to medical care, long term care, and corporate for-profit medicine. Her historical outline and her analysis of the complex forces now at work, provide an excellent basis for helping us come to terms with critical issues concerning the future of the nation's health care system.

In his provocative paper, "The New Medical-Industrial Complex," Arnold S. Relman assesses the rapid rise of proprietary institutions in health care. The trend toward providing health care services for profit through proprietary hospitals, nursing homes, diagnostic laboratories, emergency room services, hemodialysis, and a wide variety of other facilities raises a number of complex issues regarding the public interest. Dr. Relman suggests that the new "medical industrial complex" requires close scrutiny and careful monitoring in order to avoid serious abuses.

In "Rationing the Health-Care Surplus: An American Tragedy" health economist Uwe E. Reinhardt argues that Americans are rationing an oversupply of health resources according to ability to pay. He raises the critical question of whether health care is a right or a privilege. He asks how we can remedy the fact that because medical costs are so high the indigent have greatly inferior access to health care services. He points out that this is an ethical as well as an economic dilemma which has emerged from an inability or unwillingness to address the issue openly. One possible solution drawn up by Dr. Reinhardt would be a health system hierarchy that offers three levels of medical care: tourist class, business class, and designer class. He suggests that the current one-class system, which is accessible only to middle and upper income people, is not only unfair, it is absurd.

While there is general agreement that we are healthier today as a nation than ever before, we are also investing an increasing proportion of our national resources in medical care. The question is asked, What is the role of medical care in promoting health? Robert J. Haggarty urges medicine to extend its boundaries and influence beyond "illness care" to measures aimed at social and environmental factors. In "The Boundaries of Health Care," he echoes the theme that through its current more narrow focus medicine can produce only marginal gains in comparison to working in the "boundary areas" of lifestyle, housing, pollution, life stresses, and political institutions, where medicine can contribute far more to health.

There is no justification for the fact that the United States is one of only two industrialized nations failing to provide its citizens with comprehensive health care protection. The other nation is South Africa.

HEALTH CARE USA: 1984

Dorothy P. Rice

The Medical Care System: Past Trends and Future Projections

INTRODUCTION

Americans are living longer today than ever before in history. Improvements in living conditions and life-styles, and advances in science, medical technology and pharmaceutical therapies have resulted in reductions in deaths from formerly fatal infectious diseases; dramatic gains in life expectancy; and a rapid growth of the number of older Americans. Our population is aging and this demographic change has important implications for the nation's health, social and economic institutions.

The organization, delivery and financing of medical care services have evolved into a complex, pluralistic system combining private enterprise and all levels of government. As many have noted with some alarm, expenditures for medical care have been increasing at a rapid rate for many years, amounting to $387 billion in 1984, 10.6 percent of our gross national product (GNP) or $1,580 for every man, woman and child in the United States. In 1929, the earliest year for which medical care expenditures data are available, they totaled $3.6 billion, 3.5 percent of GNP. In 1950, medical care spending amounted to $12.7 billion and represented 4.4 percent of the GNP.

The private share of the American medical market has always been larger than the public one. From the end of World War II to 1966, private outlays constituted almost three-fourths of the total; within the public sector, state and local governments spent more than the federal government. The implementation of Medicare and Medicaid altered these relationships. The government's portion increased to 41 percent of the total in 1984, and federal spending was more than twice that of state and local governments. Increased public financing in the late 1960s and 70s has mitigated the earlier dominance of the private medical care market.

The continued, persistent rise in health care expenditures has led government and other third-party payors to seek limits on their spending by direct intervention in medical practice. Significant changes in payment schemes are replacing the old retrospective cost and reasonable charge arrangements.

Dorothy P. Rice, is professor in residence, Institute for Health & Aging and Department of Social and Behavioral Sciences, School of Nursing, University of California, San Francisco.

Limits are being placed on health insurance payments through benefit reductions, increased cost sharing with consumers and contractual arrangements for services with preferred-provider organizations. Health care corporations and for-profit health care are emerging as major economic forces. Competition and regulation in the medical care sector are now accepted as means of curbing its rate of growth; the specific alternatives for accomplishing this goal while preserving the quality of care are at issue.

One of the motivating forces in American medicine is the stress on maintaining and augmenting its scientific base. This concern is manifest in the increased specialization among medical personnel and the drive by hospitals to acquire increasingly sophisticated and costly medical equipment. Technological acquisitiveness is reinforced by a strong technological imperative instilled in physicians in their medical training programs, and has been encouraged in the past by the cost-based financing system.

Questions are being asked regarding the value derived from additional private and public dollars spent for medical care. We are warned that the United States will soon have to begin rationing medical care. As the elderly population grows in the future, we wishfully dream that improvements in our life-style will delay the onset of disability and result in a compression of morbidity to relieve our future society of the burden of chronic illness.

What are the critical choices that will affect the delivery, cost and quality of patient care? This paper reviews and analyzes the major trends and developments in the health of Americans and in the medical care system. The paper is divided into three parts: the first discusses the health of the population in terms of life expectancy, mortality, health status, use of medical care services, future morbidity patterns and the impact of an aging population on the medical care system. The second part examines the medical care industry: the organization, delivery, and financing of medical care services. The selected cross-cutting policy issues in the final section include changing reimbursement policies; access to medical care; long-term care; and the evolution of corporate for-profit medicine.

PART I: HEALTH OF AMERICANS

Decades of progress form the background for any discussion of the current health status of Americans. As this country and others have completed successive stages in the long transformation from rural agrarian to urban technological societies, one set of diseases has displaced another in the forefront of health concerns. As the infectious diseases were brought under control in this country in the first decades of this century, chronic diseases began to emerge as the major causes of death and disability. Life expectancy and death rates are the oldest measures of health status; these and other measures of health status are discussed below.

Life Expectancy

During this century, life expectancy in the United States has consistently increased. Since the turn of the century, more than a quarter century (27 years) has been added to life expectancy at birth and almost five years have been added at age 65. Based on mortality experience in 1900, an individual born in that year could expect to live an average of 47.3 years; by 1983 life expectancy reached 74.7 years. In 1900, an elderly person would expect to live 11.9 additional years to reach age 77; by 1983, life expectancy at age 65 increased to 16.8 years. Thus a person reaching age 65 in 1983 will survive on the average to about age 82.

Although improvements in life expectancy have been shared by males and females and by white and black persons, women and black persons have experienced the most rapid improvements. Between 1950 and 1983, women gained 7.2 years compared with only 5.4 years for men; white persons gained 6.1 years compared with 8.9 years for blacks. But the differentials in life expectancy at birth are large between men and women and black and white persons. The difference between life expectancy for males and females widened gradually by almost a year, on the average, for each decade between 1950 and 1970. The important trend that appears to be emerging since 1970 is a stabilization in the difference between male and female life expectancy—life expectancy at birth for women has been approximately 7.5 years greater than for males. Provisional data for 1982 and 1983 show a slight reduction to 7.4 and 7.3 years, respectively. It is too early, however, to forecast a trend toward reduction in the gender differentials in life expectancy.

Major gains in life expectancy at birth for blacks have occurred. From 1950 to 1983, 8.9 years were added for blacks compared with 6.1 years for whites. However, a sizable difference—5.6 years—still exists in life expectancy at birth between white and black people.

Mortality

Life expectancy is one summary measure of mortality. In 1984, 2,010,000 persons died in the United States, a rate of 8.7 per 1,000 population. Because the population has been aging, a more accurate picture of mortality trends is provided by the age-adjusted death rate, which eliminates the distortion associated with changing age composition. Thus, the crude death rate declined 11 percent while the age-adjusted death rate for the total population declined 35 percent during the 33-year period, 1950 to 1983. Examination of the trend clearly shows two separate periods: 1) a moderate decline from 1950–1970, in which the age-adjusted mortality rate declined at an average annual rate of 0.7 percent; and 2) a rapid decline from 1970 to 1983 at 1.6 percent annually.

Trends in mortality rates differ among age groups. Infant mortality rates decreased 67 percent since 1950, the largest decline for any age group. Among young people 15–24 years of age, death rates decreased about two percent per year from 1950 to 1960, but then they increased at almost the same rate during the next 10 years. Since 1970, the trend has been downward at an average annual rate of 1.7 percent. Mortality rates for persons in the age groups 25–64 years decreased 0.6 to 0.7 percent per year from 1950 to 1970, but the pace accelerated to 1.6 to 2.4 percent a year during the 1970s and early '80s.

Similarly, changes in mortality for the elderly were small from 1950 to 1970, but the rate of decline increased significantly from 1970 to 1983. This marked acceleration in declining mortality rates across the age range has significantly impacted the demographic structure of the population in the recent past and is the basis for optimistic population projections in the future.

In 1900, infectious diseases—particularly pneumonia and tuberculosis—were the leading causes of death, accounting for one-fifth of all deaths in the United States. The rapid decline in the death rates for these causes has been evident throughout the developed world. Improvements in sanitation, nutrition, housing and education contributed to the decline. Likewise, advances in medical care, such as immunization and the use of antibiotics, are associated with declining mortality. Heart disease, cancer, stroke and accidents have been the leading causes of death since 1950.

More recently, however, decreases in death rates from some of the major chronic diseases—mainly, the cardiovascular diseases, including heart and cerebrovascular diseases—have been evident. Heart disease continues to be the leading cause of death in the United States, and as such, is the predominant influence on total mortality. The age-adjusted death rate decreased 39 percent from 1950 to 1983. Some suggested explanations for the decline in heart disease mortality include decreased smoking, improved management of hypertension, improved life-styles, decreased dietary intake of saturated fats, more widespread physical activity, improved medical emergency services and more widespread use and increased efficacy of coronary care units.

The second major component of cardiovascular diseases is cerebrovascular diseases or stroke, which is the third leading cause of death in the United States from 1950 to 1970. By 1980, it became the fourth leading cause following accidents. From 1950–1970, cerebrovascular age-adjusted mortality rates decreased at an average annual rate of 1.1 percent. During the 13-year period, 1970–83, death rates from this cause were halved, declining at a rate of 3.1 percent a year. Reductions were observed for men and women, white and black people. Possible factors related to the recent decline include expanded hypertension screening programs, improved management and rehabilitation of the stroke victim and effective hypertension therapy.

Malignant neoplasms, or cancer, is the second leading cause of death in the United States. Age-adjusted death rates for this cause increased 5.5 percent since 1950. Cancer mortality has been increasing for some sites—the respiratory system, breast, colon, pancreas and bladder—and has been decreasing for others — stomach, rectum, cervix, and uterus. The highest rate of increase — almost 200 percent since 1950 — occurred in cancer of the respiratory system mainly due to the effects of smoking.

Accidents were the third leading cause of death in 1983 on an age-adjusted basis. They are the leading cause of death for the population one to 34 years of age. The major component within this category is motor vehicle accident deaths comprising about half the total deaths from accidents.

One of the largest and most persistent differences in mortality is that between white and black Americans. In 1983, blacks experienced death rates approximately 1.5 times those for whites. There are considerable differentials by age. For example, among men ages 15–24, the differential was 2.6; for men aged 25–34, it was 3.1 in 1981.

Obviously, life-style differences contribute markedly to the differentials between black and white mortality. Various forms of violence contribute to the high rate for young adult males. For older age groups, chronic diseases account for a vast majority of the deaths. Even there, life-style differences are important; a larger proportion of black people smoke than white people, and obesity is far more prevalent among black middle-aged women than their white counterparts. Furthermore, black people may be exposed to more occupational hazards than white people. Differences in access to high quality, medical care also probably account for some of the mortality differential. Black people receive considerably fewer preventive services, on the average, than do white people. Treatment is delayed until later stages of disease more frequently among black people than among white people.

Changing Demographic Structure of the Population

Improvements in mortality rates have resulted in increased longevity. The distribution of the population in e United States has shifted with considerable rapidity in both the number and the proportion of the population aged 65 and over. This population group has grown and will continue to grow at a more rapid rate for the rest of the twentieth century and is expected to continue to increase well into the next century. In the 50-year period 1930–1980, the elderly population grew twice as fast as the under age 65 population. On the basis of projection of the population by the U.S. Bureau of the Census, this differential rate of growth will be maintained during the next 50-year period, 1980–2030.

At the turn of the century, there were only 3.1 million elderly people, 4.0 percent of the total population (Forty years later the number of elderly tripled to 9 million and the proportion increased to 6.8 percent. By 1980, the elderly population almost tripled again to 25.5 million persons, representing 11.3 percent of the total population. By the year 2030, it is likely that one out of five Americans will be 65 years or older; and the total number is projected to 64.3 million, more than doubling in the 50-year period, 1980–2030.

Within the age group 65 years and over, the number and proportion of the very old have also increased rapidly. In 1900, less than 125,000 persons were 85 years and over, comprising four percent of the elderly; by 1980, there were almost 2.2 million persons in this age group, nine percent of the elderly. In the 50-year period, 1980–2030, the very old population is projected to quadruple and will comprise 14 percent of the elderly. Those aged 85 and over are projected to be the fastest growing segment of the population. Because of the growth in the number of persons who survive into their eighties and nineties, it is increasingly likely that many elderly persons will have a surviving parent.

Health Status and Use of Medical Care Services

In addition to mortality rates and life expectancy, a variety of measures can be used to depict the health of the population: their own perception of their health, limitation in their usual activities, and restricted and bed-disability days. Table I summarizes these health status measures by age. Not surprisingly, for every measure, health status declines with increasing age. In 1981, 12 percent of the noninstitutionalized population reported that their health was fair or poor compared with people their age, with the percent increasing from four percent of those under 17 years to 30 percent of those aged 65 and over. Approximately 32 million persons, 14 percent of the noninstitutionalized population, reported limitations of activity (preschool or school activities, employment or keeping house) due to chronic diseases. The number suffering limitation of activity increases with age: four percent of the total under 17 years, eight percent at ages 17–44 years, 24 percent at ages 45–64 years, and 46 percent at age 65 and over.

Restricted activity and bed-disability days also increase with age. Among the elderly, 40 days per year are restricted activity days, of which 14 are bed-disability days.

The use of all medical care services except dental care increases with age (Table I). In 1981, noninstitutionalized persons under 44 years had 4.2 physician visits (other than visits to hospital inpatients); the elderly had 6.3 visits. There were 38.6 million discharges from nonfederal short-stay hospitals in 1982 with a total of 273 million days of care. More than one quarter (27.7 percent) of all people discharged were elderly and two-fifths (39.6 percent) of all days spent in hospitals were by elderly people. Less than five percent of the civilian noninstitutionalized people were 75 years of age or older in 1982, yet they accounted for 14 percent of the discharges and 21 percent of all the days of care.

Although life expectancy for women is higher than for men, relatively more women are limited in activities of daily living, visit physicians more frequently, and are also predominant users of more days of hospital and nursing home care than men.

TABLE I Health Status and Utilization Measures by Age, United States, 1981

Measure	All Ages	Under 17 Years	17–44 Years	45–64 Years	65 Years and Over
Percent feeling fair or poor	11.8	4.0	8.3	22.0	30.1
Percent limited in activity	14.4	3.8	8.4	23.9	45.7
Percent unable to carry on major activity	3.6	0.2	1.2	6.8	17.5
Restricted-activity days	19.1	10.5	15.1	27.5	39.9
Bed-disability days	6.9	4.8	5.4	9.0	14.0
Physician visits per person	4.6	4.1	4.2	5.1	6.3
Percent seeing doctor in last year	74.3	76.2	72.1	73.5	80.1
Dental visits per person	1.7	1.6	1.7	1.8	1.5
Discharges from short-stay hospitals per 1,000 pop.	169.3	72.9*	148.7*	195.3	396.5
Days of care in short-stay hospitals per 1,000 pop.	1217.7	337.1*	769.6*	1564.0	4155.3
Average length of stay in short-stay hospitals	7.2	4.6*	5.2*	8.0	10.5
Needs help in one or more basic physical activities per 1,000 pop.	22.5**	—	5.1	20.6	90.2

*The rates for the under 17 age group are for under 15 years and rates for 17–44 age group are for 15–44 years
**Includes adults aged 18 and over

Source: US National Center for Health Statistics. *Vital and Health Statistics,* Series 10, No. 141, DHHS Publication No. (PHS) 82-1569, Series 13, No. 72, DHHS Publication No. (PHS) 83-1733, and Advance Data No. 92, DHHS Publication No. (PHS) 83-1250. Government Printing Office.

Chronic Illness

The incidence of chronic illness increases with age and becomes a major cause of disability requiring medical care. Not surprisingly, older persons who suffer from chronic and disabling conditions are high utilizers of medical resources. The elderly with chronic activity limitation had 8.7 visits to physicians per year in contrast with 4.3 visits for persons with no activity limitation. They had 41.2 hospitalizations per 100 elderly persons per year in contrast with 14.8 for those with no limitation of activity. The 46 percent of elderly people who were limited in activity because of a chronic condition accounted for 63 percent of physician contacts, 71 percent of hospitalizations, and 82 percent of all the days that older people spent in bed because of health conditions.

During a period of declining mortality rates for many of the chronic diseases, morbidity has been rising. Prevalence and limitations of activity due to chronic conditions have increased in the past 20-year period for all age groups for heart disease, hypertension, and arteriosclerosis. For cerebrovascular diseases, bronchitis and asthma, and several other chronic diseases, morbidity has risen for certain age groups. Trends in the health of middle-aged and older persons since the late 1950s suggest a paradox between longer life and worsening health. The apparent worsening health, as reflected in increasing morbidity, is attributed to people's greater awareness of their diseases due to earlier diagnosis, improved survival with more severe illnesses, and earlier accommodations to disease.

Longer life, as reflected in decreased mortality rates, may be attributed to earlier and better medical care of diagnosed cases, earlier and better self-care after diagnosis and possibly lower incidence of some chronic diseases.

Impact of an Aging Population

In their population projections, both the Bureau of the Census and the Social Security Administration assumed continued reductions in mortality and improved life expectancy to the year 2050 resulting in a rapidly aging population. Based on the population projections made by the Social Security Administration, national estimates have been made of the impact of these demographic changes in the age structure of the population on health status, health services utilization and expenditures for health care to the year 2040. The projections were based on current age-sex-specific rates of health status and utilization patterns, although it is expected that additional changes in levels of morbidity, therapies and technologies, availability, cost of care and social and economic conditions will also contribute to altered patterns and levels of utilization of medical care services. Whatever else happens, however, the projected changes in the size and age distribution of the population would alone have a significant impact on utilization and consequently on expenditures.

Table II presents the results of these projections for the 60-year period 1980–2040. The total population is projected to increase 41 percent, while the group aged 65 and over will increase 160 percent. The total number of persons limited in activities of daily living is projected to more than triple. The impact of the aging of the population on physician visits and short stay hospital days will be high. Forty percent of the hospital days of care in 2040 are projected for those aged 75 and over, compared with 20 percent in 1980.

The effect on the number of nursing home residents will be greatest, projected to more than triple (increasing from 1.5 million to 5.2 million in 2040) to meet the needs of the aging population. In 1980, 11 percent of the population aged 65 and over consumed 29 percent of total health expenditures; by 2040 the elderly are projected to comprise one fifth of the population, and almost half of the expenditures would be made in their behalf.

Short-term population projections to the year 2000 by the Bureau of the Census show significant differential rates of changes in the population of the four regions of the United States. The West and South will be the fastest

TABLE II Current and Projected Population, Limitations in Activities of Daily Living, Medical Care Utilization and Expenditures, by Age, 1980 and 2040

Characteristic and Year	All Ages	Under 65	Age 65 and Over		
			Total	65–74	75 and Over
Population (thousands):					
1980	232,669	206,777	25,892	15,627	10,265
2040	328,503	261,247	67,256	29,425	37,831
1980–2040 Percent Increase	41.2	26.3	159.8	88.3	268.5
Persons with Limitation in Activities of Daily Living (thousands):					
1980	3,142	1,362	1,780	648	1,132
2040	7,922	2,002	5,920	1,288	4,632
1980–2040 Percent Increase	152.1	47.0	232.6	98.8	309.2
Physician Visits (millions):					
1980	1,102	936	166	100	66
2040	1,621	1,193	428	187	241
1980–2040 Percent Increase	47.1	27.5	157.8	87.0	265.2
Days of Hospital Care (millions):					
1980	274	169	105	49	56
2040	549	236	312	93	219
1980–2040 Percent Increase	100.4	39.6	197.1	89.8	291.1
Nursing Home Residents (thousands):					
1980	1,511	196	1,315	227	1,088
2040	5,227	248	4,979	425	4,554
1980–2040 Percent Increase	245.9	26.5	278.6	87.2	318.6
Personal Health Expenditures (in constant 1980 billions of dollars):					
1980	$219.4	$154.9	$ 64.5	na	na
2040	369.0	201.5	167.5	na	na
1980–2040	68.2	30.1	159.7		

Source: Rice DP, Feldman JJ: Living longer in the United States: Demographic changes and health needs of the elderly. *Milbank Mem Fund Q* 6:1983.

growing regions, increasing 45 percent and 31 percent, respectively, from 1980 to 2000. The North Central population is projected to rise only 1.5 percent while the Northeast is projected to lose population during the same period. The elderly population in all regions, however, is projected to rise, ranging from a 12 percent increase in the Northeast to 60 percent in the South and West.

PART II: THE MEDICAL CARE INDUSTRY

The medical care industry in the United States encompasses a wide variety of institutions, organizations and personnel that provide the full gamut of preventive, medical, therapeutic, restorative and related services. It is one of the largest industries in the United States today. About 7.9 million persons—7.1 percent of the employed population—are health workers; more than 25,000 facilities with three million beds provide inpatient health care; and almost $400 billion—10.6 percent of GNP—was spent for health care last year. Growth in the health industry has been rapid. Since 1950, health manpower has increased five-fold, general hospital beds have doubled and health expenditures are 30 times the amount spent in 1950.

Hospital Facilities

Hospitals constitute a large segment of the medical care industry in the United States. In 1983, the hospital industry comprised 6,900 hospitals with a total capacity of 1.4 million beds. These hospitals treated 39 million inpatient cases requiring 375 million patient days and 273 million outpatient visits at a total cost of $147 billion. In terms of employment, the industry is clearly one of the largest, with 3.7 million employees and a total payroll of $80 billion.

Community hospitals—short-term general and other special hospitals—provide general medical care to the public as a whole. They represent about 75 percent of all hospital beds, handle 93 percent of all admissions and 77 percent of all hospital outpatient visits, employ 84 percent of the industry's total labor force, and account for 85 percent of the total expenses for hospital care in the nation. About 71 percent of community hospital beds are in voluntary non-profit hospitals, nine percent in proprietary hospitals and the remaining 20 percent in government hospitals.

The number of community hospitals grew rapidly following World War II and the enactment of the Hill-Burton program in 1946. This program provided Federal grants (matched in varying proportions by state and local funds) and loans for the building of hospitals. In 1950, there were about 500,000 community hospital beds, 3.3. beds per 1,000 population. By 1975, the number grew to 942,000, or 4.6 beds per 1,000 population. Although the number' of community hospital beds has continued to increase slightly, the total has not kept pace with the growth in population. In 1982, there were more than one million community hospital beds, 4.4 beds per 1,000 population, with rates ranging from 2.4 in Alaska to 7.6 in the District of Columbia. In 1976, the Institute of Medicine recommended 4.5 beds per 1,000 population with occupancy rate of 80 percent. In 1983, community hospitals operated at 73.4 percent occupancy.

A major concern in recent years is the growth of the proprietary hospitals and the rapid development of the "new medical-industrial complex" that includes for-profit hospitals and nursing homes, diagnostic laboratories, home care and emergency room services, hemodialysis and a wide variety of other services. In 1983, there were 877 proprietary hospitals in the country; most of them provide short-term general care, but some are psychiatric hospitals. Community proprietary hospitals comprised 13 percent of the total hospitals with nine percent of the beds. The major concern is the rapid growth of corporate-owned multi-institutional hospital chains, discussed below under the cross-cutting policy issues.

Nursing Homes

The skilled nursing home is a relatively new institution in the United States. Increases in the number of elderly persons, changes in patient treatment patterns resulting from advances in medical technology and changes in family living arrangements have stimulated a growing demand for limited medical and nursing care outside hospitals. In the late 1960s, the coverage of skilled nursing home care under Medicaid and the provision for extended care services under Medicare greatly stimulated the growth of the industry.

In 1963, there were 8,000 nursing homes with about 320,000 beds. By 1980, there were 23,000 nursing homes with 1.5 million beds. Unlike hospitals, these institutions are predominantly proprietary. About 70 percent of the facilities with 81 percent of the beds are under proprietary ownership. However, in six states (Alaska, Minnesota, North Dakota, South Dakota and Wisconsin), no more than half of the homes are for profit.

Nursing homes are unevenly distributed throughout the nation. The 1.5 million beds in the United States average 60 beds per 1,000 population 65 years and over. The states with the three highest averages were South Dakota (95), Nebraska (92) and Washington (91). At the other extreme, Florida (21), New Mexico (26) and West Virginia (27) had the three lowest averages. Of the 23,000 nursing homes, half had fewer than 50 beds and 95 percent had fewer than 200 beds.

Health Practitioners

During recent decades, dramatic and significant changes have occurred in the number, composition and characteristics of the nation's health personnel. Federal legislation has encouraged and promoted these changes through various means, including programs of educational subsidies to train and place health personnel as well as funds for construction of medical schools. These programs have resulted in the growth of the number and supply of health professionals and increase in the number of minorities and women in formerly white male professions.

The supply of health practitioners (physicians, dentists, optometrists, pharmacists, podiatrists, veterinarians and registered nurses) has increased greatly during the past two decades, both in absolute numbers and in relation to the population. This growth has been particularly striking during the past 17 years, although it has not been uniform among these seven professions. Estimates developed by the Bureau of Health Professions, U.S. Public Health Service, point to rapid increases in the supply of physicians in coming years. The supply of active physicians is expected to continue to increase to 706,500 by the year 2000. Although the growth in physician supply is expected to slow down during the next two decades, this growth is still expected to exceed population growth. The physician-to-population ratio is projected to increase from 199 physicians per 100,000 population in 1981 to 235 in 1990 and 260 in 2000.

Foreign medical graduates are projected to contribute less to the growth in active physician supply during the next two decades than in the previous decade. However, they will comprise a significant portion of physician supply.

The increasing supply of physicians has contributed to the growth of competition in the medical care market and is affecting changes in practice arrangements and payment mechanisms in the United States. Regardless of the method used to estimate the number of physicians needed, the general consensus is that the projected number of physicians exceeds the need; that the nation faces an oversupply of physicians; and that excessive numbers of specialists and subspecialists contribute to the high costs of the health care system. Although projections indicate an excess supply of physicians by the year 2000, an important question is whether there will be an adequate number specially trained in geriatric medicine to meet the needs of an aging population.

Private Health Insurance

The post World War II development of fringe benefits obtained through collective bargaining and the growth of union-management health and welfare funds have been instrumental in the tremendous growth of voluntary health insurance that occurred in the United States. Insurance, both private and public, has increased access to medical care and may have contributed to a healthier population. It is argued, however, that prepayment has resulted in lack of cost consciousness by patients who pay nothing or little at the time of receipt of services, thereby encouraging them to increase their use of medical care services. In addition, the historical structure of insurance benefits has encouraged use of costly inpatient rather than outpatient facilities and the overuse of tests and diagnostic and therapeutic procedures.

In 1983, private health insurance benefits amounted to $100 billion, distributed among four broad categories of insurers: commercial insurance companies — $41.2 billion; Blue Cross and Blue Shield plans — $35.2 billion; self-insured health plans — $17.5 billion; and prepaid health plans including health maintenance organizations (HMOs) and preferred provider organizations (PPOs) — $7.7 billion.

Fundamental changes have occurred during recent years in the financing and administration of private health insurance plans. Insurers increasingly provide administrative services only for many employer health insurance plans, and they no longer bear any of the risk. For many other employers, contracts have been split into self-funded and insured portions, with the insurer providing protection that is equivalent to a traditional insurance plan. Other significant changes have been the growth of HMOs, PPOs and "cafeteria plans," which offer employees choices among health insurance coverages, usually involving tradeoff between other employee benefits, including additional wages in some cases. All of these changes fundamentally affect the division of risk between employers and insurers, the responsibility for determining the amount to be reimbursed and other important aspects of insurance arrangements.

Health Maintenance Organizations. For several decades, prepaid group practice has been advocated as a logical and desirable way of arranging and paying for medical care. Group-practice prepayment plans have grown slowly, but their achievements in assuring more comprehensive care and in containing costs have drawn national attention. In more recent years, the HMO has emerged as an important alternative to traditional private health insurance. HMOs provide a comprehensive range of medical or health care services in a single organization in return for a fixed monthly or annual fee. HMOs are rooted in well-established prototypes, some of which have been in existence for 40 years or more.

The advocacy of HMOs in the 1970s to contain costs while preserving the quality of health care was based on the performance of a small number of prepaid plans in existence at that time that produced substantial savings for their patients. In three areas they differed from traditional fee-for-service health care: 1) the use of inpatient services was 40 to 50 percent lower; 2) overall costs were 15 to 20 percent lower; and 3) quality of care was better or at least equal. After a decade of further research, savings claims are still valid. In 1983, there were 280 operational HMOs in the United States with an enrollment of 12.5 million persons.

Medical Care Expenditures

The continued and persistent rise in medical care spending during recent years has generated much interest, attention and concern as it has consumed a growing share of the nation's GNP. During the 34-year period, 1950 to 1984, medical care spending increased 30 times while its share of GNP rose 2½ times. Health spending in 1984 amounted to $1,580 for every man, woman and child in America, rising from $82 per capita in 1950.

What are the factors behind the continuing increase in medical care spending and the growing burden on society? Several broad factors can be identified: population growth, inflation, product change and the increase in per capita utilization of medical care. This simple list, however, does not capture the enormous changes that have taken place in the organization, delivery and funding of medical care services. Additional economic, medical and demographic changes also affecting the increased demand for medical care services and the rise in spending include growth in private health insurance and prepayment plans; increased public support of medical care for the aged, disabled and poor; increasing population and rising proportion of elderly; a shift from care of acute to more expensive long-term illnesses; improvement and growth of high-cost technology; higher wages and salary costs in the health care industry; and growth in the supply of health manpower and facilities. The growing burden on the economy of medical care spending results from all of the above factors as well as higher medical care prices relative to general prices and a slow down in the general economy with continued growth in the health sector. Thus, in the five-year period, 1978 to 1983, the GNP rose 53 percent compared with an 87 percent increase in medical spending.

Rising prices for medical care services have been the primary force in the rise of personal health care spending in recent years. Between 1950 and 1965, price inflation accounted for 43 percent of the increase; between 1965 and 1984 it accounted for 65 percent of the increase. The effect of population growth has diminished substantially from the first period to the second. Increases in intensity of use and quality changes accounted for a larger share of the increase in the first period.

In 1984, health spending increased 9.1 percent from the previous year, the slowest annual rate of increase in 20 years. This increase compares with spending growth of 10.6 percent in 1983 and 15.3 percent in 1980, the highest single-year increase. In 1984, the GNP rose 10.8 percent, a higher rate of increase than for medical care spending. Health expenditures represented 10.6 percent of GNP, down from 10.7 percent in the prevous year and the first decrease in health spending as a percentage of GNP since 1978.

According to the Department of Health and Human Services Secretary, lower overall inflation accounted for a large measure of the reduced growth in health care spending, but the most important development was the drop in the use of hospital inpatient services: community hospital admissions fell 3.7 percent and inpatient days fell 8.6 percent, changes attributed both to the Medicare prospective payment system for hospitals and also to private sector initiatives designed to increase health care efficiency and curb rising health costs. These initiatives are discussed in more detail in Part III below.

Source of Medical Care Spending. The major portion of health care expenses has in the past been borne by the private sector. From 1950 to 1966, private outlays constituted almost three-fourths of the total. By 1984, the government's portion rose to 40 percent of the total, and federal spending was almost three times that of state and local governments. Private health insurance and philanthropy covered one-third, further reducing direct private payments to 28 percent of the personal health care bill compared with two-thirds in 1950. The rise in third-party payments tends to reduce the financial burden of serious illness and patient concern about the cost of care received, and removes the restraining influences from the physician to hospitalize patients and use high-cost technologies.

In addition to the implementation of public programs, the federal government also has influenced the health care field through tax subsidies and incentives by treatment of employers' contributions to health insurance plans as nontaxable forms of employee income. This preferential tax treatment represents a tax loss to the United States Treasury estimated at $18 billion in 1980.

Type of Expenditures. Hospital care accounted for the largest portion of health expenditures, amounting to $158 billion, 42 percent of total outlays in 1984. Hospital costs have been increasing rapidly due to a number of factors: advances in medical and hospital technology that are often costly; growth in the range of services available such as intensive care units; elaborate and costly equipment with rapid obsolescence rates; rise in labor costs, both in wages and in the number of employees per patient day; and, finally, reimbursement at cost under Medicare and Medicaid without incentives for efficiency and economy.

Health program managers and federal policy makers have become increasingly concerned about curbing inflation in hospital and medical care costs. Numerous controls have evolved, many of them in the last decade. Among these are supply limitations (certificate-of-need for capital construction), financial disincentives to the patient (insurance deductibles and coinsurance rates), authorization requirements (authorization for surgery pending second opinion), review programs (utilization and claims processing reviews), legal action (malpractice suits), regulation of rates (state hospital rate-setting commissions), and prospective budgeting (payment per discharge). The Reagan administration designed a new Medicare payment system, effective October 1, 1983, establishing separate rates for hospital admissions with different diagnoses, the diagnosis related groups (DRGS) discussed in Part III below.

Professional services—physicians, dentists and other professional personnel—totaled $109 billion in 1984 and accounted for 28 percent of expenditures. Almost two-fifths of these costs were paid by individuals out-of-pocket. Private insurance paid two-fifths and public programs one-fifth.

Nursing home care spending totaled $32 billion, accounting for 8.3 percent of expenditures. Public programs, mainly Medicaid, paid half of these expenditures and direct payments comprised the other half; private health insurance covered virtually none of these costs. Drugs and appliances accounted for nine percent of expenditures. Most of these costs—76 percent—were paid by individuals out-of-pocket.

Public Health Care Programs. During the last few decades, medical care has come to be recognized as a basic right, along with food, clothing and shelter.

The government has played a significant role in the attainment of this right, greatly enhanced by the 1965 enactment of Medicare (health insurance for the aged [the disabled were covered in 1972]) and Medicaid (health care coverage for low-income persons). Medicare and Medicaid are the two largest public programs supporting health care services and supplies, with total expenditures of $63.1 billion and $36.7 billion, respectively, in 1984. Since the inception of these programs, the gap in medical care use between low income and other persons has narrowed.

In 1982, with 28 million elderly enrolled in the Medicare program, 39 percent did not receive care paid by Medicare. Four percent received $10,000 or more each in benefits; these persons accounted for 47 percent of Medicare reimbursements. Nine percent received $3,000 to $9,999 each, accounting for 35 percent of reimbursements. Thus, 13 percent of the elderly received 82 percent of the amounts reimbursed under the Medicare program.

Of the 22 million Medicaid recipients in 1983, 15 percent were age 65 and over, accounting for 37 percent of the expenditures under the program. Fourteen percent of the recipients were blind and disabled and accounted for 35 percent of the expenditures. Seventy percent of the recipients obtained benefits through Aid for Dependent Children, accounting for 26 percent. Questions are being raised regarding relative public spending devoted to children versus the elderly, with the term "intergenerational equity" describing tradeoffs in health and social welfare allocations between the two population groups.

PART III: POLICY ISSUES

The policy issues of the last two decades ranged from the concern about equity and access to medical care to questions of control of utilization and cost, efficiency in the delivery of care; and, with increasing frequency, the efficacy of that care. National concern about the cost of health care has produced an array of options ranging from increased regulation to unfettered competition from which to choose. Policies must be chosen carefully, however, to promote consumers' incentives for healthy behavior, adequate levels of health insurance coverage and appropriate use of medical care coverage and services. Providers of medical care must also face incentives to deliver quality medical care services efficiently at competitive prices.

Discussed in this section are selected current policy issues emerging from past trends in the organization, delivery and financing of medical care in the United States, including reimbursement policies, access to medical care, long-term care and corporate for-profit medicine. These are meant to briefly highlight selected policy issues.

Reimbursement Policies

Hospital Reimbursement Policy. Cost-based hospital reimbursement had been the practice used by Blue Cross under private health insurance prior to the enactment of Medicare in 1965. The cost basis for paying hospitals was a pass-through for third-party payors, whether the Federal government or private insurer. There were no incentives for hospitals to control costs and no rewards for improving efficiency. Until October 1983, Medicare reimbursed hospitals for their "reasonable costs" of providing care, subject to a few limits and exclusions.

The Social Security Amendments of 1983 marked a major departure from cost-based reimbursement by establishing the Medicare prospective payment system. Beginning October 1, 1983, hospitals are paid a prospectively determined rate for each discharge. Patients are classified into one of 468 diagnosis-related groups and the hospital is paid a fixed predetermined payment per DRG. This prospectively determined DRG rate covers only the operating costs; excluded are costs of treating "outlier" patients, capital-related costs, medical education costs, kidney acquisition costs and bad debts, which are reimbursed on the basis of costs. The DRG payment to each hospital varies depending on the hospital's location, the area wage rate and the number of residents in training. Each of the 468 DRGs is constructed from statistical and clinical analysis of all cases treated, patient age and sex, treatment procedure, discharge status and specific diagnosis.

Implementation of the new system was phased in over a three-year period that began in October 1983. In the first year, three-fourths of the payments to hospitals were based on their own cost experience in the base year and one-fourth based on the new federal rates. By 1986, the new federal DRG prospective payment system covered all hospital payments under Medicare.

The Administration has taken steps to assure quality of care under the new prospective payment system. The first step is the establishment of Peer Review Organizations (PROs). Hospitals must contract with PROs if they are to be paid under the new system. They review the validity of diagnoses; quality of care provided; the appropriateness of admissions, transfers, and discharges; and the nature of handling outlier cases. There is one PRO in each state and each has signed a contract with the Health Care Financing Administration indicating how it proposed to undertake these functions.

The law also provides for a review of the system by a Prospective Payment Assessment Commission (PROPAC) under the aegis of the Congressional Office of Technology Assessment. The Commission's charge is to advise on setting the DRG payments, recalibrating or creating new ones; judge the rate increases built into the system; and examine coverage and technical issues concerning the DRG payment system.

Although DRGs have been in place for only a short period, we have already seen significant effects as a result of this profound change in hospital reimbursement. Early research suggests that patient classification by means of unadjusted DRGs does not adequately reflect severity of illness and that prospective payment programs based on DRGs alone may unfairly and adversely discriminate against certain hospitals.

Policy experts agree that DRGs may contain costs, but concern is expressed that they threaten to restrict access to health care and adversely affect the quality of care by premature discharges, many of whom may need long-term care services. Follow-up care may not be guaranteed, and the medical needs of patients referred to nursing homes, home health care and other forms of community care could be greater than providers are equipped to handle. It is also argued that changes resulting from the DRG payment system might increase the costs of other public programs, particularly Medicaid, as will the aged patient's costs.

The hospital industry has responded to the new payment system by making massive cuts in personnel and aggressively negotiating lower prices from suppliers. Admissions and lengths of stay were reduced in 1984 and figures for the first quarter of 1985 show continued reductions. According to the *Wall Street Journal*, hospitals began treating patients in less costly, more profitable ways. Many big urban institutions and both nonprofit and for-profit hospitals are "thriving." Some industry observers are concerned that today's profits may be at the expense of quality of care.

Physician Reimbursement. While hospitals control some of their costs through administrators' decisions about acquisition and maintenance of equipment, labor and buildings, physicians are estimated to control 60 to 80 percent of hospital costs through their medical decisions about the use of these resources—whom to admit, how long the patient will stay, the quantity of ancillary services used, whether or not to perform surgery. . . . In making these decisions, physicians are influenced by financial factors, especially third-party reimbursement rates. The amount paid by Medicare to physicians has a major impact on the number of services that beneficiaries receive and on the amount paid for each service.

Medicare's method of paying physicians is based on "customary, prevailing, and reasonable charges." The amount paid for each procedure is called the "reasonable charge." It represents the lowest of three factors: 1) the price charged by the physician for the service; 2) the customary charge by that physician for the procedure; and 3) the prevailing charge defined as the 75th percentile of charges of all physicians in that specialty and geographic area for that procedure during the preceding year. After the beneficiary has paid a $75 annual deductible, Medicare pays 80 percent of the reasonable charges for any service. The remaining 20 percent is the responsibility of the beneficiary, who may have supplementary private insurance that covers it.

Access to Medical Care

In the two decades since the enactment of Medicare and Medicaid, impressive strides have been made in ensuring more Americans access to the benefits of the health care system. More people attained regular access to health services, and a backlog of long-neglected needs, especially among the elderly and the poor, was specifically addressed.

Medicaid also has been successful in improving access to physician services for the population it covers. Evidence suggests, however, that those poor not covered by Medicaid continue to lag well behind others in the use of services. Significant gaps still exist between subgroups of the population by income, race and place of residence. Since the poor tend to be sicker than the nonpoor, the higher medical care use rates among the poor do not necessarily indicate that they get more care given similar health status. After adjustment for health status, persons who report their health as fair or poor have significantly fewer visits than those in the highest income groups. The use-disability rate, a measure of the number of physician visits per 1,000 disability days, shows a wider differential between income class.

The recent focus of policy analysts, states, hospital associations and private foundations has been on the uninsured population. The inability of large public hospitals to shift the cost of uncompensated services to patients with insurance has complicated the issue.

Estimates of the uninsured population range between 30 and 35 million — 12 to 15 percent of the population. Both the number and percent of the population without health insurance today have grown in the last few years.

The health care financing and delivery system is undergoing rapid and profound changes. The adoption of DRGs and other prospective payments for hospital care, the growth of for-profit health care, the adoption of business-oriented approaches by health care providers and the growth of competition in the medical care market may result in greater vulnerability to access barriers for our neediest citizens. The issue of how to provide and finance medical care for the 35 million uninsured must be actively addressed by both private and public interests.

Long-Term Care

In addition to medical care, many persons who have lost some capacity for self-care due to chronic disease or who suffer disabling physical or mental conditions require a wide range of social, personal and supportive services. Services may be continuous or intermittent, but are delivered for a sustained period to individuals who have a demonstrated need to enable them to be maintained at their maximum levels of health and well-being. Long-term care is defined as physical care over a prolonged period for those incapable of sustaining themselves without this care, a spectrum of services responding to different needs along a trajectory of chronic illness and disability. To address the multiple and varied long-term care needs of the aged, services must cross the boundaries between income maintenance, and health, social and housing programs.

While 29 percent of the long-term care population reside in an institutional setting, 71 percent are in the community. Residents of institutions are generally more disabled than dependent elderly in the community. However, for every person 65 years of age and over residing in an institution, there are twice as many living in the community requiring similar levels of care.

With the growing numbers of chronically ill elderly and disabled adults, increasing consideration is given to alternatives in long-term care services and in preventing institutionalization. Recent years have seen the development of a variety of community services such as day care, home health, meals-on-wheels, respite care. Most of these services aim at maintaining the independence of the aged or disabled person at home to avoid institutional placement, often viewed as a measure of last resort.

Despite the availability of this vast array of health and social services, families, friends and neighbors still provide the bulk of long-term services to the aged and disabled in the United States. It is estimated that as much as 60 to 80 percent of the care presently received by the disabled and aged stems from this source.

Although the debate surrounding what to do about long-term care has intensified in recent years, there is little, if any, consensus regarding how the disparate elements that constitute the long-term care financing and delivery system should be brought together to fashion a coherent set of national policies. The unique characteristics of the people needing long-term care, the vast numbers of public and private entities involved in the policy-making service delivery processes and the many unknowns regarding the most efficient and effective way to deliver care all pose formidable barriers to needed change. Moreover, inflationary pressures and budgetary short-falls have made cost considerations a paramount concern to policy makers of all levels of government and inhibited new initiatives in this area to a significant degree.

Corporate For-Profit Medicine

In 1980, Arnold Relman sounded the alarm that a "new medical-industrial complex" had emerged in the prior decade. He defined this phenomenon as "a large and growing network of private corporations engaged in the business of supplying health-care services to patients for a profit — services heretofore provided by nonprofit institutions or individual practitioners."

Coupled with the emergence of the for-profit sector has been the growth of investor-owned chains which continue to expand their holdings through the purchase, lease or management of existing not-for-profit hospitals. The movement toward for-profit centralized ownership has progressed from acute-care hospitals to nursing homes, psychiatric hospitals, dental care, home health care, health maintenance organizations, freestanding surgi-centers and emergi-centers, alcoholism and drug dependency clinics, primary care centers, and medical equipment suppliers.

Various predictions are being made regarding the growth of corporate for-profit medical care. One estimate is that by 1990, about 2,000 corporations will be responsible for the nation's health care, as compared with 5,000 in 1980. Another forecast is that by the end of this decade, we are likely to have 20 to 30 national chains and 200 or 300 medical groups providing most of the nation's health care. Other health care experts predict that within a decade, health care will be in the hands of 10 to 15 giant conglomerates. Under this theory, all the nation's physicians, nurses and other health care practitioners could be working for large conglomerates.

Of special concern is the future economic viability of teaching hospitals. Investor-owned chains are actively acquiring teaching hospitals with important public policy ramifications for medical education, biomedical research and the development and testing of new medical technology. A major concern is that profits from operating teaching hospitals will no longer be used to cross-subsidize the societal contributions of teaching hospitals but instead will revert to investors.

Another vexing issue is the preservation of academic and professional values in a profit-making setting. A moral dilemma is created when physicians act as patient advocates and as corporate employers or investors in for-profit health care. Several agreements have been made in the past three years between academic health centers and investor-owned corporations for the operation of university teaching hospitals. Whether such ventures can be structured in ways that continue to safeguard the values and traditional functions and responsibilities of academic health centers remains to be seen.

CONCLUSION

Americans are healthier now than ever before. High quality medical care has contributed substantially to improvements in our health status over the years. A variety of social, economic and historical forces have significantly affected medical practice in the United States. These are complex developments that have led us to the organization, delivery and financing of health services that are in place today.

The burden of illness is large and multifaceted. The dimensions presented here have significant implications for investments in efforts to solve the health, disease and medical care problems that beset our society. They are legitimate considerations essential for planning to meet the future demand for medical care services and for priorities in biomedical and health services research.

A recent survey of 415 health system leaders responding to questions about the future of the United States health system is informative and optimistic. Respondents expected life expectancy and health status to improve in the next 20 years, but at a lesser rate than in the past 20 years. Almost all respondents believe the public's greatest concern about personal health services had shifted from access in 1962 to cost in 1982. Two out of every five respondents said "cost" is the most important problem of the health system today. Half of these respondents wanted to implement competition or cost-containment, or encourage alternative delivery systems; the remainder described other changes. Respondents' visions of the most significant change that would occur in the United States health system in the next 20 years included improved life-styles, the corporatization of health care; a national health care system; competition among providers; and advances in technology.

Some policy analysts have characterized the current era as a period of revolution focused on containing medical care costs. According to Fuchs we are in the midst of the third revolution in health care financing since the end of World War II. The first revolution took place between 1945 and 1960 with the rapid growth of private health insurance; the second occurred in 1965 with creation of Medicare and Medicaid and the explosion of health care costs. Since the late 1970s, the primary goal of the revolution is to contain costs. Reinhardt characterizes this cost containment with health providers and policymakers on opposite sides of the battle line. "Providers believe that policymakers seek to constrain health-care expenditures without any regard to the quality of care. Policymakers, on the other hand, believe that the providers' manifest concern over quality is just a smokescreen put up to defend a habit of reckless spending (and opulent life-styles) without regard to economic efficiency. At the moment there are recriminations all around and nary an attempt at constructive dialogue."

In the eighth decade of our century, an increasing number of enquiring minds are dissatisfied with the results of bigger and better analyses. They realize that most children born now will grow to maturity. However, when they become adults, physical pains and emotional miseries will probably be so severe that they cannot live without sedatives and tranquilizers.

IDA ROLF

Arnold S. Relman

The New Medical-Industrial Complex

In his farewell address as President on January 17, 1961, Eisenhower warned his countrymen of what he called "the military-industrial complex," a huge and permanent armaments industry that, together with an immense military establishment, had acquired great political and economic power. He was concerned about the possible conflict between public and private interests in the crucial area of national defense.

The past decade has seen the rise of another kind of private "industrial complex" with an equally great potential for influence on public policy—this time in health care. What I will call the "new medical-industrial complex" is a large and growing network of private corporations engaged in the business of supplying health-care services to patients for a profit—services heretofore provided by nonprofit institutions or individual practitioners.

I am not referring to the companies that manufacture pharmaceuticals or medical equipment and supplies. Such businesses have sometimes been described as part of a "medical-industrial complex," but I see nothing particularly worrisome about them. They have been around for a long time, and no one has seriously challenged their social usefulness. Furthermore, in a capitalistic society there are no practical alternatives to the private manufacture of drugs and medical equipment.

The new medical-industrial complex, on the other hand, is an unprecedented phenomenon with broad and potentially troubling implications for the future of our medical-care system. It has attracted remarkably little attention so far (except on Wall Street), but in my opinion it is the most important recent development in American health care and it is in urgent need of study.

THE NEW MEDICAL-INDUSTRIAL COMPLEX

Proprietary Hospitals

Of course proprietary hospitals are not new in this country. Since the past century, many small hospitals and clinics have been owned by physicians,

Arnold S. Relman, M.D., is editor-in-chief of the *New England Journal of Medicine*, Waltham, Massachusetts.

primarily for the purpose of providing a workshop for their practices. In fact, the majority of hospitals in the United States were proprietary until shortly after the turn of the century, when the small doctor-owned hospitals began to be replaced by larger and more sophisticated community or church-owned nonprofit institutions. The total number of proprietary hospitals in the country decreased steadily during the first half of this century. In 1928 there were 2435 proprietary hospitals, constituting about 36 per cent of hospitals of all types; by 1968 there were only 769 proprietary hospitals, 11 per cent of the total. However, there has been a steady trend away from individual ownership and toward corporate control. During the past decade the total number of proprietary hospitals has been increasing again, mainly because of the rapid growth of the corporate-owned multi-institutional hospital chains.

There are now about 1000 proprietary hospitals in this country; most of them provide short-term general care, but some are psychiatric institutions. These hospitals constitute more than 15 per cent of nongovernmental acute general-care hospitals in the country and more than half the nongovernmental psychiatric hospitals. About half the proprietary hospitals are owned by large corporations that specialize in hospital ownership or management; the others are owned by groups of private investors or small companies. In addition to the 1000 proprietary hospitals, about 300 voluntary nonprofit hospitals are managed on a contractual basis by one or another of these profit-making hospital corporations.

The proprietary hospitals are mostly medium-sized (100 to 250 beds) institutions offering a broad range of general inpatient services but few outpatient facilities other than an emergency room. Some are smaller than 100 beds and a few are larger than 250 beds, but none would qualify as major medical centers, none have residency programs, and few do any postgraduate teaching. Most are located in the Sunbelt states in the South, in the Southwest, and along the Pacific Coast, in relatively prosperous and growing small and medium-sized cities and in the suburbs of the booming big cities of those areas. Virtually none are to be found in the big old cities of the North or in the states with strong rate-setting commissions or effective certificate-of-need policies.

Although there are no good, detailed studies comparing the characteristics and performance of proprietary and voluntary hospitals, there is a generally held view that proprietary hospitals have more efficient management and use fewer employees per bed. It is also said that fewer of the patients in proprietary hospitals are in the lower income brackets and that fewer are funded through Medicaid.

Proprietary Nursing Homes

Proprietary nursing homes are even bigger business. In 1977 there were nearly 19,000 nursing-home facilities of all types, and about 77 per cent were proprietary. Some, like the proprietary hospitals, are owned by big corporations, but most (I could not find out exactly how many) are owned by small investors, many of them physicians.

Laboratory and Other Services

The number of laboratory tests performed each year in this country is huge and growing at a compound rate of about 15 per cent per year. About a third of the diagnostic laboratories are owned by profit-making companies. Most of these are relatively small local firms, but there are a dozen or more large corporations currently in the laboratory business, some with over $100 million in sales per year. Some of these corporations operate laboratories in the voluntary non-profit hospitals, but most of the proprietary laboratories are outside hospitals and use an efficient mail or messenger service.

A large variety of services are being sold by newly established companies in the medical-industrial complex. Included are mobile CAT scanning, cardiopulmonary testing, industrial health screening, rehabilitation counseling, dental care, weight-control clinics, alcohol and drug-abuse programs, comprehensive prepaid HMO programs, and physicians' house calls. Two markets that deserve special mention are hospital emergency-room services and long-term hemodialysis programs for end-stage renal disease.

With the decline in general practice and the virtual disappearance of physicians able and willing to make house calls, the local hospital emergency room has become an increasingly important source of walk-in medical and psychiatric services in urban and suburban areas. The use of emergency rooms has increased rapidly in the past two decades and has stimulated the development of emergency medicine as a specialty. Most third-party payers reimburse for services rendered in hospital emergency rooms at a higher rate than for the same services provided by physicians in their private offices. The result has been a vigorous new industry specializing in emergency services. Many large businesses have been established by entrepreneurial physicians to supply the necessary professional staffing for emergency rooms all over the country, and this has proved to be a highly profitable venture. In some cases, large corporations have taken over this function and now provide hospitals with a total emergency-care package.

Hemodialysis

Long-term hemodialysis is a particularly interesting example of stimulation of private enterprise by public financing of health care. In 1972 the Social Security Act was amended to bring the treatment of end-stage renal disease under Medicare funding. When the new law was enacted, only about 40 patients per million population were receiving long-term hemodialysis treatment in this country, almost entirely under the auspices of nonprofit organizations. Forty per cent of these dialyses were home based, and renal transplantation was rapidly becoming an alternative form of treatment. The legislation provided for reimbursement for center-based or hospital-based dialysis without limit in numbers. The result was an immediate, rapid increase in the total number of patients on long-term dialysis treatment and a relative decline in home dialysis and transplantations. The number of patients on dialysis treatment in the United States is now over 200 per million population (the highest in the world), and only about 13 per cent are being dialyzed at home.

Proprietary dialysis facilities began to appear even before public funding of end-stage renal disease but the number increased rapidly thereafter. These facilities were usually located outside hospitals and had lower expenses than the hospital units. According to data obtained from the Health Care Financing Administration, nearly 40 per cent of the hemodialysis in this country is now provided by profit-making units.

INCOME AND PROFITABILITY

This, in barest outline, is the present shape and scope of the "new medical-industrial complex," a vast array of investor-owned businesses supplying health services for profit. No one knows precisely the full extent of its operations or its gross income, but I estimate that the latter was approximately $35 billion to $40 billion last year—about a quarter of the total amount expended on personal health care in 1979. Remember that this estimate does not include the old medical-industrial complex, i.e., the businesses concerned with the manufacture and sale of drugs, medical supplies, and equipment.

The new health-care industry is not only very large, but it is also expanding rapidly and is highly profitable. New businesses seem to be springing up all the time, and those already in the field are diversifying as quickly as new opportunities for profit can be identified. Given the expansive nature of the health-care market and the increasing role of new technology, such opportunities are not hard to find.

The shares of corporations in the health-care business have done exceedingly well in the stock market, and many Wall Street analysts and brokers now enthusiastically recommend such investments to their clients.

WHY HAVE PRIVATE BUSINESSES IN HEALTH CARE?

Let us grant that we have a vast, new, rapidly growing and profitable industry engaged in the direct provision of health care. What's wrong with that? In our country we are used to the notion that private enterprise should supply most of the goods and services that our society requires. With the growing demand for all kinds of health care over the past two decades and the increasing complexity and cost of the services and facilities required, wasn't it inevitable that businesses were attracted to this new market? Modern health-care technology needs massive investment of capital—a problem that has become more and more difficult for the voluntary nonprofit institutions. How appropriate, then, for private entrepreneurs to come forward with the capital needed to build and equip new hospitals, nursing homes, and laboratories, and to start new health-care businesses. The market was there and a good profit ensured — the challenge was simply to provide the necessary services efficiently and at an acceptable level of quality.

In theory, the free market should operate to improve the efficiency and quality of health care. Given the spur of competition and the discipline exerted by consumer choice, private enterprise should be expected to respond to demand by offering better and more varied services and products, at lower unit costs, than could be provided by nonprofit voluntary or governmental institutions. Large corporations ought to be better managed than public or voluntary institutions; they have a greater incentive to control costs, and they are in a better position to benefit from economies of scale. We Americans believe in private enterprise and the profit motive. How logical, then, to extend these concepts to the health-care sector at a time when costs seem to be getting out of control, voluntary institutions are faltering, and the only other alternative appears to be more government regulation.

That, at least, is the theory. Whether the new medical-industrial complex is in fact improving quality and lowering unit cost in comparison with the public or private voluntary sectors remains to be determined. There are no adequate studies of this important question, and we will have to suspend judgment until there are some good data. But even without such information, I think that there are reasons to be concerned about this new direction in health care.

SOME ISSUES

Can we really leave health care to the marketplace? Even if we believe in the free market as an efficient and equitable mechanism for the distribution of most goods and services, there are many reasons to be worried about the industrialization of health care. In the first place, health care is different from most of the commodities bought and sold in the marketplace. Most people consider it, to some degree at least, a basic right of all citizens. It is a public rather than a private good, and in recognition of this fact, a large fraction of the cost of medical research and medical care in this country is being subsidized by public funds. Public funds pay for most of the research needed to develop new treatments and new medical care technology. They also reimburse the charges for health-care services. Through Medicare and Medicaid and other types of public programs, more and more of our citizens are receiving tax-supported medical care.

The great majority of people not covered by public medical-care programs have third-party coverage through private insurance plans, most of which is provided as a fringe benefit by their employers. At present almost 90 per cent of Americans have some kind of health insurance, which ensures that a third party will pay at least part of their medical expenses.

There are other unique features of the medical marketplace, not the least of which is the heavy, often total, dependence of the consumer (patient) on the advice and judgment of the physician. Kenneth Arrow, in explaining why some of the economist's usual assumptions about the competitive free market do not apply to medical care, referred to this phenomenon as the "informational inequality" between patient and physician. Unlike consumers shopping for most ordinary commodities, patients do not often decide what medical services they need—doctors usually do that for them. Probably more than 70 per cent of all expenditures for personal health care are the result of decisions of doctors.

All these special characteristics of the medical market conspire to produce an anomalous situation when private business enters the scene. A private corporation in the health-care business uses technology often developed at public expense, and it sells services that most Americans regard as their basic right—services that are heavily subsidized by public funds, largely allocated through the decisions of physicians rather than consumers, and almost entirely paid for through third-party insurance. The possibilities for abuse and for distortion of social purposes in such a market are obvious.

Health care has experienced an extraordinary inflation during the past few decades, not just in prices but in the use of services. A major challenge—in fact, *the* major challenge—facing the health-care establishment today is to moderate use of our medical resources and yet protect equity, access, and quality. The resources that can be allocated to medical care are limited. With health-care expenditures now approaching 10 per cent of the gross national product, it is clear that costs cannot continue to rise at anything near their present rate unless other important social goals are sacrificed. We need to use our health-care dollars more effectively, by curbing procedures that are unnecessary or inefficient and developing and identifying those that are the best. Overuse, where it exists, can be eliminated only by taking a more critical view of what we do and of how we use our health-care resources.

How will the private health-care industry affect our ability to achieve these objectives? In an ideal free competitive market, private enterprise may be good at controlling unit costs, and even at improving the quality of its products, but private businesses certainly do not allocate their own services or restrict the use of them. On the contrary, they "market" their services; they sell as many units as the market will bear. They may have to trim their prices to sell more, but the fact remains that they are in business to increase their total sales.

If private enterprise is going to take an increasing share of the health-care market, it will therefore have to be appropriately regulated. We will have to find some way of preserving the advantages of a private health-care industry without giving it free rein and inviting gross commercial exploitation. Otherwise, we can expect the use of health services to continue to increase until government is forced to intervene.

THE ROLE OF THE MEDICAL PROFESSION

It seems to me that the key to the problem of overuse is in the hands of the medical profession. With the consent of their patients, physicians act in their behalf, deciding which services are needed and which are not, in effect serving as trustees. The best kind of regulation of the health-care marketplace should therefore come from the informed judgments of physicians working in the interests of their patients. In other words, physicians should supply the discipline that is provided in commercial markets by the informed choices of prudent consumers, who shop for the goods and services that they want, at the prices that they are willing to pay.

But if physicians are to represent their patients' interests in the new medical marketplace, they should have no economic conflict of interest and therefore no pecuniary association with the medical-industrial complex. I do not know the extent to which practicing physicians have invested in health-care businesses, but I suspect that it is substantial. Physicians have direct financial interests in proprietary hospitals and nursing homes, diagnostic laboratories, dialysis units, and many small companies that provide health-care services of various kinds. Physicians are on the boards of many major health-care corporations, and I think it is safe to assume that they are also well represented among the stockholders of these corporations. However, the actual degree of physician involvement is less important than the fact that it exists at all. As the visibility and importance of the private health-care industry grow, public confidence in the medical profession will depend on the public's perception of the doctor as an honest, disinterested trustee. That confidence is bound to be shaken by any financial association between practicing physicians and the new medical-industrial complex. Pecuniary associations with pharmaceutical and medical supply and equipment firms will also be suspect and should therefore be curtailed.

What I am suggesting is that the medical profession would be in a stronger position, and its voice would carry more moral authority with the public and the government, if it adopted the principle that practicing physicians should derive no financial benefit from the health-care market except from their own professional services. I believe that some statement to this effect should become part of the ethical code of the AMA. As such, it would have no legal force but would be accepted as a standard for the behavior of practicing physicians all over the country.

The AMA's former Principles of Ethics, which has just been superseded by the new set of principles adopted by the House of Delegates at its last meeting, did include a declaration on physicians' financial interests, but it was directed primarily at fee-splitting and rebates.

If the AMA took a strong stand against any financial interest of physicians in health-care businesses, it might risk an antitrust suit. Its action might also be misconstrued as hostile to free enterprise. Yet, I believe that the risk to the reputation and self-esteem of the profession will be much greater if organized medicine fails to act decisively in separating physicians from the commercial exploitation of health care. The professional standing of the physician rests no less on ethical commitment than on technical competence. A refusal to confront this issue undermines the moral position of the profession and weakens the authority with which it can claim to speak for the public interest.

Critics of the position argued here will probably point out that even without any investment in health-care businesses, physicians in private fee-for-service practice already have a conflict of interest in the sense that they benefit from providing services that they themselves prescribe. That may be true, but the conflict is visible to all and therefore open to control. Patients understand fee-for-service and most are willing to assume that their doctor's professional training protects them from exploitation. Furthermore, those who distrust their physicians or dislike the fee-for-service system have other alternatives: another physician, a prepayment plan, or a salaried group. What distinguishes the conflict of interest that I have been discussing are its invisibility and a far greater potential for mischief.

OTHER PROBLEMS

The increasing commercialization of health care generates still other serious problems that need to be mentioned. One is the so-called "cream-skimming" phenomenon. Steinwaid and Neuhauser discussed this problem with reference to proprietary hospitals 10 years ago, when the new health-care industry was just appearing on the scene. "The essence of the cream-skimming argument," they said, "is that proprietary hospitals can and do profit by concentrating on providing the most profitable services to the best-paying patients, thereby skimming the cream off the market for acute hospital care and leaving the remainder to nonprofit hospitals." According to these authors, there are two types of "cream-skimming": elimination of low-frequency and unprofitable (though necessary) services, and exclusion of unprofitable patients (e.g., uninsured patients, welfare patients, and those with complex and chronic illnesses). The nonprofit hospitals could not employ such practices, even if they wished to do so, because they have community obligations and are often located in areas where there are many welfare patients. Another form of "skimming" by proprietary hospitals, whether intentional or not, is their virtual lack of residency and other educational programs. Teaching programs are expensive and often oblige hospitals to maintain services that are not economically viable, simply to provide an adequate range of training experience.

Although these arguments seem reasonable, there are no critical studies on which to base firm conclusions about the extent and implications of the skimming phenomenon in the proprietary sector. One has the sense that the larger teaching institutions, particularly those that serve the urban poor, will be feeling increasing competitive economic pressure not only from the proprietary hospitals but also from the medium-sized community hospitals in relatively well-to-do demographic areas. Their charges are generally lower than those of the teaching centers, they take patients away from the centers, and they put the centers in a difficult position in negotiating with rate-setting agencies.

Another danger arises from the tendency of the profit-making sector to emphasize procedures and technology to the exclusion of personal care. Personal care, whether provided by physicians, nurses, or other health-care practitioners, is expensive and less likely to produce large profits than the item-by-item application of technology.

A final concern is the one first emphasized by President Eisenhower in his warning about the "military-industrial complex": "We must guard against the acquisition of unwarranted influence." A private health-care industry of huge proportions could be a powerful political force in the country and could exert considerable influence on national health policy. A broad national health-insurance program, with the inevitable federal regulation of costs, would be anathema to the medical-industrial complex, just as a national disarmament policy is to the military-industrial complex. I do not wish to imply that only vested interests oppose the expansion of federal health-insurance programs (or treaties to limit armaments), but I do suggest that the political involvement of the medical-industrial complex will probably hinder rather than facilitate rational debate on national health-care policy.

SOME PROPOSALS

The new medical-industrial complex is now a fact of American life. It is still growing and is likely to be with us for a long time. Any conclusions about its ultimate impact on our health-care system would be premature, but it is safe to say that the effect will be profound. Clearly, we need more information.

My initial recommendation, therefore, is that we should pay more attention to the new health-care industry. It needs to be studied carefully, and its performance should be measured and compared with that of the nonprofit sector. We need to know much more about the quality and cost of the services provided by the profit-making companies and especially the effects of these companies on use, distribution, and access. We also must find out the extent to which "cream-skimming" is occurring and whether competition from profit-making providers is really threatening the survival of our teaching centers and major urban hospitals.

I suspect that greater public accountability and increased regulation of the private health-care industry will ultimately be required to protect the public interest. However, before any rational and constructive public policies can be developed, we will need a much greater understanding of what is happening. A vast amount of study is still to be done.

The private health-care industry is primarily interested in selling services that are profitable, but patients are interested only in services that they need, i.e., services that are likely to be helpful and are relatively safe. Furthermore, everything else being equal, society is interested in controlling total expenditures for health care, whereas the private health-care industry is interested in increasing its total sales. In the health-care marketplace the interests of patients and of society must be represented by the physician, who alone has the expertise and the authority to decide which services and procedures should be used in any given circumstance. That is why I have urged that physicians should totally separate themselves from any financial involvement in the medical-industrial complex. Beyond that, however, physicians must take a more active interest in assessing medical procedures. Elsewhere I have argued for a greatly expanded national program of evaluation of clinical tests and procedures. Such a program would provide an excellent means by which to judge the social usefulness of the private health-care industry, which depends heavily on new technology and special tests and procedures.

If we are to live comfortably with the new medical-industrial complex we must put our priorities in order: the needs of patients and of society come first. If necessary services of acceptable quality can be provided at lower cost through the profit-making sector, then there may be reason to encourage that sector. But we should not allow the medical-industrial complex to distort our health-care system to its own entrepreneurial ends. It should not market useless, marginal, or unduly expensive services, nor should it encourage unnecessary use of services. How best to ensure that the medical-industrial complex serves the interests of patients first and of its stockholders second will have to be the responsibility of the medical profession and an informed public.

The century just passed may well be examined by future historians as a period during which humans explored their world with a tool, or if you will a microscope, of specialization; as a period when people thought that by increasing the detail known about the enveloping universe, they could have their world under control. The fallacy of this is now increasingly apparent. Even specialists in a field now sense that they are becoming fixed in a limited area, and that they have lost not only the sense of movement, but that of perspective and orientation. Consequently, many thinkers are now spending time and effort to understand and lessen this cultural imbalance.

IDA ROLF

Uwe E. Reinhardt

Rationing the Health-Care Surplus: An American Tragedy

We Americans hold this truth to be self-evident: Our health-care system is the best in the world. This assertion is recited as a form of incantation whenever we meet to discuss health policy. To question the claim would be a rude breach of etiquette.

Actually, much evidence supports that boastful claim. The rigor and thoroughness of American health education probably rank second to none. The products of our health research community are the marvels of the world. Our hospitals and clinics are repositories of the most sophisticated technical know-how imaginable, and they attract the rich and famous worldwide. We have more than enough physicians and nurses to cater superbly to our citizens' health-care needs. And we have a veritable glut of hospital beds — about three for every two actually needed.

The glory, however, comes at a stiff price. To bring us the marvels of modern health care, our providers exact from us a pretty penny. The nation now spends almost 11% of its Gross National Product (GNP) on health care. Few nations hand over such large slices of their national pies to their health-care providers.

And more vexing problems abound. Because health-care costs are so high, middle- and upper-income Americans are increasingly reluctant to purchase health services for low-income families. The nation is redirecting health resources from poor individuals who desperately need care to well-to-do individuals who not only do not need such resources but may even be harmed by the abundance of resources requiring fiscal investment.

Our current dilemma — that is, the rationing of abundant resources — grows out of this nation's inability to agree on the distributional ethics that should be imposed on health.

Uwe E. Reinhardt, Ph.D., is James Madison Professor of Political Economy at Princeton University, Princeton, New Jersey.

FINANCING U.S. HEALTH CARE

In principle, a nation as wealthy as ours could easily afford to spend 11% or more of its GNP on health care. For example, if between 1980 and 2000, health-care expenditures grew at an annual compound rate of 13% and the GNP increased only 9%, then fully 20% of the GNP would go to health care in the year 2000. However, in real (inflation-adjusted) terms, the remaining 80% of the GNP (on a per-capita basis) would still be about 35% higher than its 1980 value! There could still be a chicken and a videocassette recorder in everybody's pot, and our Pentagon could spend, not $700 per toilet seat, but $1,000 or more—perhaps to silver-line toilets or to equip them with FM stereos. In short, there is absolutely no danger that health-care expenditures by themselves will push the nation to the brink of economic ruin in the foreseeable future.

Social role of health care. Unfortunately, what is true for the nation as a whole is not necessarily true for the individual citizen. The degree to which a given national outlay on health care burdens an individual clearly depends on the manner in which that burden is shared.

If the individual's share of total national health expenditures was related strictly to his or her ability to pay, and not to his or her health status, then an outlay tolerable at the national level also should be tolerable at the individual level. Such an arrangement would imply the socialization of health-care expenditures through national health insurance. Fundamental to this arrangement would be the ethical precept that health care, like jurisprudence and basic education, is a *social good* that should be collectively financed.

However, if health care is viewed as a *private consumption good* that should be financed primarily by its individual recipients, then even a relatively modest overall national outlay on health care can translate into considerable fiscal agony for individuals who are both sick and poor.

For better or for worse, Americans have never quite agreed on the social role of health care. Individuals on the left of the political spectrum tend to believe health care is a social good; individuals on the right tend to believe health care is a private consumption good. Most people in between develop a view on the issue only when they are seriously ill. Prior to that, they live along happily, occasionally joining the chorus that our health-care system is the best in the world.

Health insurance coverage. Unable to reach a consensus on the ethics of health-care delivery after decades of public debate, we have developed a complicated health-care financing system which has absurd parts. Some types of health services (such as acute hospital care) are now extensively covered by health insurance while others (such as preventive ambulatory care, prescription drugs, and long-term custodial care) are minimally covered. Some population groups (such as powerful labor union members, business executives, and the well-to-do aged) have excessively generous health insurance policies while others (such as small business employees and the unemployed) have very thin insurance coverage or none at all. Census data from the early 1980s show that as many as 15% of Americans do not have any health insurance whatsoever, with lack of insurance coverage heavily concentrated among the poor and near poor, particularly among minorities.

"Reasonable" fees.   What happens to uninsured, poor Americans when they become ill? During the financially flush 1970s, we used the following approaches with such people. For mild to semi-serious illness, we left these people to fend for themselves, thus effectively rationing health care to them on the basis of price and ability to pay. For critical conditions, however, we extended to them whatever acute, inpatient care was deemed necessary and available nearby. Those who provided that care did not have to absorb the cost of doing so because insurance policies made it easy for providers to shift the cost of charity care to paying patients.

It was only a matter of time before this financial dream house collapsed. To tell physicians and hospitals to scoop up in the sundry insurance treasuries whatever they deemed "reasonable" and then to expect that the "reasonable" would remain modest was patently absurd. "Reasonable" came to mean that American physicians should receive fees three times as high as the fees paid for the same procedures in Canada. And "reasonable" in the hospital sector has meant that charges per day could escalate from year to year and exceed the general price index for the economy as a whole.

Buyer's versus seller's market

Eventually, the government (which pays almost 40% of all U.S. health-care expenditures), the business community (which pays for another third), and patients (which pay the balance directly out-of-pocket) tired of the relentless escalation of health-care prices. They tired of it because sometime during the 1970s, our health-care sector metamorphosed from a seller's market (in which there was a pervasive shortage of health resources) to a buyer's market (in which there is surplus of health resources). In a seller's market, providers can write their own economic tickets, and they did. In a buyer's market, health-care purchasers will now seek to write their own tickets. They can do so by playing off one potentially underemployed provider against the other in a quest for price concessions. That strategy is now being implemented throughout the nation.

Thus, in the early 1980s, both the government and the business community began to switch to what is euphemistically called "prudent purchasing." The government shifted from retrospective, full-cost reimbursement of the individual hospital to prospective compensation by defined medical case. Eventually, flat fees will be applied nationwide with only minor adjustments for local circumstances. The business community is shifting to preferred provider organizations (PPOs) under which price concessions are sought from physician and hospital panels in exchange for the promise to channel patients to these panels. Both forms of prudent purchasing ultimately aim to procure services and products from providers at substantially reduced prices. Because there is no end in sight for the growing surplus capacity in our health-care sector, this form of pressure can be expected to intensify for decades to come.

From the perspective of paying patients, the newly emerging buyer's market in health care will be delightful. Ultimately, more health services will be available for the same expenditures or, alternatively, less of a slice of the GNP will be offered to providers for the same level of services.

For the uninsured poor, however, this buyer's market creates an entirely new problem. If payers apply economic pressure, providers will be less willing to provide charity care through the hidden cross-subsidies referred to as "cost shifting." Cost shifting raises prices for paying patients to cover the costs of treating nonpaying patients. Yet when prices are fixed prospectively, charity care costs can only be shifted backwards to the provider's own bottom line, and the incentive for providing charity care is removed. A price-competitive health-care market means nice guys tend to finish last in the financial race.

The American public must realize that financing indigent care through hidden cross-subsidies does not make sense within the context of price-competitive prudent purchasing. If price-competition is what Americans want in health care, then they must condone the prospect that these cross-subsidies will be squeezed from the system like water from a sponge. Americans must be prepared either to pay explicitly for the health care of poor fellow citizens, or to let the latter wither on the vine.

Free lunch in health care

Yet the public refuses to make a choice. Americans still want both prudent purchasing and the imaginary free lunch in charity care, with no thought given to the unconscionable inconsistency inherent in that posture. And thus in 1985, we spent almost 11% of the GNP on health care while allowing millions of Americans to remain uninsured.

If we are "the most generous people on earth" (as we tend to consider ourselves), lack of insurance coverage would hardly deprive a woman from health care during pregnancy. There is, after all, such a thing as the Hippocratic oath, which apparently cannot always prevent disaster.

It may be added parenthetically that in 1984, the profit margins (revenues minus expenses as a percentage of revenues) of American hospitals soared to their highest levels in 20 years. Profits generally soared in both the for-profit and the "not-for-profit" hospital sector—a misnomer if there ever was one. This illustrates my earlier point: Financial incentives alone can trigger the denial of care even if the level of compensation is generous.

Technical versus moral dimensions

The best health-care system in the world? Perhaps so, if we ignore the moral quality of that system. Although health-care providers in other nations might protest, a case could possibly be made that, in terms of the purely *technical* dimension of health care, our system is best. However, that assertion, even if it were valid, is overly narrow and rather smug. If we consider the moral dimension of health-care systems, the ranking of alternative systems becomes more arguable.

We would have to be complete health-care chauvinists to assert that, in terms of its moral quality, the American health-care system ranks above or equal to Canadian or Western European systems. The vignettes cited previously simply are not heard of in those countries. To be sure, the British health system is so tightly budgeted that elective surgery is rationed by queues (waiting lines), and some procedures (such as renal dialysis) are said to be rationed by age. But where such rationing occurs, it involves allocating limited physical resources on the basis of medical judgment, with the limit on physical resources being determined by an open, democratic, political process. By contrast, we Americans deny poor citizens acutely needed health care within sight of empty hospital beds and idle physicians, strictly because of patients' inability to pay. We literally are rationing our oversupply of resources!

Our current approach to rationing does not reflect a careful design, but rather, our perennial ambivalence over the distributional ethics we desire in health care. Before we can sensibly allocate health resources, we must openly debate what these distributional ethics should be. Once the debate is settled, we should be able to design a health-care system that will not progress to become the laughing stock of the world.

SOME OPEN QUESTIONS ON SOCIAL ETHICS

Americans are still grappling with the following questions:

1. Is health care to be viewed primarily as a *private consumption good* or as a *social good* (such as jurisprudence or elementary education)?
2. Is access to at least a basic set of health services an American citizen's *basic right*, or is the provision of such care merely an implicitly understood *moral obligation* on the part of physicians and hospitals?
3. If access to basic health care were declared a *right*, should it be defined and enforced by the *national* government, or should that task be left to local communities?

Private consumption good

The nation's ambivalence over the first question has been discussed earlier. American physicians appear traditionally to have defended the view that health care is a private consumption good. Clearly, not all American physicians hold this view. However, through lobbying, American physicians have steadfastly advanced the proposition that health care should be traded in free markets like any other normal consumption good. That position, for example, was the philosophical underpinning for organized medicine's tenacious fight against the introduction of the Medicare program for the elderly.

Entitlements to health care

Regarding the second question, most Americans would probably agree that access to *life-saving* medical intervention is an American's fundamental entitlement. In fact, many states have statutes to that effect. However, the debate focuses on the question of how far from life-threatening situations such a right should extend. Some argue that providing needed health care to indigents should be accepted as a moral obligation of society, but should not be legislated as the indigents' *entitlement* (Blumstein, 1985). This viewpoint appears most popular today.

Several reasons exist for this nation's aversion to the establishment of entitlements. First, by international comparison, Americans harbor a particularly deep suspicion of "big government." In probably no other democracy are distrust and even outright contempt for "government bureaucrats" more openly taught than in the United States. The realization of entitlements, however, can be enforced only by government. Therefore, not surprisingly, when Americans face a trade-off between establishing tax-financed entitlements and visible social pathos among the poor, they often choose the latter as the lesser of two evils.

Accompanying this nation's suspicion of "big government" are ingrained beliefs about the origin of poverty that create barriers to poor entitlement grants.

America is a country for self-starters. In contrast to Europe, where the individual is fairly well-protected from myopic economic planning (where "economic planning" includes education and training), America demands a high degree of economic self-discipline from its citizens. Individuals are expected to engage voluntarily in prudent life-cycle planning or suffer the consequences of early improvidence.

Because this country tends to view both wealth and poverty as somehow "deserved," programs for the poor, including entitlements to basic health care, consistently encounter resistance.

Aside from the belief that poverty tends to be self-inflicted, the racial and ethnic heterogeneity of this country tends to amplify this nation's hard-nosed attitude toward its poor. Although the majority of the American poor are white, a disproportionate number of black and Hispanic Americans are poor. Because poverty is often identified with groups alien to the better-off majority, poverty may not evoke as much empathy in the United States as in more ethnically homogeneous societies.

Government's responsibility

Finally, is access to health care — whether considered a right or merely a moral obligation — the responsibility of the federal, state, or local governments? Should residents in one state be concerned about the health care accorded sick fellow Americans in another state? We clearly do care fiercely about the health care received by fellow Americans held captive in distant lands. But what of fellow Americans who are hostages to poverty and sickness in neighboring states? Here the answer is less clear.

Evidenced by the federal Medicare program, residents in one state obviously do care about the health care of Americans in neighboring states if these Americans are aged 65 or over. By virtue of large federal subsidies to the state-administered Medicaid program, residents in one state do express at least some concern over the welfare of American women and their children in other states, although the standards of care offered by Medicaid vary by state. For numerous other Americans, however, we have no national standards.

Our ambivalence on this issue dates back to our nation's creation. Since then, our domestic policy has emerged as a tug of war between two distinct conceptions of nationhood: the view that this nation is one community that should observe national standards for basic human rights, and the view that ours is a nation of distinct communities each having the prerogative to establish its own social policy standards. This latter perspective is most popular today.

What Next, Medicine?

Our general responses to the previously raised questions are:

1. Health care is a private consumption good.
2. Health care is not a right.
3. The provision of access to health is a moral obligation of local communities, not the federal government.

These answers and the social ethic from which they emerge are incompatible with a one-tier health system. They imply a two-tier or multi-tier health-care system. The best that system champions of the poor can hope for may resemble this hierarchy:

Tourist class care: Publicly financed health care paid for primarily through competitively bid, prepaid capitation plans with rationing similar to the British model.

Business class care: Health care financed through employer-paid health insurance and delivered under a mixture of prepaid capitation plans, PPOs, and the traditional fee-for-service system.

Designer care: Health care delivered in luxury hospital suites or health-care resorts, and paid for privately by the well-to-do.

From the public sector's perspective, financing health care for the poor could be best accomplished through competitive bids solicited from competing health maintenance organizations (HMOs). That approach, already widely tried in several states (such as Arizona and California), endows the public purchaser of health care with market power previously absent in public health programs. No longer will the government have to surrender the key to the public treasury to secure health care for the nation's poor.

Whether the bottom tier would render lower quality services would depend, in the first instance, on the funds allocated by the public sector to that tier. Delivery of lower quality care would depend, however, on the professional ethics of the providers working in that tier. Indeed, the development of such a bottom tier health-care system will clearly differentiate the two types of providers who have always worked side-by-side in our health system: those whose primary motive is service to their fellow citizens, and those who view their profession essentially as an outlet for profit-oriented entrepreneurship.

If a sufficient number of providers propelled by the service motive could be found, the choice-constrained lower tier described previously could represent a decided advance over the imaginary one-tier system the nation fancies itself to operate at this time. That system has only been accessible to the uninsured poor in the form of unpredictable acts of condescending charity on the part of some health care providers. Predictable access to at least some services as a matter of right would endow the uninsured poor with a measure of dignity now absent from their health-care transactions. This would be the chief virtue of the bottom tier.

Thousands upon thousands of persons have studied disease. Almost no one has studied health.

ADELLE DAVIS

Robert J. Haggerty

The Boundaries of Health Care

National priorities have now been set for health services in our country: they are to increase access, to moderate cost, and to maintain or increase quality. Most of the current efforts are directed to the first two of these goals — getting existing types of services to those who do not now receive them and reorganizing and financing care to improve efficiency and contain costs. Solutions to these first two goals are in sight although considerable struggles still lie ahead before they are achieved.

While the public and the professions are most concerned with these two issues today, I suspect that the next crisis will center around the issue of quality — and by quality I mean effectiveness of the whole process of health services and what factors produce health. I will review a few studies that bear on this and then discuss what role medicine can play in the production of health as opposed to merely providing health services. This will lead me on into several areas not now a part of traditional medical care. This future oriented area, I think, is appropriately titled "The Boundaries of Health Care."

I. HEALTH SERVICES AND THEIR EFFECT ON HEALTH

First, I would like to review . . . the effectiveness of health services in changing health. Health itself is difficult to measure, but there can be little argument that it is somehow the reciprocal or absence of mortality, morbidity, disability and distress. . . .

In the absence of our ability to show much reduction in death, disease and only occasionally in disability as a result of medical care, most of us have turned to measure other factors that we felt might be more responsive to care — costs, utilization of services such as hospitals, office visits and compliance with preventive or curative regimens. Here the evidence that different types of medical care have different effects is much better.

Robert J. Haggerty, M.D., is president of the William T. Grant Foundation, New York City, and the author of *The Health Care System* and *Community Child Health*.

. . . There is not much evidence that illness care (which is what most medical care consists of) reduces mortality or morbidity very much. When well organized, it can reduce utilization of expensive facilities such as hospitals and emergency rooms and can reduce other costs such as laboratory and pharmacy without any measurable difference in health status. In other words, the effect of illness care after a point produces only marginal gains in health.

I need to make perfectly clear that I am well aware that we do have some data on the effectiveness of specific aspects of curative medicine — penicillin for pneumonia, antimicrobial treatment of meningitis, drug therapy for essential hypertension and a few other conditions that have been shown by controlled clinical trials to be positively affected by modern therapy. And I certainly do not wish to belittle the very important effects of our role as relievers of pain and distress. Individuals and society need someone who provides hope by not giving up when the outcome is death. They need the comfort that there is access to such people as physicians even for conditions that will be self-limiting. Medicine satisfies a deep human need for someone else to provide help. I need also to make clear that I, as a clinician who has spent my entire professional life caring for children and their families, like to practice medicine. I am not disillusioned, bitter or tired of practice. But I also believe that we need to be humble about what we clinicians accomplish and raise our sights a bit to see if there may not be other things that we or someone in society could do to improve health much more than we are doing today. . . .

David Mechanic, who expresses so many things so well, said that "medicine has three principal tasks: (1) to understand how particular symptoms, syndromes or disease entities arise, either in individuals or among groups of individuals; (2) to recognize and cure these or shorten their course or minimize any residual impairment; and (3) to promote living conditions in human populations which eliminate hazards to health and thus prevent disease." The first of these tasks has generally been the province of biomedical research, the second of curative medicine and the last of public health and social medicine. The time is now at hand to join these three and to move into what I like to call the boundaries of health care.

The problem is simply stated. Where do health services end and other human services begin? Or, what factors affect health? The answers are far from clear. Let me first discuss the evidence.

II. SOCIAL AND ENVIRONMENTAL FACTORS' EFFECT ON HEALTH

On a superficial level it is easy for everyone to accept that the way, we live, our diet, our pace of life, our housing, our political and social structure, all contribute to health — perhaps sharing only with our genes predominance as the factor most responsible for our state of health. In comparison, what we as doctors do for people is rather insignificant. Let me spend just a few moments documenting this bold statement since it is said with a good deal more conviction than the facts often allow.

A. Lead poisoning   is an easy example with which to start. Most lead poisoning in children results from ingestion of paint from housing with high lead content paint. The outcome of therapy, once symptomatic poisoning occurs, is bad—mortality and especially late intellectual morbidity are high. We can now diagnose body lead burdens above normal before symptoms appear and have fairly good chelating agents to accelerate its elimination, although we still do not know the long term consequences of asymptomatic lead burdens. But the poisoned child usually must remain in his same environment where he will continue to ingest lead. To date no cure for his desire to eat paint has been found to be successful. We must remove him from the lead. Even if we move him, however, another family with a small child is likely to move into the same house and become poisoned. Getting landlords and even parents to remove the paint from the housing has been disappointing—it is costly, time consuming and, with absentee landlords and poorly prosecuted housing codes, often impossible to accomplish. What is medicine's role? Should it stop at treatment of the symptomatic child? At surveillance programs to detect and then treat the asymptomatic child? At getting social workers to move the child to a new home? At enforcing housing codes that may require the physician's attendance in court if he pushes hard enough? At promotion of building new, safe housing for his community? At political action? At building the new housing himself? Clearly, each of us stops somewhere along this spectrum, usually before building the new housing himself. But until new housing has been built to replace all the old, or complete renovation of the old achieved, there will not be a solution to lead poisoning, any more than there was a solution to the problem of rickets until vitamin D was put in all milk.

B. Environment: A second example of the effect of physical environment on health is the . . . work of H. Sultz and W. Winkelstein. . . . They showed that on days when there was high air pollution, there were also many more asthmatic children having acute attacks and coming to physicians. What role should we as clinicians play in air pollution control when it directly affects the health of our patients?

One of the most strikingly successful stories of such a role in altering environment by a physician is that of L. Colebrook, a surgeon in Britain, who became incensed that little girls were frequently severely burned by standing close to open hearth fireplaces and catching their clothes on fire. He collected data, presented it and got legislation passed requiring that every fireplace have a grate six inches in front of the fire. Such burns were significantly reduced as a result. As a clinician he contributed more to health by this move than by all his surgical skills.

C. Way of Life: Let me now take a third example from adult medicine. L. Breslow and his colleagues in California have been engaged for some years in the Human Population Laboratory conducting a longitudinal study of the health status of a random sample of people and correlating this with various aspects of life style. He found that five factors in the way people live—the amount of sleep (less than six hours/night vs. 7–8), diet (erratic or regular), alcohol consumption (less or more than five drinks per day), regular exercise and tobacco use—were significantly associated with health. Good health practices were associated with good health, and the relation was cumulative—the more of these factors that were "good" the better the health. In fact, people of 55–64 who had had these "good" habits had the health, as determined by their functioning, of 25–34 year olds who had these "bad" habits. To the epidemiologists there are, of course, many missing links. Most important to the clinician is the question, can such "bad" habits, if present, be changed and how; and if changed, will that alter a person's health? For the purpose of this discussion the issues I would like to have you think about include, "Is it medicine's job to educate people on how to sleep, eat, drink, exercise and smoke?" Is this within or beyond the boundary? The implications are that if we could change men's function this much by altering life habits, we would accomplish more than through all of our therapeutic medicine.

D. Schools and Health: The next example I would like to mention is the role of medicine in schools. Traditional school health programs of "laying on of hands," inspections, referrals without follow-up have been shown to be a waste of time. But at the same time one quarter of the referrals of children to our pediatric clinic are now sent for "school learning problems." We find very few traditional medical problems among such children. But the suffering of the child and family with such problems is still just as real, and the management requires that we alter the child's environment—the school and the home. We have been quite unsuccessful, even after doing rather complete work-ups in the clinic, if we only make recommendations or treat with drugs. When we have moved out of our offices into the schools, we have achieved greater success. We need to join with teachers to help them understand how children grow and develop, with psychologists to understand how they learn, and sociologists to learn how the organization of the school affects learning. While the data to support the effectiveness of such new programs are not all in, we as doctors either have to decide that we do not have anything to offer such parents and children or we have to join forces with other professions to seek solutions to the problems by crossing the boundaries of traditional health services.

The schools also offer remarkable settings for health education to achieve more healthy patterns of living that may then affect health. The boundary between medicine and education is not difficult to accept, but few of us have crossed it.

III. POPULATION VS. INDIVIDUAL HEALTH CARE

Most of these examples could be thought of as in the range of traditional public health—that is population medicine—and the clinician would be quite correct to say that the boundary problem is largely one between population medicine, where responsibility for such things as housing, group health in schools and community-wide health education is the province of the public health physician, while the provision of curative medicine of individual patients is his domain.

One of our own studies illustrates that the problem of boundaries exists even for the clinician dealing with individuals. For some time we have been interested in the clinical observation that family-life stress seemed to be positively related to illness and also to the timing of seeking health care related to such stress. We have studied two types of family stress—long term or chronic, such as poverty, divorce, poor housing, unemployment, and short term, such as quarrels in the family, deaths in near relatives, loss of jobs, moves and interpersonal problems outside the family. . . . Long term or chronic stress is very strongly associated with illness—in fact it accounts for as much as 20 per cent of all illness in families with children. Likewise short term stress has a strong association with illness, but little over-all relation to when people seek health care. There are interesting and important differences in the relation of stress (controlling for the amount of illness) and where care is sought. Telephone, emergency room, and OPD contacts are two to three times more likely if there is family stress, while office visits show no difference.

There is a considerable body of other data in this field of stress and illness. L. E. Hinkle's documentation of the greater occurrence of illness in workers in a telephone company at times of stress, and a study by R. H. Rahe, J. D. McKean, and R. J. Arthur of navy men's greater illness at times of life changes (moves, deaths of close relatives, job changes) give credence to our view that life stress is an important cause of physical illness.

The important point is again the boundary problem. If this type of family-life stress and life change is a major factor in causing illness and in determining when and where people seek care, what should be the physician's role in helping families to avoid or learn to cope in more healthy ways with stress? What is the physiologic pathway by which such stress works its havoc? What could social changes, such as income maintenance, or various educational efforts, such as operant conditioning (to teach families how to manage life crises without the stress that leads to illness), do to improve health? What should be the doctor's role in these boundary problems? Should we become engaged in these areas? I think it is clear that, as a society, we must find ways to manage boundary problems if we are to improve health. As physicians we do have another reason for involvement.

G. Caplan many years ago proposed the crisis intervention theory. In brief, he postulates that at these times of crisis, people are more amenable to changing ways of life that are unhealthy than at more stable times. If this is so, and we obviously need data to prove or disprove it, then crisis-related illness and crisis-related use of health services bring the clinician into the middle of social medicine.

By working in these boundary areas it seems likely that we will contribute more to health than we will by sticking purely to our curative, traditional medical care. . . .

Perhaps the major thing medicine has to contribute is the ability to meld biology and social sciences — drawing people from both disciplines to work on the complex problems of social and family life and how they affect health. We and society may then end up by developing new helping groups or professions that actually deal with or deliver the care at these boundaries. . . .

The boundaries of medical care offer exciting challenges to the future oriented biosocial physician. By successful blending of social and biologic research we may finally, as physicians, contribute to improved health and not merely to the production of health services.

We Americans hold this truth to be self-evident: Our health-care system is the best in the world. This assertion is recited as a form of incantation whenever we meet to discuss health policy. To question the claim would be a rude breach of etiquette.

UWE E. REINHARDT

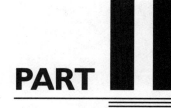

PART II

Health Policy: A Framework for Action

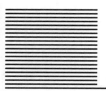

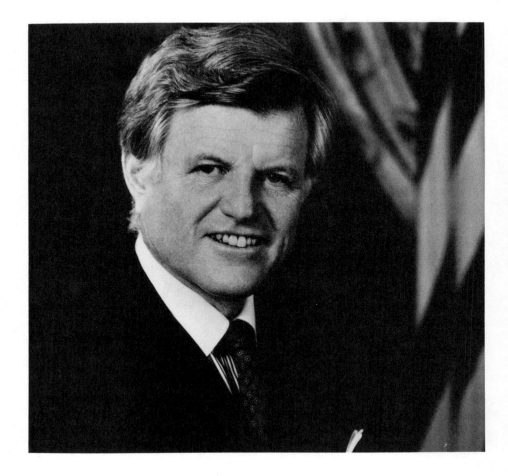

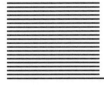

3

The Politics of Health

A MERICANS place great trust in their physicians, nurses, dentists, and other health care providers, in the insurance companies that pay for much of their care, and in the government that regulates, oversees, and to a great extent finances the system. In Part II, we take a look, in one sense, at the underbelly of this system: the struggle for power, money, and control of various aspects of health services by a variety of groups. Underneath the regulation and legislation is a power struggle, the outcome of which ultimately determines the quality of services we receive. It decides who will care for us when, where, and how, the method by which we will pay for care, where hospitals will be located and the size and scope of these facilities. It has great influence on health professions education, and it determines the scope and direction of research.

On the surface, it appears that these decisions emanate from the government. But in reality policymakers take their cues for health care legislation and regulation from a variety of sources. Historically, some special-interest groups, such as physicians, have been able virtually to dictate policy in specific areas. This dominant role has changed in recent years as more and more interest groups appeared on the scene, as consumers took a more active role in attaining public accountability, and as the stakes escalated to sky-high proportions. The four most powerful interest groups are physicians, hospitals, insurance companies, and the drug industry. There are also lobbying groups for dentists, nurses, and many other health professions; for nursing homes and other such institutions; for labor and business groups; and for most other participants in the health care arena. While these groups participate in the high-quality care we receive, they also are helping to ensure that their own interests are served.

The making of health policy across several levels of government and hundreds of programs is complex. Policy students have identified five characteristics of the policy process in the United States: (1) the relationship of government to the private sector; (2) the distribution of authority and responsibility within a federal system of government; (3) pluralistic ideology as a basis of politics; (4) the relationship between policy formulation and administrative implementation; and (5) incrementalism as a strategy for reform. These characteristics are considered from a variety of perspectives in this chapter.

It is only fitting that we open this discussion with the words of a policy-maker—in this case, Richard D. Lamm, who served as governor of Colorado for twelve years, 1975–1987. Mr. Lamm's ten commandments of health care at first glance may appear to be a deceivingly lighthearted view of current health care policy, but on closer investigation we see that they highlight some of the most treacherous hazards we face. He looks at the 11 percent of the national budget spent on health care with a view toward stretching those resources to provide better services to more people with less waste. Ultimately, he suggests, health care is too much of a dominating factor in the nation's economy, and he has recommendations for liberating some resources that now are swallowed up by health so that they can go to work for us in fiscally neglected areas.

In an article written for the British medical journal, *The Lancet*, U.S. health policy analysts Philip R. Lee and Lynn Etheredge address the current movement in the United Kingdom toward privatization of health services. The authors point to the U.S. experience as a model for what happens when there is no national health policy and when no national system exists to provide health care services to all citizens. In particular, they discuss the fragmentation in financing and provision of care, current crippling cost escalations, the high cost of administration, the commercialization of medicine, the trend toward defensive medicine, the erosion of physician authority, and the lack of access for many citizens.

In "Government and Health: The Political Aspects of Health Care—A Sociopolitical Overview" Theodor J. Litman provides historical background for government health policy. He documents the growth of the federal government's role in health care contrasted with the role of state governments and ends with an outline of lessons that can be learned from the past.

Contrary to Mr. Lamm, Vicente Navarro, a veteran health policy analyst, recommends an expansion of health expenditures and a strengthening of government interventions. To support his contention that class influences determine economic and social policy, and they eventually define the distribution of health care services, Dr. Navarro provides a historical analysis of U.S. health policy. He states his case that the current austerity policies in health and social programs are a result not of the wishes of the American people but of the political structure that ultimately determines policy.

In "American Medical Policy and the 'Crisis' of the Welfare State: A Comparative Perspective," Theodore R. Marmor addresses the connection between medical policy concerns and the development of welfare states in the advanced industrial democracies. He relates the debate about the crisis of the welfare state to U.S. concerns about medical care and points out that during the 1980s the national debt, defense spending, and the population's unwillingness to pay higher taxes have paralyzed medical care policy. The result is that the only government programs that can gain favor are those that promise to save the government money. Thus, those with an interest in health services are in a position of devising methods to insure the survival of current programs, rather than participating in a period of growth and creativity.

Good health is a basic part of a large dream of opportunity.

EDWARD M. KENNEDY

Richard D. Lamm

The Ten Commandments of Health Care

Our nation must reassess its health care priorities
if it is to meet the needs of future generations

An admiral in the navy was on the high seas when, all of a sudden, a little blip showed up on his ship's radar screen. The admiral told his ensign, "Tell that ship to change its course fifteen degrees." A message came back on the radio, "You change your course fifteen degrees." The admiral said, "Tell that ship that we're the United States Navy and to change its course by fifteen degrees." The word came back on the radio, "You change your course by fifteen degrees." At this, the admiral himself got on the radio and said, "I am an admiral in the United States Navy. Change your course fifteen degrees." The word came back, "You change your course fifteen degrees. I am a lighthouse."

It's a perfect parable, at least for my views. I believe the United States is heading for shoals. It's true that this can be prevented; we can change our course. But if we don't change our course, we are heading for shoals. The only way to really avoid those shoals is to take on some sacred cows, to address some political taboos, and to really get involved in some areas that in the past have been too sacrosanct. We must crawl into the no man's land of politics where, I believe, unfortunately, a lot of the solutions lie.

It's a vastly different America we are seeing right now from when people of my generation graduated from high school. When we graduated from high school, most of us took the generational baton from our parents, looked over our shoulders, and saw that there was nobody else in sight. The United States had 44 percent of the world's economy when I graduated from high school in 1953. When my son graduated from high school this past June, he got out to an America that is now the world's largest debtor nation. The United States has the slowest rate of productivity growth of any of the industrialized nations. Its politicians borrow twenty cents out of every federal dollar they spend. It has massive back debts. I believe very strongly that, if we are going to rejuvenate America, we must, in fact, deal with some of these sensitive subjects.

Richard D. Lamm, L.L.B., served three terms as governor of Colorado (1975–1987) and now directs the Center for Public Policy and Contemporary Issues at the University of Denver.

What types of things are we talking about? The average enlisted person in the military retires at the age of thirty-nine; the average officer retires at forty-three. Both retire with indexed pensions and health care coverage. You can't retire people at the age of thirty-nine when they live into their eighties! In the United States, incredible amounts of money are spent not only on service-connected disabilities but on nonservice-connected disabilities for veterans. Eleven cents out of every dollar in America is spent on health care. If capital is the stored flexibility we possess with which to build our children and our grandchildren a better life, then you have to look at where that capital goes. It's the Willie Sutton theory of bankrobbers: you go where the money is.

Consequently, like a lot of other people in public policy, I have simply looked at the health care area and asked, "How can we make it more efficient? Where is the money going? How do we use this capital that we have to build our children a better life?" It is my own personal opinion that my generation — those of us in our fifties and beyond — have been prodigal parents. I believe that, in fact, we have built up systems that are unsustainable for the indefinite future, whether it's pension systems, health care, or whatever else. To me, it is almost a moral issue: how can one generation heap that kind of burden and moral debt on another generation?

Schopenhauer says, "Every man confuses the limits of his mind with the limits of the world." Perhaps I do, too. But nevertheless, from the viewpoint of somebody who has been in public policy for twelve years and to illustrate my concern, I would like to offer you what I consider to be the "Ten Commandments of Health Care."

I. HUMANS CANNOT LIVE BY HEALTH CARE ALONE

Just as people cannot live by bread alone, a society cannot live by health care alone. But that is almost exactly where we seem to be going in the United States. We have other, desperately important functions in which we must invest to create the kind of world we want to leave for our children and our grandchildren. We must invest in education, infrastructure, and retooling America. Where are we going to get the jobs for our children? Yet, this problem is ignored while our whole system is tilting toward health care and toward the military.

When I entered high school in 1950, health care represented 45.9 percent of what our society spent on education. This past year, it was over 100 percent. We have many important things to do with our limited societal resources. Health care is certainly one of them, but it isn't the only one. Yet, it is the one to which we give so much precedence that it almost dominates all the others. One of the governors calls health care the Pac Man of his budget. In my opinion, like the fading southern family in a William Faulkner novel that takes sick and ceases to work, we are treating illness at the expense of our livelihood.

We spend more than a billion dollars a day for health care while our bridges are falling down, our teachers are underpaid, and our industrial plants are rusty. This simply can't continue. There is something fundamentally unsustainable about a society that moves its basic value-producing industries overseas yet continues to manufacture artificial hearts at home. We have money to give smokers heart transplants but no money to retool our steel mills. We train more doctors and lawyers than we need but fewer teachers. On any given day, 30 to 40 percent of the hospital beds in America are empty, but our classrooms are overcrowded and our transportation systems are deteriorating. We are great at treating sick people, but we are not very great at treating a sick economy. And we are not succeeding in international trade. When you really look around and try to find the industries the United States is succeeding in, you discover that they are very few and far between.

I believe one of the challenges of America's future is to invest our scarce resources wisely. To do this, we must be realistic, we must ask heretical questions, and we must question the sanctity of sacred cows. We simply cannot stand back and let one segment of our economy — no matter which one it is — dominate all the others. When you look at where America is spending its resources, you see health care.

Like the person who carries a first aid kit, the weight of which gives him or her blisters, our health care system has become part solution, part problem. We wouldn't want to be without it, but it has become a heavy burden. It is definitely interfering with the public's ability to invest in our public goods and with private industry's ability to retool itself. Health care insurance now costs U.S. corporations approximately $125 billion per year, which is 50 percent of their profits before taxes. That's money that is desperately needed elsewhere.

II. HONOR NOT ONLY THY DOCTOR AND THY HOSPITAL BUT THY PUBLIC HEALTH NURSE AND THY SEWAGE DISPOSAL PLANT WORKER

This is startling, perhaps, but, when you start looking at how you buy health for a society, you do not start with doctors and hospitals. With all due respect to doctors and hospitals, which are immensely important, there is little correlation between how much money is spent on doctors and hospitals and how healthy a society is. We are too easily seduced into thinking that health care means doctors and hospitals, when actually the great advances in health care have been made in sanitation, pasteurization, chlorination, and refrigeration. Screen windows to keep out mosquitoes were an incredible health advancement. Public health officials have saved more lives than hospitals.

If we look at how we can improve the health of the average American, we find a similar figure. The greatest causes of *premature* mortality, not of total mortality, are very simple: smoking, drinking too much, eating the wrong things, and not wearing a seat belt. If you really want to know how to make America healthy, start attacking those things. Those are four things an individual has within his or her control, and three of them are things you do with your mouth. The mouth is the most dangerous organ in the body.

It becomes clear that there are many paths to health, and certainly doctors and hospitals are one of them. I would rather have a dollar-per-pack tax on cigarettes than I would another $100 billion put into health care. The number of people in America who die from smoking is equivalent to the number who would be killed if a 747 crashed every day. Look at the alternatives available. Give me some of those empty hospital beds in return for locking up some drunk drivers and I'll save more lives than the hospitals would. A mandatory seat belt law would probably save more lives than most medical procedures.

America has to look at what it is getting for its money. The United States spends $2,000 per capita on health care, Great Britain spends $500 per capita, Singapore spends $200, and all three have the same mortality and morbidity rates. You're going to say that these figures don't include cataract operations and hip replacements, and you're right. But I'll tell you again, mortality and morbidity rates are an immensely important yardstick. There is an inverse correlation in our industrialized world between how many doctors there are and how healthy that society is. West Germany has the largest number of doctors per capita; they've got the worst health statistics. The Japanese have the least number of doctors per capita; they're the healthiest. There are many ways to attain health, and society has to look objectively and ask how we can get the most bang for our buck.

III. LOVE THY NEIGHBOR

But one cannot bankrupt America by giving to one's neighbor all of the medicine that is technologically available. We are not wealthy enough to base our health care system on the assumption that we can give everything that medical genius has invented to all of the people in our country. I believe strongly that the United States must ration medicine. We already ration health care. In the comic strip *Peanuts*, Linus says, "There's no issue so big you can't run away from it."

But the genius of medicine has outpaced America's ability to pay; *The Painful Presumption* by William Schwartz and Henry Aaron tells us that. Rudolf Klein, a very thoughtful observer from England, says, "Rationing is inherent under any health care system." Representatives from Oregon Health Decisions, a statewide health policy group, say:

> We cannot live under the idea that we can give everybody all the health care that they need. Rationing of health care is inevitable because society cannot or will not pay for all of the services modern

medicine can provide. People in this state must search their hearts and their pocketbooks and decide what level of health care can be guaranteed to the poor, the unemployed, the elderly, and others who depend upon publicly funded health services.

They point out that we already ration medicine. We ration it chronologically, economically, geographically, politically, scientifically, and by disease.

In short, rationing is not a future possibility—it is a present reality. The ancient Greeks said, "To know all to ask is to know half " I believe that, if we start asking the right questions, we vastly improve our chances of coming up with the right answers. If we ask ourselves how to avoid rationing, I believe that we do our society an injustice. If we ask how we might allocate finite resources to meet an infinite demand and do it compassionately and justly, then I believe we can increase rather than decrease medical care in our most basic areas. In short, rationing can be described in the same words Mark Twain used about Wagner's music: "It's not as bad as it sounds."

IV. SPEND THY HEALTH MONEY WHERE IT WILL BUY THE MOST HEALTH CARE

I believe very strongly that in certain instances we are looking for ways to maximize our health care dollars. Humana Hospital's budget for the artificial heart is roughly equivalent to what society spent on eradicating smallpox. Consider the difference between the two. The fact is, we have a system that seems to give the health care dollar to highly dramatic technology while a third of the children in America have never seen a dentist and 20 percent of them haven't had their polio shots. In 1982, the Robert Wood Johnson Foundation found that 12 percent of all Americans—one in eight—have serious problems with access to health care. In the same year, the foundation also found that one millon families had at least one member who had been refused health care.

Lester Thurow talks about an exercise for doctors in which every time an expensive procedure is ordered, the doctor responsible for making such an order would have to pick an American worker to be sentenced to a period of slavery long enough to pay the medical bill for that procedure. Victor Fuchs suggests that physicians have always practiced within constraints and, as long as rationing was implicit, they were tolerant. Rationing at the individual patient's bedside can continue to remain implicit if the patient-physician-family nucleus has accepted the economic, social, and moral importance of national restraint. All of society must understand that we can't do everything for everybody. Theologian Harvey Cox says, "Not to decide is to decide." So, in fact, by avoiding these issues, we *are* deciding.

V. NEITHER OVER-DOCTOR NOR OVER-LAWYER SOCIETY

Forty percent of the Rhodes Scholars in this country go to law school. Japan trains one thousand engineers for every one hundred lawyers. We train one thousand lawyers for every one hundred engineers. Which society in a technologically based, information-based market is going to succeed? The one that trains lawyers? I've read a little bit of history and I have yet to find an example in history in which a nation has sued its way to greatness. But the same thing applies to the field of medicine. It is estimated that there may be as many as 145,000 more physicians than needed by the year 2000. A study by Duke University points out the fact that every excess doctor, or every doctor in practice, increases the nations health care costs by $300,000 annually. Thus, on an average career spanning forty years, a single physician would create health care costs of some $12 million. We've got to limit the number of people going into medicine and law.

Likewise, defensive medicine hangs like a sword of Damocles over the medical profession. Hospital bankruptcies in a lot of areas in America ought to be put under the "Good News Today" column of the newspapers. There are 200,000 excess hospital beds in the United States. That's equivalent to at least 1,000 hospitals out there that we don't need, that we've overbuilt. Some studies show that one-third of the people in hospital beds don't need to be there.

I really believe that there is no way we are going to come to grips with this problem until we also look at some of these areas that aren't going to go away. One of the toughest of these is what Victor Fuchs calls "flat-of-the-curve-medicine" — those medical procedures which are the highest in cost but achieve little or no improvement in health status. He says that they must be reduced or eliminated. We must demand that professional anxieties and licensing authorities establish norms and standards for diagnostic and therapeutic practice that encompass both costs and medicine. We're going to have to come up with some sort of concept of cost-effective medicine.

VI. DO NOT KILL NOR STRIVE OFFICIOUSLY TO KEEP ALIVE

We must look much more maturely at these sensitive issues. Victor Fuchs says that, in a number of areas, one of our assumptions is that we should spend any amount of money if a life is at stake. I governed a state that has many plane crashes because of its high mountains. There were 101 crashes in Colorado in 1985. Was I supposed to close the schools and penitentiaries and send people out looking for crash survivors because a life might be at stake? It sounds so good, but, in fact, when you're faced with that situation, what you have to do is the best you can. You must balance the tragedy to be averted with the resources available.

Consequently, I think we need to discuss death and dying much more candidly and openly. We treat death as if it were optional. People talk about the right to die as if they have the right to refuse to die. Shakespeare said, "We all owe God a death." Once we stop treating death as an enemy and start recognizing it as an inevitability, we can save massive resources. Today, patients with massive strokes are saved from death but live for years in a comatose state. Others with metastatic cancer are subject to a myriad of studies and therapies that add little to their longevity.

I think we must look rationally at the phenomenal amount of resources we spend on the last few weeks of people's lives, only to prolong suffering. We simply cannot afford a system in which, on the way out the door, we take $100,000 to $200,000 of our children's limited resources to give us a couple of extra days of pain-wracked existence. If you can make people better, terrific. But in American medicine, it often seems to be against the law to die in peace. Most elderly don't fear death as much as they do the pain and suffering and degradation and loss of economy that our Faustian bargains have brought to them.

VII. HONOR THY MOTHER AND FATHER, BUT ALSO HONOR THY CHILDREN

The way the whole health care system is slanted toward the benefit of my generation is another sensitive subject. When my wife and I bought our first home, our house payments were forty-nine dollars per month. A recent congressional study concluded that less than 50 percent of the people under thirty are going to be able to buy their own homes. I would suggest that one of the great issues of the future is going to be intergenerational equity. Our children are going to wake up one day and find out how badly we screwed things up.

I don't question the need to give both the young and the elderly access to preventative and primary care, but, when it comes to limited resources that cannot be made available to everyone, I approach the problem in a very personal way. I have a fifteen-year-old daughter. If there is a limited resource and you have to decide between my fifteen-year-old daughter and me, give it to my daughter. I'm not being a hero, but my daughter has 60.4 statistical years ahead of her and I have 28.1 statistical years ahead of me. Such a policy is not age discrimination; it's a common sense answer to the question of who should get any limited resources.

This leads me into the question of Medicare, an ultimate sacred cow. When Medicare was passed in 1965, the elderly were disproportionately poor. There was every good reason in Congress to vote for Medicare then. But the elderly are no longer disproportionately poor. In 1970, 23 percent of the elderly were poor and 12 percent of the children were poor. Today, 12 percent of the elderly are poor and 23 percent of the children are poor. Yet, we give 254,000 millionaires Medicare while we're closing well-baby clinics.

The aged are not a static group; it is a status through which we all will go one day. We cannot change our gender or our race, but we all age daily. In a marvelously egalitarian way, time takes its toll on all of us. The elderly are the same people – at a different stage of their lives – about whom we worry while we deny prenatal care to pregnant women. I believe we must weigh the marvels of our health care technologies against other less visible but more cost-effective strategies. Everybody pulls for the Barney Clarks and the Baby Fayes and the marvelous technology that helps them. But we don't hear about the 33 percent of American women who don't receive prenatal care in their first trimester. Stalin was horribly right when he said, "One man's death, that's a tragedy. A million men's death, that's a statistic." We look at the individual and we ignore the statistics. The money we spent on the heart transplant for Mr. Schroeder could have been far more productively spent on the replacement of heart valves for two hundred patients or for prenatal care for that one-third of American women who currently receive none in the first trimester of pregnancy.

VIII. DO NOT COVET THY NEIGHBOR'S WIFE'S ARTIFICIAL HEART

In the area of artificial organs, I would announce right now that, until other needs are met, no taxpayer money should be spent on artificial organs. Are we going to wait until a politically active group of chronic heart patients – many of them smokers – wheel a bunch of artificial heart recipients before a congressional committee, their hearts literally and figuratively in their hands, and plea for the taxpayers to save their lives by providing publicly paid artificial hearts? Is that how we want to set our health care priorities?

I am not a medical Luddite. I admire the miracles of medicine. But I contrast cornea transplants, cataract operations, and hip replacements – all of which add tremendously to the quality of life for many elderly people – to artificial hearts. We should continue to experiment with artificial hearts; medical science must not be stifled or hampered from experimenting. Medical science has made some of its greatest discoveries from the unexpected. I object only to the taxpayers being forced to pay for this at the expense of other, more beneficial health care programs. This occurred in California in 1985 when it was decided that organ transplants would be funded while 200,000 low-income people were knocked off Medi-Cal. That is not a good trade.

The National Institutes of Health called for greatly expanded federal research efforts to develop a fully implantable permanent artificial heart. Such devices, it said, "could provide a significant increase in lifespan, with an acceptable quality of life, for 17,000 to 35,000 patients below the age of 70 annually." The group estimated its annual cost would be up to $5 billion!

This would be a staggering price to pay for the few people who would benefit. It would add significantly to the cost of health insurance premiums for all of us. It would eat into the budgets for Medicare and Medicaid. But, most significantly, it wouldn't do a thing to prevent heart disease in the first place. And if we think we would be able to add availability of the artificial heart to other programs and still pay for them all, we are tragically mistaken.

IX. DO NOT WORSHIP GRAVEN IMAGES OF HIGH TECHNOLOGY

My criticism is not of high technology. There certainly are high technologies that deserve to be worshipped and certainly deserve to be respected. My criticism is aimed at the mindless way in which we invent certain high technologies and then are forced to use them while foregoing many more high-benefit procedures and technologies that could save so many more lives. An artificial heart is a high-technology, low-benefit invention because its cost is very high and it only benefits a few people.

The ultimate goal to which this society should apply its high technology is the understanding of the mechanisms that are the underlying causes of disease. In Medusa and the Snail, Lewis Thomas wrote that the diseases that were the greatest menace to human health when he was a medical student on the wards of Boston City Hospital fifty years ago were, "in the order of degree of fear they caused in the public mind, tertiary syphilis of the brain, pulmonary tuberculosis, and acute rheumatic fever. Also, of course, poliomyelitis." He points out that because of classical clinical research, they "have nearly vanished as public health problems, and the vanishing involved the expenditure of pennies compared to what we'd be spending if they were still with us."

Now, *that* is true high-technology medicine.

But just as we would never have cured polio by putting all our money into artificial lungs, so also we will not understand and cure heart disease if we put our money into artificial hearts. In a world of limited resources, such choices become clear.

I do not have a tenth commandment. But let me conclude with an anecdote. I am reminded of a story that came out of the Second World War when rationing was widespread. A man went into a restaurant, ordered a cup of coffee, and then asked for more sugar. The waitress cast a cynical eye on him and said, "Stir what you have." I believe that is what America must do with its medical care expenses: we must stir better the more than $1 billion per day that we put into health care already. There is not enough money, and we can buy an incredible amount of health if we utilize our resources better.

The great genius of democracy is that, once we start asking the right questions, we can all get together to come up with the answers. We really do have to develop a concept of appropriate care or some sort of cost-effective medicine. I know that is difficult. I know that when a doctor is treating a patient at the bedside he or she is not required to balance the federal budget — total dedication to the patient is the first priority. But this doesn't mean that we still can't find ways to set standards, perhaps through professional organizations, which can develop cost-effective medicine.

Clearly, we can stop training so many doctors and lawyers. We can, via tort reform, give some protection to the physicians against the incredible cost of malpractice insurance. Let me share with you a curse that comes out of Mexico to be used only if you hate somebody very much: "May your life be filled with lawyers!"

We can close hospitals and reduce the number of hospital beds and intensive care units. We can regionalize some of the high-technology medicine. We can push for alternate delivery systems. There are many things we can do, but the issue boils down to this: what kind of world are we going to leave our children and grandchildren? Health care *is* a very high priority, but it isn't the *only* priority. It can't be a monopoly. By working together, we can find ways to deliver more health care to more people at a lower cost.

Supposedly we have the highest standard of living in any country in the world. Do we, though? It depends on what one means by high standards. Certainly nowhere does it cost more to live than here in America. The cost is not only in dollars and cents but in sweat and blood, in frustration, ennui, broken homes, smashed ideals, illness and insanity. We have the most wonderful hospitals, the most gorgeous insane asylums, the most fabulous prisons, the best equipped and the highest paid army and navy, the speediest bombers, the largest stockpile of atom bombs, yet never enough of any of these items to satisfy the demand. Our manual workers are the highest paid in the world; our poets the worst. There are more automobiles than one can count. And as for drugstores, where in the world will you find the like?

HENRY MILLER

Philip R. Lee/Lynn Etheredge

Clinical Freedom: Two Lessons for the U.K. from U.S. Experience with Privatization of Health Care

In the United Kingdom (U.K.), politicians and policy analysts seem increasingly eager to apply lessons from the United States (U.S.) to the National Health Service (NHS). It is clear that the Thatcher Government strongly favors increased marketplace competition and privatization of health services. There has been support for increased competition, for creation of internal markets within the NHS, and for managed care. There has been a rapid increase in U.S.-style employer-provided health insurance benefits. There has been a substantial increase in the number of proprietary hospitals outside the NHS and in the contracting of hospital services through competitive bidding. There has been a transformation of regional and district management within the NHS, with a system of general management replacing consensus management. And, since the liberalization of consultant contracts in 1980, the number of consultants engaging in private practice has increased substantially, as has their income from private practice.

These developments reflect an ideology that has strongly influenced health care policies in the U.S., particularly during the almost eight years of the Reagan administration. Yet today there are growing concerns, among physicians and others in the U.S., about the impact of the policies on medical care costs, on the commercialization of medicine, and on physician autonomy. As a result of these new market-oriented policies, physicians in the U.S. are now the most litigated-against, second-guessed, and paperwork-laden physicians in western industrialized democracies. Physicians' day-to-day clinical decision-making — commonly referred to as clinical freedom — is increasingly subject to review and approval by "case managers" working for employers, insurance carriers, and government financed and regulated professional review organizations. Malpractice suits and administrative costs are multiplying. The growing adversarial relationship with private and public payers and

Philip R. Lee, M.D., is professor of social medicine and director of the Institute for Health Policy Studies, School of Medicine, University of California, San Francisco. Lynn Etheredge is a private health care consultant, Chevy Chase, Maryland.

loss of physician autonomy are closely related to the growing view that medical care should be treated like any other private business. The long-term consequences of these trends for the medical profession and medical care in the U.S. are very serious: will medicine continue as an autonomous profession, or will it become increasingly influenced by large purchasers and the ethics of the marketplace? What will be the effect on the clinical freedom of physicians and on the quality of medical care?

What would be the consequences for the U.K. of adopting a more competitive model for the NHS and expanding the role of private health insurance and private practice? Of a growing commercial influence? The dangers to the NHS of following the mixed public-private model of the U.S. have been pointed out by others. There is a risk that a U.S.-style approach could result in the overuse of technology services at the expense of primary care and in a two-class system of care. If the Government succeeds in diminishing, or perhaps even eliminating, the NHS, British physicians may suffer the same fate that awaits their American colleagues. A recent review of private health care in Britain detailed current developments in the U.K. and defined many of the critical issues of privatization facing the NHS.

We believe that the dangers to the medical profession of a growing private sector in the U.K. have not been sufficiently appreciated by physicians. We address here two major dilemmas that have arisen from an increasing emphasis on the marketplace, competition, and commercialization in medical care in the U.S.: first, diminishing physician autonomy and clinical freedom; and second, the leaping administrative costs and burdens, including those in the physician's office.

DIMINISHING PHYSICIAN AUTONOMY

The Role of Lawyers, Courts, and Regulatory Agencies

The issue of malpractice is a growing concern in the U.S. and the medical profession is sinking in public esteem. When public regard for the medical profession is low, physicians are more likely to be the target of malpractice suits. The number of suits has lately been increasing substantially: studies by the American Medical Association show that the rate of malpractice suits against private practice physicians more than tripled in the first five years of this decade. 37% of U.S. physicians have had a medical malpractice suit against them in their career, and more than ten malpractice claims per hundred physicians were filed in 1985. For some specialties, such as obstetrics and orthopedic surgery, these rates are much higher.

These developments have resulted in a rapid increase in the cost of malpractice insurance premiums. Professional liability premiums for private practice physicians in the U.S. increased by 22% annually from 1982 to 1986.

By 1986, annual premiums were an average of $12,800 per physician; premiums for obstetrician/gynecologists were more than double this amount ($29,300) and were even higher for orthopaedic surgeons ($35,200). In some areas, orthopedic surgeons and obstetrician/gynecologists pay annual premiums of nearly $100,000.

Because of these trends, defensive medicine—i.e., more laboratory tests, more patient investigations, more consultations, and more follow-up visits to guard against malpractice suits—is now a consideration in clinical practice for private physicians. In one study, the costs of defensive medicine were more than 3–5 times the cost of malpractice insurance premiums and accounted for almost 15% of the total U.S. expenditures for physicians' services.

The courts, in their interpretation of antitrust laws, also have had a role in substituting the competitive process of the market for professional self-regulation. The concept of private sector peer review was challenged in the courts as a result of a suit filed in Astoria, Oregon. The Supreme Court of the United States supported a district court ruling that the professional review conducted by physicians in disciplining a member of the community hospital staff was anticompetitive and that it was subject to antitrust laws. The decision was based partly on the fact that the peer review process was done entirely in the private sector, without government review. The courts have further intruded into professional decisionmaking and standards of care in the applications of technology, particularly for the very young, the very old, and the terminally ill.

The Federal Trade Commission (FTC) has been active in extending general economic theories about competition to physicians. Medical care has become a focus for antitrust litigation, and the FTC is involved in several of those suits. Such developments are relevant for U.K. health care professionals in view of the recent consultative document *Review of Restrictive Trade Practices Policy* issued by the Department of Trade and Industry in the U.K. The document states that there will be no exemptions for professional services "without the merits of each exemption having been established afresh," even though the Restrictive Trade Practices Act of 1976 specifically exempts medical services.

The Role of the Payers

The most intrusive day-to-day pressures on clinical freedom have resulted from the Reagan administration's use of the government's purchasing power to change the conduct of physicians and hospitals and also from the rapid expansion in private payers' review programs designed to contain ever-rising medical costs.

The federal Medicare program, which insures 30 million elderly and disabled persons, was the subject of a new prospective payment system for hospitals in 1983. This system introduced fixed payments per admission based on diagnosis-related groups which encourage hospitals to decrease inpatient lengths of stay and to reduce the resources used in providing care. Hospital administrators suddenly were concerned not only with their traditional area of responsibility — the price of inputs (capital, labor) — but also with the volume and types of services. Also, there was a requirement by Congress for new Medicare contracts with peer review organizations (PROs) designed to control the use and quality of care. These contracts include negotiated objectives between the federal government and PROs for review and change of medical practices.

Pressure on hospitals and physicians by the Medicare program have influenced clinical decisions about the care of the elderly. There was a 9% decrease in hospital admissions from 1984 to 1987 for those aged 65 years and over, and the average length of stay for elderly inpatients decreased by more than a day to 8.9 days. Within 2 years, 1983–85, the proportion of Medicare's surgical charges in hospital outpatient departments increased from 6.7% to 20.5% with corresponding decreases in inpatient surgical procedures.

The Medicare program has also started to apply new financial pressures on physicians' charges (e.g., a fee freeze in 1984) and has stepped up its medical practice reviews. In 1987, Medicare paid less than was charged on 82% of physicians' bills, and reduced charges per bill by more than 25%. The Reagan administration has requested an increase in Medicare's medical review budget for physicians' services from $65 million in the fiscal year 1988 to $127 million in the fiscal year 1989.

The increasing attempts by the Medicare program to influence clinical decisionmaking have been paralleled by a "managed care revolution" among private sector payers. Managed care, defined as insurer programs that require previous approval by insurance companies for hospital admissions and concurrent review of lengths of stay, grew from 4% of the private health care market in 1984 to 60% in 1987. Enrollment in health maintenance organizations (HMOs) grew from 9.1 million in 1980 to 29.3 million in 1988, and enrollment in preferred provider organizations (PPOs) increased from 1.3 million in 1984 to 17.5 million in 1987. Both HMOs and PPOs, which are part of the managed care revolution of the competitive market, use various methods to monitor and regulate physician conduct.

GROWING ADMINISTRATIVE COSTS AND BURDENS

Clearly, the economic record of the competitive market in the U.S. health care system during the Reagan administration necessitates a re-examination of the anticipated benefits from privatization of health services. National health care spending in the U.S. has more than doubled from $248,000 million in 1980 to over $500,000 million this year — a spending increase of over $1000 percapita. Adjusted for inflation, health care expenditures have been growing at near-record levels. Competition has not been the answer to cost containment: a recent study found that for hospitals, greater competition led to higher prices. Because the cost of health insurance premiums has risen and because increasingly competitive insurance companies have dropped "bad risks" (i.e., people who most need health insurance), the numbers of uninsured have increased from 30 million in 1980 to approximately 37 million in 1987; millions more are underinsured.

Not so well recognized is the vast amount of paperwork, complexity, administrative burdens, and costs—for physicians, hospitals, patients, and payers—that are involved in the U.S. market-driven medical care review and bill-paying system. Uwe Reinhardt, professor of economics at Princeton University, refers to these issues as the B (bureaucratic) factor in medical care. Among his bureaucrats, Reinhardt includes civil servants, health insurance company employees, medical review firms, and others who process paper. He contends that the U.S. now has the highest B ratio of health care bureaucrats to health caregivers in the industrialized world and notes that the B factor in the U.S. is rising rapidly. Although overall health care expenditures increased by 85% between 1980 and 1986, Reinhardt found that, according to the official government accounts of national health spending (which include only payers' administrative costs), the administrative expenses of the U.S. health system increased by 186% from $9,200 million to $24,500 million; most of the increase was in the administrative costs of private health insurance which more than tripled from $5,100 million in 1980 to $17,800 million in 1986.

Overhead expenses for the U.S. health care system must also take account of physicians' "business" costs that are part of operating private medical practices. Office practice expenses, in addition to malpractice premiums, were an average of $86,000 per physician in 1986. These costs included an average of 2.7 full-time employees per physician, of whom 1.7 were clerical and administrative personnel to handle bills and other paperwork, while 1 was a nurse or medical assistant. Many physicians already devote 1.2 hours a day to administrative matters, and even more of their time is now being taken up in appeals and discussions of fee issues with patients. The total costs of practice, including malpractice, are now about 50% of most physicians' practice incomes. This contrasts with 36% in Canada and 29% in the U.K. Himmelstein and Woolhandler calculated that, in 1983, the total U.S. health care administrative costs were $77,700 million (22% of all health care spending). Their estimates included insurance program administration, and also hospital and nursing home administration and physician office overheads. They projected savings of approximately half of these administrative expenses, about $38,400 million annually, if the U.S. adopted a U.K.-style national health service.

CONCLUSIONS

During the Reagan era in the U.S., health care policies have emphasized competition to control costs. However, the market-driven policies in the U.S. have not controlled the public's costs, but they have produced an increasingly frustrated, alienated, and angry medical profession. Physicians, policy analysts, and politicians in the U.K. would be well advised to carefully and critically evaluate the U.S. experience before adopting piecemeal, policies for the privatization of the NHS.

You would be surprised at the number of years it took me to see clearly what some of the problems were which had to be solved. . . . Looking back, I think it was more difficult to see what the problems were than to solve them.

CHARLES DARWIN

Theodor J. Litman

Government and Health: The Political Aspects of Health Care—A Sociopolitical Overview

When the Eighty-ninth Congress adjourned in 1966, its record of legislative accomplishments made it the most health-minded Congress in U.S. history. Not only had more national health legislation been enacted into law during its first session than had been passed in both sessions of all Congresses in the past decade, but it had appropriated more money for health in the last 2 years of its term than its predecessors had in the previous 168 years. Never before had one session of Congress produced legislation of such far-reaching implications for the health, education, and socioeconomic welfare of the American people than had been enacted in 1965. So extensive was the legislative activity in terms of the number and scope of health actions taken that one observer depicted the period as a turning point in health law.

As far as health care financing was concerned, the issue was no longer that of public versus private enterprise. According to Anne Somers, that issue had seemingly been settled in favor of the nation's or the United State's unique pluralistic health care economy with its programmatic amalgamation of public and private activities. What had changed was the nature of the mix, which seemed to lean markedly in favor of the public sector. Moreover, with the passage of the National Planning and Resources Development Act (PL 93-641) in 1974, the question of the federal government's right to interfere in the private practice of medicine appeared to be decided, for all intents and purposes, in favor of government.

The role of the federal government in the organization, financing, and delivery of health care services in the United States at mid-decade seemed assured, and the prospects for adoption of some form of national health insurance seemed imminent, if not a foregone conclusion.

But although the federal initiative of the past 20 years or so had been seen by many as a sociopolitical watershed in which the powers and machinery of government were mobilized to improve access to services, to further distribute

Theodor J. Litman, Ph.D., is professor of health services administration, School of Public Health, University of Minnesota, Minneapolis.

justice and equity, and to redress social and economic wrongs, times and circumstances change. The heady optimism and faith in the unbridled growth and intervention of the federal establishment of the 1960s and 1970s soon gave way to suspicion, distrust, and disillusionment with government programs. Thus, in spite of a number of notable accomplishments—such as demonstrated gains in access to care and health status among the poor and the elderly, greater rationalization of the health planning process, and increased production of health personnel—skepticism and dissatisfaction with such initiatives began to grow in the face of rising costs, economic stagflation, limited revenues, diminished financial resources, programmatic cutbacks, indifferent if not hostile central administration, and bureaucratic insensitivity to the infringement of federal policies, directives, and regulations on state and local prerogatives, culminating in the Reagan election in 1980.

The response was sudden and pointed. The new chief executive, who had ridden to victory on a promise to get government off the backs of the American people, moved quickly and decisively. Within 6 months of taking office, through the deft and imaginative use of the budgetary process and with the support of a group of conservative Democrats (known as the Boll Weavils) who were ideologically closer to the Republican party than their own, the president succeeded in gaining congressional approval of a package of budget cuts that repealed and modified scores of programs that had become integral parts of the nation's social and economic fabric while reversing the federal expansion of the last half-century and reducing the size and scope of government.

And so, as the United States entered the new decade, it seemed to be embarking on a different course, one reflected in the president's commitment to less social planning and regulation, a smaller public and larger private sector in health as well as other aspects of life, and an abrupt reduction in government, especially in federal funding for social programs. Whether the results of the 1980 election marked a major shift in sociopolitical thought in the United States vis-à-vis the relationship of government to the individual and his or her health care, as many early editorial writers suggested, or was merely an aberrational interlude in the United States' continuing flirtation with the adoption of some form of national health program, remains to be seen. Suffice it to say, however, that the answer is likely to lie in an understanding of the peculiar nature and role of government and politics in American life, with the decision reached, the product of a deliberative political process.

GOVERNMENT AND HEALTH IN THE UNITED STATES

A number of years ago, the noted British social historian T. H. Marshall observed that no modern government could disdain responsibility for the health of its people nor would it wish to do so. Policies, he noted, differ not so much in the aims pursued as in the methods adopted in pursuit of them. But although the notion of a national system of health services has long been a well-established fact in much of the rest of the world, it has been slow to take hold in the United States. Since the first governmental system of health care was established in Germany under Bismarck in 1883, the provision of health and medical care to an entire population on a nationwide basis through some form of national health service or insurance mechanism has been adopted in nearly half of the world's sovereign nations, including most of those in Western Europe. On the whole, this development has generally come about through an evolutionary rather than revolutionary process, a function of the social, cultural, political, and economic fabrics of the various countries involved. In most cases, government programs for the financing of health care services have evolved as part of a broader system of social benefits. To a large extent, each nation's health care system is a reflection of its own particular legacy of traditions, organization, and institutions, and the American experience has been no exception. Thus, to understand where the United States is and may be heading, it is necessary to know something of the past and the nature of the governmental system.

THE UNITED STATES SYSTEM OF GOVERNMENT

As most students of government are aware, ours is a limited system of federalism predicated on the notion of representative government with an emphasis on minority rights, majority rule, and the preservation of individual liberty. Historically, the American conception of freedom has taken the guise of rights to be protected from restraint, rather than duties to be performed, and a suspicion of established authority. Thus, largely in response to government oppression experienced in Europe, the framers of the Constitution provided an extensive system of checks and balances upon the federal establishment. Although Madison and others recognized the need for national supremacy — earlier attempts to rest sovereignty in the state or colonial legislatures as called for under the original Articles of Confederation had proven unsuccessful — they were also aware of the need for protection from the arbitrary use of power by the national government. To pit sovereignty against sovereignty, however, was seen as a formula for disaster.

As set forth under Article 1, Section 8 of the Constitution, the relationship between the states and the federal government was fairly well drawn, with the federal government given certain prescribed delegated powers, other powers reserved for the states, and still others left to be exercised jointly.

But the framers were also farsighted and realized that the United States was bound to change over time. As a result, the Constitution was envisioned to be a flexible document, confined neither in time nor place. Thus, the role of government in American life has evolved over the past 200 years or so in large part through judicial interpretation and response to executive initiatives and legislative action.

The Nations Health

32⁵⁰

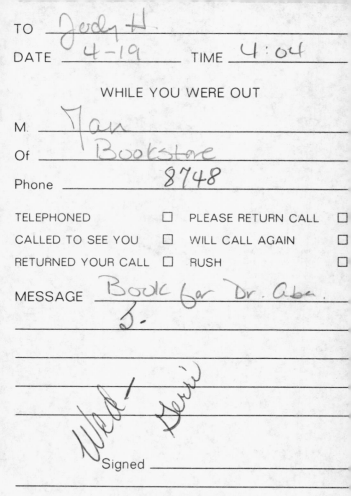

TO **Jody H.**

DATE **4-19**   TIME **4:04**

WHILE YOU WERE OUT

M. **Man**

Of **Bookstore**

Phone **8748**

TELEPHONED	☐	PLEASE RETURN CALL	☐
CALLED TO SEE YOU	☐	WILL CALL AGAIN	☐
RETURNED YOUR CALL	☐	RUSH	☐

MESSAGE **Book for Dr. Aba.**

Signed

The Standard Register Company

FEDERALISM AND THE CONSTITUTIONAL RELATIONSHIP BETWEEN THE NATIONAL GOVERNMENT AND THE STATES

The question of the proper role of government in general, as well as the relative distribution of powers among the national, state, and local governments in particular, has been the subject of prolonged philosophical debate in the United States, with the line in any given controversy ultimately drawn by the courts. Such deliberations have ranged from Marshall's Doctrine of National Supremacy (*McCulloch v. Maryland*) to the Doctrine of Dual Federalism of the Taney court (*Cooley v. Board of Wardens*) with the states having concurrent powers in those matters considered to be truly local in character, to the Cooperative Federalism of the Cardozo court (Steward Machine Company case) to the concept of Creative Federalism under President Johnson and the New Federalism and new New Federalism of the Nixon and Reagan administrations.

Before the 1930s, both federal and state legislation in the field of social welfare were invalidated by the courts on the basis of the due process clause. In 1937, however, the Supreme Court reversed itself (*West Coast Hotel Company v. Parrish*) and repudiated the old doctrine that the due process could be used to crush social welfare legislation. Nevertheless, it was Marshall's interpretation of the commerce clause and the supremacy of the central government that served as the basis for much of the legislative initiatives of the New Deal (Roosevelt), the Fair Deal (Truman), the New Frontier (Kennedy), and the New Society (Johnson).

State-Federal Regulations

The role of the states in the U.S. political system has changed dramatically over the past 200 years as events and trends have altered the fiscal, functional, and political balance within the federal system and rekindled debate over the proper division of powers and responsibilities among the constituent units.

The expansion of the federal government's role in U.S. life has been neither an historical accident nor an altogether noxious historical legacy, but has come about for good historical reasons.

Over the course of the past few years, however, under both the Nixon and Reagan administrations, increasing interest has been expressed in the importance of the relations among the various levels of government. At issue has been how large the federal government's role should be in its relations with its state and local counterparts. The answer has been caught up in philosophical differences that separate not only Democrats and Republicans but also conservatives and liberals within each party.

Beginning under Roosevelt's New Deal and continuing under the Democratic administrations of the sixties, a fairly broad agreement was reached in Congress that the federal government should play an active role in areas traditionally within the province of state and local governments, particularly regulation where state laws were either nonexistent or failed to conform to one another. There was also broad agreement that the federal government should have a role in providing financial assistance to states and localities for a variety of purposes, such as fighting poverty, pollution control, local law enforcement, and housing. The issue was no longer legitimacy of whether the federal government should be involved in such areas but rather how it should go about assisting the state and local governments.

Traditionally, federal assistance has been in the form of categorical grants-in-aid made to a variety of governmental and other public and private entities for specific purposes. Such grants-in-aid enable state and local governments to preserve their autonomy within a framework of federal assistance; to assure minimum levels of services regardless of income inequities among states and localities; and to help achieve national objectives that states and localities may be unwilling or unable to pursue as well as stimulate, through federal matching, increased investment of state and local funds. Moreover, since federal taxes are generally more progressive than their state and local counterparts, federal grants help reduce interstate inequities both in the level of government services and the tax burden. As a matter of fact, one of the major reasons for the proliferation of categorical grants programs was that not only could the federal government tap far more revenue sources than the states and localities, but the latter officials could not or would not provide funds to deal with certain problems.

On the other side of the coin, the expansion of federal power at the expense of state and local government is inherent in such revenue-sharing mechanisms, leading to federal domination or control. It was in reaction to just such concerns, as well as the trend toward centralization of government authority in Washington, D.C., that the concept of block grants was developed. Block grants, which are federal payments to states or local governments for specified purposes such as health, education, or law enforcement, were pushed by Republicans in Congress and the executive branch since the 1960s as a way of returning federal decision making to state and local officials. In contrast to categorical grants, which can only be used for specific programs directed by Congress, with block grants state or local officials may make the decisions on how the money is used within the general program area.

The New Federalism   The debate continues with President Reagan's efforts to return many government programs to the states. His proposal, however, although clothed in the mantle of the "New Federalism," represents less a sorting out of functions among the various levels of government than opposition of fiscal conservatives to large-scale public sector spending on particular domestic activities regardless of the level of government. Moreover, although the Reagan proposal to return power and responsibilities to the states has been viewed by some as a watershed in the history of U.S. federalism, critics see the president's New Federalism and Economic Recovery Act as a device to reduce federal expenditures for key domestic activities, and as an abandonment of the national commitments to certain costly social programs, involving the transfer of responsibility to the states and their political subdivisions without adequate funding.

As states and local units of government have been forced to struggle with the need to provide more human services in the face of ever diminishing financial resources, proposals to return such functions to their control, without a commensurate transfer of funds, have tended to lose much of their aura and appeal, while the debate over the proper role of government in U.S. life continues.

THE GROWTH IN THE GOVERNMENT'S ROLE IN HEALTH AND HEALTH CARE IN THE UNITED STATES

Evolution Not Revolution

It has long been a truism of U.S. political life that government is only permitted to do that which private institutions either cannot or are unwilling to do. The basic economic justification for government intervention, Blumstein and Zubkoff note, is as a remedy for some market failure. In essence, the traditional basis for government involvement has been a remedial one, that is, when, for whatever reason, the market does not achieve an efficient allocation of resources.

In the area of health and welfare, such a view was perhaps best expressed by a 1965 U. S. Chamber of Commerce Task Force on Economic Growth and Opportunity recommendation on the role of government: "Government programs should be used to help the sick, disabled and aged only if voluntary and private means — truly tried and tested — cannot adequately meet society's needs."

A related corollary to the above would add that with the exception of those powers delegated to it by the Constitution, the growth of the federal government's involvement has generally come about in those areas in which the states have also been found wanting. The Interstate Commerce Act of 1887 was passed only after the states had failed to control the spiraling interstate railroad networks, and enactment of the New Deal came after 4 years of economic collapse that found the states broke, with only 17 having old age pension plans, most of which were woefully underfunded.

The expansion of government or public intervention in health and health care in the United States has essentially been one of evolution rather than revolution, a function of social, economic, and political forces as well as judicial interpretation.

HISTORICAL DEVELOPMENT

Over the course of the past 200 years, the role of government in the organization, financing and delivery of health care services in the United States has evolved from that of a highly constricted provider of services and protector of public health to that of a major financial underwriter of an essentially private enterprise whose policies and procedures have increasingly encroached on the autonomy and prerogatives of the providers of care, as he who pays the piper calls the tune.

Although extensive and, at times, seemingly pervasive, such growth has come about neither capriciously nor because legislators or bureaucrats have had any great desire to interfere in this area of endeavor, but rather because the parties primarily involved—the providers (with the notable exception of organized medicine), consumers, insurance carriers, and politicians—realized and came to recognize the need for assistance and government involvement.

NATURE OF THE GOVERNMENT ROLE IN HEALTH AND HEALTH CARE IN THE UNITED STATES

Both traditionally and historically, responsibility for the medical care of recipients of public assistance, veterans with service-connected disabilities, and other special populations such as Indians and the armed forces and for public health in the United States has rested with government, whereas responsibility for the cost of facility construction and health personnel training has been shared among various levels of government and the private sector. The provision of direct personal health services, on the other hand, is and has been essentially a private endeavor.

For the most part, government intervention in the health care system has tended to embrace the following features:

1. Financial underwriting in order to assure the availability to all in the population through either contributory insurance (e.g., Medicare), general tax revenues (e.g., Medicaid), or both
2. The development and establishment of various standards and procedures to safeguard the quality of services financed through public funds
3. The provision of services wherever possible through nongovernmental practitioners and institutions
4. Extension toward comprehensiveness in publically financed services
5. Direct financial support for the modernization, construction, and equipment of health care facilities and for the education and training of needed personnel

Federal Role

As indicated earlier, the federal role in health throughout much of U.S. history has tended to be a constrained one, limited to crisis intervention, the control and prevention of disease in public health. Typically, as Blumstein and Zubkoff have noted, federal intervention in the health area has been on an ad hoc basis without an overall plan, formulation of objectives, or theoretical underpinning. Moreover, in the absence of any specific formulation, national health policy in the United States has been more or less an amorphous set of health goals, derived by various means within the federal structure, with little overall concordance or coordination.

Health Policy at the Federal Level.   For the most part, the legislative initiatives in health at the federal level over the course of the past 20 years rested on a set of assumptions and presumptions, many of which were well meaning and seemed to embrace the conventional wisdom of the period but have proven to be overly optimistic, idealistic, or unfounded.

To a large extent, according to Brown of the Brookings Institution, federal health care policy in the United States has tended to embrace two essentially antithetical models or approaches that today are "nurtured in tension." Thus, while "mainstream" equalizing programs continue to receive strong public support, they are challenged by a set of federal proposals based largely on "revisionist" premises concerning constraints on supply and demand for services. As a result, U.S. health care policy has tended to be discontinuous, inconsistent, and at times, contradictory. Brown goes on to note that by avoiding hard choices and by reconciling in public policy such seemingly contradictory models, we have tended to institutionalize our ambivalence, while preserving the claims of equality of medical services on one hand and delimiting its scope on the other.

Role of the States

In contrast to their federal counterparts, whose influence over health stems in large measure from its enormous fiscal power, the states have rather broad, comprehensive legal authority for a wide variety of programs. As a result, their role in health has taken a number of forms: (1) financial support for the care and treatment of the poor and chronically disabled, including the primary responsibility for the administration of the federal and state Medicaid program; (2) quality assurance and oversight of health care practitioners and facilities, for example, state licensure and regulation; (3) regulation of health care costs and insurance carriers; (4) health personnel training, that is, states provide the major share of the cost for the training of health care professionals; and (5) authorization of local government health services.

Similarly, although historically the power of the governor has been limited, a throwback to the colonists' distrust of the royal governor in the area of public taxation, the states' chief executive appears to exert considerable influence in determining health policy via the power of appointment. A recent review of the statutory authority governing public health decision making in the 50 states found the governor responsible for the appointment of about 91 percent of the 427 positions on the states' boards of health. In 11 states, the members of the board sit at the pleasure of the governor. Moreover, turnover among state health officials has been reported as "brisk" with about 60 percent of them being replaced every 2 years.

State Expenditures for Health.   State spending and responsibility in health have traditionally been directed toward broad public health activities, institutional care of the mentally ill, and the purchase of health care services for the economically disadvantaged. During the past 35 years, state spending in health and other human services has been increasingly shaped by federal prescriptions and initiatives, including a variety of apportionment formulas and project grants. As a matter of fact, a familiar characteristic of the U.S. federal system is that many of the programs that carry out national policies are created and operated by the states under rules established by federal legislation and regulations. Moreover, variable methods of federal funding related to purpose, budgetary limits, formulas, and duration impose similar variability on the states' application of funds to the counties.

Like their federal counterpart, state expenditures for health are provided through direct provision of services and indirect purchase of services and have been the subject of considerable political debate over the scope, cost, level of funding, and appropriateness of such expenditures. For all this costs money, and the funds may not be readily available in times of economic recession. Thus, while many states found themselves with expanding treasuries during the late 1960s and early 1970s, fueled by inflation and aided and abetted by increased federal revenue sharing and a thriving economy, in the face of a serious economic downturn nationally, declining state revenues, reduced federal aid, rising costs, a heightened demand for health and welfare services, threatened taxpayer revolts, and bulging budget deficits, they were forced to cut back greatly on their programs and allow more and more of the burden to fall back on their local counterparts.

The Impact of Federal Initiatives in Health on States and Localities.   Finally although the evidence on the extent of the impact of federal initiatives on state and local priorities in health is limited, the key to understanding the ways in which federal aid influences state health goals and programmatic activities appears to lie in the political environment of the state. In a study of six states and four public health programs, for example, Buntz et al. found that although federal programs facilitate rather than inhibit the attainment of state health goals, federal influence tends to be secondary to that of the state's political environment. A federal program, they note, may elevate an issue to the state's active policy agenda but need not necessarily lead to formulation of a state policy or goals unless interests within the state are receptive. Moreover, the federal influence on state health policy appears to be both state and program specific, reinforcing changes supported at the state level and altering state goals at the margin. Such changes in state goals, however, are likely to occur only when the political environment of the state is receptive to change. For although the federal government has the power to force states to pay attention to certain national goals, it cannot force them to sift their goals in any fundamental way nor to accept those goals as legitimate.

Public and Private Financing of Health Care in the United States

Although initial consideration of the adoption of some form of national health insurance in the United States occurred at about the same time as in Europe — at the turn of the century — and in reaction to similar forces — industrialization, urbanization, the demise of the extended family, and employment practices and policies that heightened the threat of work-related injuries and disease as well as unemployment — unlike Europe, the implementation of social security in the United States came through selected income maintenance programs and the preservation of the voluntary sector.

Thus, the provision of third-party health insurance coverage in the United States developed primarily on a voluntary basis through Blue Cross-Blue Shield and the commercial insurance industry. The attendant mixture of approaches resulted in a complex pattern of health care financing in which (1) the employed are predominantly covered by voluntary insurance provided through contributions made by their employers and themselves; (2) the aged are insured through a combination of coverages financed out of Social Security tax revenues and voluntary insurance for physician and supplementary coverage; (3) the health care of the poor is covered through Medicaid via federal, state, and local revenues, and (4) special population groups such as veterans, merchant seamen, Indians, members of the armed forces, Congress, and the executive branch have coverage provided directly by the federal government.

According to Kramer, private health insurance primarily has been a collection of payments mechanism that supports and reinforces existing patterns of health services. Government spending for health, on the other hand, has been largely confined to filling the gap in the private sector, that is, environmental protection, preventive services, communicable disease control, care for special groups, institutional care for the mentally and chronically ill, provision of medical care to the poor, and support for research and training. The high cost of public medical care programs, Kramer reminds us, owes its genesis to the markedly unique division of risk taking and responsibility between the public and private sector that has thrust upon government the cost of caring for those segments of the population with the highest incidence of illness and greatest need for care, that is, the aged, poor, mentally ill, retarded, chronically ill, and disabled.

Finally, the use of fiscal stimuli through grants-in-aid, the commitment of major financing programs to retrospective reimbursement of costs on a fee-for-service basis, and reliance on peer review for quality assurance reflect a preference for the achievement of public objectives through strategies that offer inducements, persuasion, and positive rewards to providers for compliance rather than impose penalties or costs for failure to comply. Such strategies, however, have been inherently expansive, tending to minimize the need for deliberative allocative choices by increasing the flow of resources into the health care system. Once costs rise and revenues become short, such choices no longer can be put off and questions of constraint and costs are raised.

Problem of Cost Versus Services in Government Programs.   The amount of money that a nation spends for its health services, Anderson and Newhauser noted in 1969, tends to be a product primarily of a political process arrived at by implicit and explicit public policy decisions within the body politic. An equally appropriate maxim, however, is that whatever government giveth, it can taketh away. In other words, although public programs often initially are enacted on essentially altruistic grounds, for example, increased accessibility to health care services by removing financial barriers to care while defraying costs over a wide segment of the public, once this is done and the costs that originally were borne by patients, their families, and/or the private sector and are now assumed by government rise, there is a strong tendency on the part of the latter to cut back on its commitment by reducing coverage, that is, who and what is covered and increasing the amount paid by those who use the services.

Thus, as costs rise, the tendency is to cut back on the coverage especially if the constituency being served is not a very powerful or influencial one, such as the poor, the socially and economically disadvantaged and, up to the 1960s, the elderly. For as commendable and needy as a service may be and as legitimate as government involvement is, the question ultimately gets down to a fundamental economic one: the cost of the service given the limited funds (however defined) available for it.

Therefore, beginning in the latter part of the 1960s–early 1970s, the federal government and the states, confronted by escalating costs and depleted resources, began to cut back on the Medicare and Medicaid programs. Thus in contrast to 20 years ago when the dual programs were first enacted and the primary policy concern was increased access to health care services for more U.S. citizens, ostensibly the aged and economically disadvantaged, the programs were so successful that the budget soon became incapable of containing them. As a result, the policy has taken a 180-degree turn toward greater restriction and control, with often devastating consequences on the provision and receipt of services, in many cases proving to be "penny cheap and pound foolish."

Case of Medicaid.   This conflict between costs and services has been especially true of the Medicaid program, whose expenditures tend to be particularly susceptible to the forces of unemployment and inflation. For not only does the size of its clientele, that is, recipients of public assistance and "the medically indigent," vary with the level of unemployment, but the services it renders are purchased in the general medical marketplace and are susceptible to the impact of inflation. In addition, the negative effect of reduced tax receipts on state and local revenues as a result of a national economic recession tends to place both levels of government in a whipsaw as the demand for services on them rises because of heightened unemployment while their capacity to pay for them diminishes.

CONCLUSION

The growth in government's involvement in health has been an evolutionary one, a response to changes in times and circumstances. Over the past 40 years, there have been major shifts in the role and posture of the federal government in the organization, financing, and delivery of health care services and its relationship with the states in which the following have occurred:

1. The traditional federal role of sharing the cost of health care gradually has been expanded to include programs of care purchased by the government itself as well as the use of federal funding to initiate and develop new forms of delivery, for example, neighborhood health centers and health maintenance organizations (HMOs).
2. An increased use of categorical and project grants in health found the federal government involved in the budget funding of local programs and bypassing local governments considered unresponsive to the needs of the poor.
3. The federal focus has shifted from encouraging the expansion of state programs to assuring their integrity and from concern over improving access to services to control over their costs with both patients and providers often caught in the middle.

The progression in such involvement has been a slow and steady one, a function of the nature of the nation's political process and social and economic systems. Incrementalism, rather than fundamental changes in the structure of the health care delivery system, has been the hallmark of federal policies. What has evolved then, as Anderson has aptly observed, has been a partnership—

sometimes rather tenuous and strained—between government (federal and state) and the voluntary system, working together, not as rivals but as partners—not necessarily equally or smoothly, but as partners nevertheless.

Given the experience of the United States over the past half-century with various government entreaties in health, what lessons can be learned? The following are suggested for future consideration:

1. Reform of the health care system in the United States is likely to be incremental, a compromise involving the resolution of a number of interests.

2. National programs require consideration of regional and local problems and needs.

3. Regional variations and the diversity and voluntary-private nature of the health care enterprise make the imposition of national fee schedules, reimbursement formulas, and facility guidelines difficult if not impossible to achieve.

4. Equality in financing is not sufficient to guarantee equal access to medical care.

5. All third-party coverage, whether private or public, such as Medicare and Medicaid, contributes to inflation.

6. All modern national health care systems, predicated as they are on sophisticated technology, are inherently costly.

7. Open-ended reimbursement to providers on the basis of cost is inflationary, whereas unrealistic or picayune controls tend to be self-defeating, leading providers to opt out of the system and leaving recipients a limited range of choices of care.

8. Although any government system is likely ultimately to impose restrictions on the autonomy and prerogatives of providers, such controls can neither be arbitrary nor capricious but should seek the cooperation of professional interests and the use of financial incentives and rewards.

9. A conflict between cost and services is inherent in government programs.

10. Government efforts to reduce expenditures for health services programs by transferring their costs without appropriate financial safeguards to lesser levels of government or recipients of services does not effectively reduce the overall costs of the services but merely shifts the financial burden to those least able to bear it while depriving those most in need.

11. Utilitarianism, that is, "put people back to work" and "get them off the welfare rolls and onto the taxpaying rolls," rather than humanitarianism and altruism, underscore the ultimate adoption of most government human services programs.

12. Protection against the financial burden of health and medical care is impossible without the placement of a ceiling on the patient's financial responsibility. Unless the family is guaranteed that its share of the cost of care will not exceed some reasonable fraction of income, the goal of

preventing or protecting against the financial burden of health care services cannot be achieved. While what that level of income or ceiling is or should be is open to debate, it should be noted that artificial financial barriers or income cutoffs tend to be highly susceptible to the tyranny of inflation, that is, as dollar amounts soar, real value and purchasing power decline.

13. The use of administrative and regulatory controls, such as Medicare's requirement of a three-day hospital stay before a patient may be authorized to be admitted to a nursing home, second opinion requirements, inadequate reimbursement to providers, reduction of the tax deduction for health and medical expenditures, and elimination of deductibility for health insurance premiums, rather than civil or criminal penalties, tend to be misdirected, self-defeating, and ineffective.

14. Programs covering only poor people must be carefully designed so as to avoid adverse incentives and inequities in which some people receive substantial assistance and others equally in need or deserving, that is the near or working poor, receive nothing or practically nothing.

15. Assumptions that the elderly are protected against the cost of long-term care by Medicare are ill-founded and wrong. The only government-provided protection the elderly have against the cost of catastrophic illness is Medicaid — a welfare program.

16. Geographic inequities are bound to occur when states have a major role in setting eligibility and benefit levels.

17. Government health care programs predicated on the virtues of competition and the free marketplace and a preferred single delivery system ignore the fact that one of the major sources for the high cost of hospital care in the United States has been the virtually unfettered costly competition between health institutions for staff, equipment, and so on, which results in a duplication of services, minimize the value of a diverse pluralistic system of delivery and the variable needs and demands of consumers as well as providers.

18. Whatever the future role of government in health in the United States is to be, it will be the product of a deliberate decision made in the political arena and will likely embrace the unique features of the nation's social, political, economic, and health care system.

Health care is as much a component of American goods and products and services as are raw materials. The U.S. spends eight times more than many of its international competitors on health care.

RICHARD D. LAMM
Governor of Colorado
1975–1987

Vicente Navarro

Federal Health Policies in the United States: An Alternative Explanation

One of the most important characteristics of the policies of the current Republican federal administration has been an unprecedented (in peace time) growth of military expenditures and an equally unprecedented reduction of social (including health) expenditures. From 1980 to 1985, the federal military expenditures rose from 7.2 percent to 9.9 percent of the gross national product (GNP), with a projected rise to 10.5 percent of the GNP in 1988. By 1990, the United States government will have spent, during the period of 1980 to 1990, $2,500 billion, which is more than the whole United States military expenditure from 1946 to 1980 ($2,001 billion). On the other hand, federal social expenditures (including Social Security) declined for the period of 1980 to 1985 from 11.2 percent to 10.4 percent of the GNP. Federal funds for health and medical programs have also been reduced from 44.9 percent of all social welfare expenditures in 1980 to 42.4 percent in 1983. And the rate of growth of federal health expenditures has fallen from 16.5 percent per year in 1980 to 10.1 percent in 1983. The U.S. Council of Economic Advisors in its 1984 report to the president refers to such shifts of federal resources as "absolutely unprecedented."

The explanations given for these federal policies are many. A widely held interpretation attributes these policies to a popular mandate received by the Republican administration in the 1980 and 1984 presidential and congressional elections. Instances of this interpretation in the health and medical care bibliography are many. For example, the leaders of the Robert Wood Johnson Foundation, in an article in the *New England Journal of Medicine*, referred to the 1980 election as a "powerful mandate to decrease taxes and non-defense expenditures." In the same issue, J. K. Iglehart, reporting on a major conference attended by leading exponents of the medical establishment, wrote of a quasi-consensus among participants that cuts in federal health expenditures had to be made in response to a popular mandate.

Vicente Navarro, M.D., Ph.D., is professor of health policy and management at Johns Hopkins University, Baltimore, Maryland, and editor of the *International Journal of Health Services*.

That popular mandate was perceived to be a result of popular disenchant-ment with government, and a popular desire to reduce government interven-tion in the health sector. Again, examples of this interpretation of the popular-mandate argument in the medical care bibliography are many. For instance, Paul Starr in his influential *The Social Transformation of American Medicine*, interprets the victory of Reagan in 1980 as a result of people's belief that the government was *the* problem. This popular belief was based on the perception that, as David Mechanic approvingly put it, "the heavy hand of government causes more problems than it solves." Consequently, and as indicated by the publisher and the editor of *Health Affairs*, a major health policy forum in the United States, Americans wanted the size of their government reduced and its interventions in the health sector diminished. These are not solitary voices. Far from it. These are representative voices of prevalent interpretations of current federal health policies.

The accumulated evidence for all of these years does not, however, support this interpretation of a popular mandate for these federal health policies. Quite to the contrary, a survey of all major opinion polls from 1976 to the present shows that there has been a constant and undiminished support for an expansion rather than a reduction of health and social expenditures (and for keeping and/or strengthening government interventions to protect workers, consumers, and the environment). Similar evidence exists to show that the reduction of social expenditures, as well as other domestic policies carried out by the current administration, such as the transfer of federal funds from the social to the military sector, are not popular policies. Even Senator Paul Laxalt, a close friend of President Reagan and the chairman of the Republican National Committee, has recently referred to "the strange phenomenon that most Americans express approval of Ronald Reagan, although they are opposed to much of what the President supports." Lipser, Ferguson and Rogers have shown that the majority of Americans remain more liberal than the president on economics, defense, foreign policy, and social questions. A survey of popular opinion regarding federal health policies shows that the same is true for health questions.

In light of this evidence, a question that needs to be raised and answered is why did people vote both in 1980 and in 1984 for a candidate whose commitment to carry out those unpopular policies was clearly stated? Indeed, a major assumption made by the authors who believe in the popular mandate as the force behind those federal social policies is that *electoral behavior and antipopular opinion are synonymous*. The answer to the question needs to be given at different levels. One explanation is that the overwhelming majority of United States presidents have been elected by a minority, not a majority, of potential voters. And President Reagan, elected by 32.3 percent of the potential electorate in 1984 and 27.2 percent in 1980, was no exception to this reality.

Still, the question may be asked again. How is it that so many people voted for candidate Reagan despite the fact that they did not support his social

(including health) policies? The answer involves the nature of Western democracy and its limitations. The act of voting is based on a totalizing interpretation of policy. In other words, in the act of voting (except in referendums),
people are asked to vote for totalities, not for sectional choices. One votes either
Republican or Democratic. But one cannot vote selectively, i.e., one is not
offered the chance of voting for the many components of those policies (such
as education, health services, transport, and employment policies). The vote is
everything or nothing.

Thus, representative democracy is insufficient. It does not measure, nor
does it reflect, the popular will on the many dimensions of public life. *Electoral
behavior and popular opinion are not synonymous.* Consequently, there is no
contradiction or schizophrenia involved in Reagan's winning the election
while the majority of the people (including his voters) have different and even
opposite views on many and even the majority of Reagan's policies.

In summary, there is no evidence to support the thesis that the current
federal social (including health) policies respond to a popular mandate. Thus,
the original question of why these policies remain. I postulate that in order to
answer this question we have to analyze these policies within the social,
political, and economic context in which they take place. In other words, in
order to understand these federal health policies—the tree—we have to understand the actual distribution of social, economic, and political power in the
United States today—the forest.

CLASS AS EXPLANATORY VALUE IN HEALTH POLICY

One of the most striking areas of silence in the analysis of health policy in the
United States is the absence of class as a category of power. Class, in health
care bibliography, seems,to be an "un-American" category. In most of this
bibliography, the citizens and residents of the United States are divided
according to biological (e.g., gender, race) or cultural (e.g., Hispanic, ethnic)
categories, but rarely, if ever, according to class categories. Thus, the United
States is the only major country in the Western industrialized world in which
health and social statistics are not recorded according to class. An elementary
observation needs to be made, however. The United States has classes. This
observation bears repeating in light of dominant discourse in which class as a
category of analysis and bearer of power relations is rarely mentioned. Aside
from references to the United States as a middle-class society (a society in
which the majority of United States citizens are supposed to be in the middle,
between the rich and the poor), the power category of class never, or very
rarely, appears in the major media in general or in the medical literature in
particular. This definition of the United States as a middle-class society takes

place, incidentally, in spite of the fact that more United States citizens define themselves as members of the working class (48 percent) than of the middle class (43 percent).

Actually, the size of the working class is even larger than that based on people's self perception of themselves as part of the working class. Erik O. Wright has shown how the actual size of the working class is over 60 percent of the United States population. The middle class, which has always been smaller in size than the working class, has been further reduced in size recently owing to the changes in the occupational structure of the United States. Most of the major media, however — including the medical media — never refer to the majority of the United States population as working class. Rather, they define it as middle class. The United States capitalist class is the most powerful capitalist class in today's world. In a truly Gramscian fashion, the interests of this class have been presented (and accepted) as the universal interest. To be anticapitalist, for example, is to be perceived as anti-American. Indicative of the power of this class to define the dominant discourse is the fact that classes never appear in that discourse. The capitalist class, however, is the most class conscious of all classes in the United States. And the current leadership of the Republican administration represents the most "class conscious" stratum within that class.

United States health services are largely paid for by work-related health benefits achieved through a bargaining process in which each sector of labor tries to get as much as possible for its own constituency. As a result of this situation, we find that different sectors of the working population in the United States have different types of health coverage, with manufacturing having better coverage than other workers, and sales and service workers being the least protected.

The consequence of this "interest group" behavior is that, while the coverage is comprehensive for some sectors of the working population, the coverage for the whole class is rather limited. As an average, United States citizens still pay in out-of-pocket and in direct expenses larger percentages for health benefits than any other Western industrialized nation. Another consequence of relating health benefits to employment (besides reinforcing the resource disparities arising from pay differentials) is that it weakens the popular demand for improving governmental programs. Thus, those who remain unprotected through the work place are more isolated politically, decreasing the popular pressure for government to meet their needs.

This focus on work-related benefits (assured by collective private bargaining) rather than benefits assured by the state (which may be paid through general revenues or payroll taxes) is the primary difference between the expansion of health services coverage in the United States and in western Europe. While the working class in western Europe has conducted its struggle for expanding health services coverage primarily through the state, its counterpart in the United States has struggled (not as a class but as an interest group) primarily through the bargaining table at the work place.

CLASS, TAXES, AND HEALTH LEGISLATION

The point that needs to be emphasized is that federal expenditures (including health expenditures) are based on taxes coming from labor rather than from capital, i.e., the welfare state is paid for to a very large degree by the working population. Here, it is important to clarify a much debated and misunderstood issue: the overall level of taxation. It is true that the total United States tax level is relatively low compared with other countries. In 1974 it was 27.5 percent of the GNP, placing the United States 14th out of 17 major industrial capitalist nations. Only Switzerland, Japan, and Australia had lower overall tax levels. But, if instead of looking at overall levels one focuses on levels of taxation by occupational groups, it then emerges that for an average production worker the United States ranked 8th highest in the tax burden. The American tax system is indeed highly regressive.

This regressiveness is further highlighted if we look at what the average citizen gets in return for his or her taxes. The average European gets more from government than does the United States citizen. For the most part, the European citizen gets free or almost free health care (very low out-of-pocket expenses), generous family allowances, and better unemployment insurance, pensions, and disabilities than his or her American counterpart, as well as many other social benefits that increase individual income. The United States welfare state is underdeveloped compared with western Europe. In the health sector, for example, the United States citizen still pays 27 percent in direct costs compared with 8 percent in Sweden, 5 percent in Great Britain, 12 percent in West Germany, and 19 percent in France. And no other country among Western industrialized nations has 38 million inhabitants (representing 16 percent) uncovered by any kind of insurance. Fifty-six million people under the age of 65 are either uninsured for health care during the entire year, uninsured for a part of the year, or significantly underinsured. For the 30 million people over the age of 65, Medicare covers only 49 percent of total health care costs, costs which average $4,200 per year. The average American taxpayer gets comparatively little from his or her taxes. A large percentage of taxes goes for military expenditures that return very little economic benefit to the average citizen.

This measure of regressiveness explains why the average citizen feels, under a heavy tax burden and strongly opposes increasing taxes. People are against increasing taxes because they are not getting much in return. But (and it is an extremely important but), they are willing to pay higher taxes if they are assured that they will benefit from them. This explains why: (1) Social Security taxes (the taxes that have increased most rapidly in the last ten years) are the least unpopular taxes; (2) the majority of Americans would be willing to pay higher taxes if they could be assured that those revenues would pay for health services (such as a national and comprehensive health program) from which *all* citizens would benefit. People are not willing to increase taxes, however, to resolve the deficit problem. Their anti-tax sentiment is highly selective. Thus, it is wrong to state, as is frequently done, that people are against paying taxes. How people feel about paying taxes depends on what they will get in return. It is as simple and logical as that; and (3) there is more support for New Deal types of programs (aimed at the whole population) than for Great Society programs (aimed at specific populations).

In brief, the average United States citizen is getting less in return for his or her taxes than the average citizen in major western European countries, a situation that is in large degree explained by the highly skewed nature of the tax system of the United States (falling heavily on the middle- and low-income levels of the working population) and by the large proportion that military expenditures represent within federal government expenditures. Since social expenditures are, for the most part, financed by taxes imposed on the working population, these transfers of government funds have not had a redistributive effect from the capitalist class to the working class. Rather, there has been a redistributive effect within the working population, with some sectors of the working class paying for others. This situation explains why Great Society programs have been somewhat less popular than New Deal types of programs. They have frequently been used to divide the working class, pitting whites against blacks, men against women, young against old, the middle-income families against low-income families, and so on. The identification of the Democratic party with the Great Society (e.g., Medicaid) rather than the New Deal (e.g., Medicare and Social Security) has contributed to the weakening of the popularity of the party.

It is in those countries in which class practices within the working class do not exist and in which labor operates as one more interest group (highly divided into different subgroups, each one looking out for its own), that we also find a depoliticization of the population, with low voter turnout and a fragmentation of politics. This is precisely what is happening in the United States today.

The lack of polarization of American politics and the conventional wisdom that parties have to move to the center to attract the middle class are producing a depoliticization of American life, with increasing disenchantment toward the two major political parties.

AN EXAMPLE OF A NEW DEAL PROGRAM: A COMPREHENSIVE AND UNIVERSAL TAX-BASED HEALTH PROGRAM

There is today a large problem in the health care sector of the United States. By whatever health indicator one can think of (infant mortality, low birthweight, life expectancy, etc.), indicators in the United States do not compare favorably with those in other developed industrialized countries. And the situation is deteriorating in many important areas. For example, the decline of infant mortality has slowed down since 1981. This is a result, among other factors, of the 1979 to 1982 recession and of the reduction of social expenditures, a reduction that affected primarily but not exclusively the low-income groups within the working class. Those cuts were carried out with bipartisan support, following a nonexistent popular mandate. This reduction of social expenditures further increased the number of people who did not have any form of private or public insurance coverage. This problem also affected the majority of the population that did have some form of coverage, since the most common form of coverage is not comprehensive and still requires substantial payments by the patient.

These major problems explain why people in the United States want to see changes in the health sector. In 1983, 50 percent of polled Americans indicated that "fundamental changes are needed to make the health care system work better" and another 25 percent felt that "the American health care system has so much wrong with it that we need to completely rebuild it." These percentages increased in 1984 to 51 percent and 31 percent respectively.

If the United States does not have a national health program it is not, as Victor Fuchs wrongly indicates, because Americans do not want it. Nor is it because, as Reinhardt has indicated, we Americans face a moral crisis, "an apparent unwillingness of society's will to pay for the economic and medical maintenance of the poor." (Reinhardt assumes, as many others do, that whatever occurs in federal health policy is the outcome of people's wishes. This assumption perceives the American political system as fully responsive to people's wishes. This assumption ignores the accumulated evidence that shows that popular opinion is not always the determinant of federal executive and legislative behavior.) Actually, in a 1984 ABC News-*Washington Post* poll, an unprecedented 75 percent of the respondents indicated that "the government should institute and operate a national health program," a demand preferred by the majority of the American population for the last fifteen years.

Nor is the absence of such a program due to lack of resources; the United States spends 10.8 percent of the GNP on health services. The problem is in the channels (i.e., the institutions) through which those resources are being spent. Indeed, the problems of insufficient coverage and high costs are rooted in the private, for-profit character of American medicine. An international analysis of health services shows that those countries with government control of the funding and administration of health services have better coverage, lower costs, and better distribution of health resources than those countries that have large for-profit private sectors in the health services — such as the United States.

The funding of a comprehensive and universal health program could be based on different but highly popular interventions:

1. Changed priorities within the health sector, not only through incentives but also active government interventions. The current reliance on highly technological medicine is neither good medical care nor good health care. Although high-technology curative medicine has a role to play, it should not be the dominant form of intervention. For example, the state of North Carolina has about the same number of deliveries per year as Sweden, but twice as many low-birth-weight babies and neonatal deaths, due to poverty and malnutrition. In 1978 and 1979 there were only 30 ventilator-equipped neonatal intensive-care-unit beds in Sweden compared to 60 or so in North Carolina, where even further expansions are now proposed. It would be cheaper and more humane to provide food and other social services rather than curative technology. The laissez-faire approach to medical care enables and stimulates a sophisticated technological approach to medical problems, but does not serve well a broadly based preventive approach capable of diminishing both the problems and the need for expensive technology. In summary, there is a need to shift the priorities away from hospital, curative, personal, and highly technological medicine toward preventive, community, environmental, occupational, and social interventions. This shift of priorities will not occur by continuing reliance on the for-profit private sector; it requires an active government intervention and active popular participation.

2. A shift of resources within the public sector, away from the military and back to social expenditures, reversing a trend that threatens the survival of the United States population. These funds are spent, in official rhetoric, to make American children more "secure" from external enemies. Meanwhile, from 1980 to 1985, during the Reagan administration, more American children died from poverty than the total number of American battle deaths in the Vietnam War. It is estimated that, until 1990, 22,000 American babies will die per year because of low birth weight. Poverty is the greatest child killer in 1985 in the affluent United States. None other than President Eisenhower indicated that "the problem in defense is how far you can go without destroying from within what you are trying to defend from without." Here again, we find that Americans do support the reversal of this trend, with the shifting of resources from military to social and health expenditures. The level of popular support for health and social expenditures is much, much higher than the level of support for military expenditures.

3. Increases in the level of taxation of the corporate class and upper-middle class, a level that has declined dramatically and is even imperiling the functioning of the American economy. The overall size of tax cuts aimed at the corporate class was $220 billion in 1984. The entire federal cost of a

comprehensive health program was estimated by the Carter administration to be $20 billion for 1984, less than 10 percent of the revenues lost to the federal government because of tax cuts for the corporate class. A comprehensive health program has to be redistributive, based on authentically progressive revenues. It should increasingly rely on general revenues rather than Social Security taxes, which would also allow for shifting revenues among sectors. This situation is particularly important in light of the demographic transition, which is usually presented as a major reason for the rise of health expenditures. To have more elderly means to have more health consumption. The absolute and percentage growth of the numbers of the elderly is presented as one of the reasons for the crisis in the Western systems of health care. Due to the repetitiveness of this argument, let me clarify two points. First, the enormous growth of expenditures in the federal program for the elderly—Medicare—for the period 1978 to 1982 was not caused primarily by an increase in the numbers of elderly. The major cause of that growth in expenditures was price inflation, i.e., price inflation of hospital and medical services that benefit providers and suppliers but not the patients. Second, the same demographic transition leads to fewer young people, with a freeing up of public funds for education, transportation, and recreation that could be shifted to health services. For example, the Organization for Economic Cooperation and Development secretariat has shown that, in the seven major industrialized countries, the estimated saving for public education due to the demographic transition could ensure a 0.7 percent annual growth of real social expenditures until 1990, more than sufficient to cover the expanding demands of the elderly in health services.

4. Government funding and administration of the health care services and institutions, with active worker and community participation in the running of these institutions. Himmelstein and Woolhandler have documented the ideological biases of most cost-control measures that are being researched in the United States, and that are being implemented by the American government. A majority of these measures involved a cut of benefits to the working population. A progressive agenda will have to focus on cost controls that enlarge these health benefits and further empower the patient and potential patient population, i.e., the citizenry. These authors estimated that if the United States had had a national health insurance in 1983, it would have saved the population $42.6 billion annually ($29.2 billion in health administration and insurance overhead, $4.9 billion in profits, $3.9 billion in marketing, and $4.6 billion in physicians' income). If the United States had had a national health service, the population would have saved $65.8 billion ($38.4 billion in health administration and insurance overhead, $4.9 billion in profits, $3.9 billion in marketing, and $18.6 billion in physicians' income). Complete nationalization of the health services, with nationalization of the drug and

supplies industries, would save $85.3 billion (one third of all health expenditures). And most important, these savings would occur while expanding rather than reducing the health benefits for the whole population.

All of the points presented in this article bear repeating in light of current arguments about the "crisis" of the welfare state and the health and social austerity policies that are being followed, which attribute that crisis to the growth of public expenditures (assumed to be out of control), and which explain and justify those austerity policies as responding to a popular mandate. Evidence presented in this article questions each one of these positions. These policies of austerity respond to the correlation of forces, including class forces, that exists in the United States today. The resolution of the major health problems, such as insufficient coverage and high costs, requires a change in the political practices and assumptions of the two major parties, with further development of the New Deal by the establishment of a national health program. Contrary to what is widely reported, there is, indeed, evidence of popular support for this health policy intervention by the federal government. The creation of such a program depends not only on that popular support but on the practices of the political and economic instruments through which class interests are expressed.

The U.S. has one of the most inefficient health care systems in the world, as well as one of the most expensive.

RICHARD D. LAMM
Governor of Colorado
1975–1987

Theodore R. Marmor

American Medical Policy and the "Crisis" of the Welfare State: A Comparative Perspective

Most policy debates in most countries are parochial affairs. They address national "problems," cite historical and contemporary national developments in a particular domain (e.g., pensions, urban affairs, transportation), and embody conflicting visions of what policies the particular country should adopt. Only rarely are the experiences of other nations seriously considered. When cross-national examples are employed in such parochial struggles, their use is typically part of policy warfare more than of policy understanding.

So it was in the United States during the postwar period that Britain's "socialized medicine" became a familiar epithet in discussions of national health insurance and, later, Medicare. For others, the "advanced" welfare state of Sweden has been a model of how pensions should be structured. In child welfare, the universal child allowances of many European nations have been the exemplary instances — or criticized symbols — of what family policy should include. Historically, the focus is national and programmatic; cross-nationally, the emphasis on similar problems or policies abroad. Only very rarely in social policy debates has the agenda included a broad review of other national experiences with a set of related, but distinct, policies. Where such review takes place, it more typically occurs in economic policy, where the cross-national treatment of fiscal, monetary, and industrial policy issues is far more developed.

This article takes as its focus the connection between medical policy concerns and the postwar development of welfare states in the advanced industrial democracies. First, I discuss the widespread cross-national questioning of the welfare state in the wake of the stagflation of the post-1973 period. For the past decade and a half, the "crisis" of the welfare state has become a staple of policy discussion in otherwise quite varied regimes. Exactly what is alleged to have occurred? Second, I examine the evidence about what in fact happened during this period — the information crucial to understanding

Theodore R. Marmor, Ph.D., is professor and chair of the Center for Health Studies, Institution for Social and Policy Studies, Yale University, New Haven, Connecticut.

the response of different polities to the common strain of lower growth rates, inflation, increased unemployment, and large welfare state claims on public expenditure. Finally, I explain how the argument about crisis and the facts about adjustment relate to American concerns about medical care.

This paper's agenda is broad and its commentary summary, but its argument is straightforward. Our medical policy disputes have been substantially changed by the fear that our nation cannot afford its present social programs; attention to the broader welfare context is therefore crucial to understanding American medicine and its politics. It is as if our debates have centered on the distribution and character of an area's fires, without much attention to the direction and velocity of the prevailing wind.

THE ALLEGED CRISIS

The claim of crisis in the welfare state that arose in the 1970s and continues to be voiced in the 1980s calls for the radical restructuring of the set of social programs that emerged in the Depression and postwar period. In America, that aim is very much identified with the election of Ronald Reagan in 1980 and the subsequent attacks on federal social spending. In Europe, it is certainly associated with the triumph and continued political victories of Margaret Thatcher of Great Britain and with shifts to the right in a number of other political regimes.

The claim of the welfare state's crisis has been a cliché of political debate over the last fifteen years. That claim is, however, quite ambiguous. Contemporary discussions, relying on unclear and often misunderstood terms, provide a clue to the confusion about exactly what the "troubles of the welfare state" are. Are the social policies of the modern state in crisis, or is the state in crisis because desirable welfare commitments overwhelm fiscal capacity? What exactly is meant by "the welfare state"? Does it refer to the major spending programs of contemporary governments? If so, leaving defense aside, we are talking about pensions, medical care, education, and housing in different mixes in different countries. Or is legitimacy, rather than expenditure, the issue? Measured by popular support, the major spending programs in health and pensions are cross-nationally popular. Is the crisis then one of finding the means to finance crucial and popular commitments? Or does the problem include governmental extension of authority into disputed policy areas such as abortion and busing in the United States, redistribution towards French-speakers in Canada, "guest workers" in Germany and Sweden, and the like? Simply put, there is no agreement about what the topic is.

The wide body of literature concerning the welfare state falls into three categories. Some analysts regard the welfare state's growth as the main cause of many contemporary political troubles. Most often associated with the apocalyptic right, those who espouse this belief focus on restraining the overreaching state and redeveloping the institutions of the market and the hegemony of individual choice.

Others see the modern state's experience with slowed economic growth as the source of strains *for* social welfare programs. In the middle politically, these center incrementalists are preoccupied with the way in which fiscal strain and stagflation required cutbacks. They view the current crisis as caused by fiscal strains on welfare state programs rather than as a result of any inherent feature of welfare state institutions. They assume that if and when economic growth resumes, the crisis will abate.

A third group stresses the controversies over particular social programs (usually not fiscally important ones) that reach to issues of legitimate governmental purpose. The proponents of this view see the strains on the welfare state as evidence of the contradictions of modern capitalism, and the crisis in the modern welfare state as a portent of future troubles along the way.

There are, of course, overlaps among these three approaches, and the first two can, without heroic effort, be tightly linked. But there are differences, and they make a difference in mapping the subject.

Approach #1: From social welfare programs to the state's crisis. There are two different versions of this approach. Both share the view that social welfare programs played a major role in the poor economic performance of the 1970s. At the theory's simplest level, social programs compete with other budget outlays, preventing the proper balance between investment and consumption. Some critics call this the "bankrupting" of the state; they insist on the importance of budgetary competition and the unfortunate consequences of welfare state expansion. The second form of argument stresses the indirect consequences of many social programs for the mobility of capital and labor. This argument gives us something worth pondering. But it is important to notice that the causal arguments very differently interpret the undeniable growth of spending in this sector during the 1960s and early 1970s. The first argument treats spending as the problem. In the second argument, the rigidities are not centrally involved with the largest spending programs, though unemployment insurance is certainly both important and moderately prominent in budget terms.

Approach #2: From the fiscal crisis of stagflation to welfare state troubles. From this point of view, the problem is that the worldwide recession of the mid-1970s critically threatened the welfare state. The combination of low rates of economic growth, increasing levels of unemployment, and worrisome levels of investment produced strain for the programs that grew rapidly in the earlier decade. In the short run, the welfare state programs appropriately cushioned the effects of recent recession. But because inflation and unemployment increased outlays when recession reduced government revenues, the fiscal strain became quickly apparent. For the longer run, the prospects of unavoidable pressures in medical care and pensions are evident and are sometimes used to prod present action through panic mongering. For the United States, the crucial strains in pensions lie in the twenty-first century, when the baby-boom generation will be old. There is thus ample time to adjust taxes, benefits, and retirement conventions. But it is important to see the difference between the short-term effects of stagflation and the structural-demographic prospects for major spending programs over time. It is difficult to exaggerate the fearfulness of these discussions in the United States, and thus it is important to consider the range of reactions to common stresses.

Approach #3: Welfare state strains and governmental legitimacy.   The two perspectives just outlined need not attack the fundamental purposes of major social welfare programs. The elimination of want, ignorance, squalor, disease, and idleness are aims that are compatible with either the view that remedial programs have grown too costly for economic health or the view that, with less means, more efficient ways to established ends are required. But a third perspective on the social policy strains of the 1970s and 1980s is in one sense more fundamental. It is the view that welfare state programs include some efforts that are wrong—public means that should not be employed even if funds are available or the effects on economic vitality are not worrisome. This is what I mean by criticisms of legitimacy.

WHAT ACTUALLY HAPPENED

The differing views just outlined charge in one way or another that the critical flaws of the welfare state programs and thus of the welfare state itself were not of a general dissatisfaction with the modern institutions of government. The assumptions rest on factual mistakes. Cross-national evidence from the 1970s—a time when government revenues were restrained by stagflation and the burdens on the welfare state increased—supports the notion that the major social spending programs remained quite broadly popular. In the United States the major programs—pensions, medical care, and education—never lacked public or political support. Both public opinion polls and the public reaction to attempted cutbacks by the Reagan administration testify to the popularity of these programs. The most vehement criticism of the welfare state has largely concentrated on its more fiscally trivial programs.

It is quite clear, however, that the future of the welfare state in countries with large, settled programs cannot possibly replicate the extraordinary growth in social spending that marks the postwar experience. It is equally clear that the slow growth of social spending in the 1970s and 1980s is due to the combination of slower economic growth and the overwhelming fact that large, mature programs simply cannot continue to grow rapidly without imposing steadily increasing opportunity costs. Further sharp increases in already-large government programs would, for instance, impose additional tax burdens on those already at the bottom of the income distribution. The defensible argument for selectivity in program-growth and spending arises therefore not from ideological rejection of their earlier purpose but from the reality that these very large, settled programs in pension, health care, and education reduce the margins for continued growth in the future.

Klein and O'Higgins use the most recently published OECD data (1985) on social expenditure trends from 1960 to 1981 to analyze the overall patterns as well as the the country-by-country and program-by-program variations. Their analysis yields a number of significant conclusions. First, from 1975 to 1981, all the OECD countries reduced the rate of increase in social spending, but none actually reduced real total social expenditures. They all exhibited the capacity to steer their welfare states to hold down spending increases in response to the adverse economic environment. Second, the reactions of different countries varied both in the extent to which they reduced spending growth and in the priorities accorded different spending programs.

AMERICA'S DISTINCTIVE RESPONSE

By the mid-1970s, the United States had moved considerably from its postwar position as the laggard in the scope and financing of social welfare programs toward being a mature welfare state, with a large, fully indexed (after 1972) pension scheme. Our governmental health insurance for the poor and the elderly, although not on the universal scale of other countries, had expanded considerably and contributed to that growth. We had an apparatus of social welfare programs that covered a wide range, and the key spending components — old-age pensions and medical care — were inflating just as in the rest of the world. The predictable result was fiscal stress as stagflation increased program outlays and as lowered economic growth reduced governmental revenues. This much was common across the world of industrial democracies. Where the United States differed was in the more limited degree of acceptance of the welfare state's purposes and clarity about its aims. The growth of the early 1970s had largely come from unexpected inflation and pension indexation, not from a fundamental reexamination of purpose. The result was that the maturing American welfare state had fewer means to cushion the strains macroeconomic developments brought. It was all too easy to confuse economic problems facing the welfare state with problems within the programs of the American welfare state.

The reasons for this mismatch between scale of effort and national understanding have much to do with the structure of American politics and the nature of its typical policy developments. The fragmentation of American politics puts an enormous premium on consensus, on gaining agreement so that the multiple veto points of the polity can be avoided. But agreement on the existence of a problem is far easier to secure than agreement on an appropriate policy response. The result is that American politics moves by fits and starts, with long periods of gestation and sudden bursts of political action when issue majorities are assembled. This also means that as long as the question is whether sufficient support exists for taking action, the political incentives direct reformers to concentrate on problem symptoms and the broad legitimacy of desirable remedies.

So it was that in the long battle over Medicare contending parties debated endlessly whether the medical troubles of America's aged warranted anything like a social insurance response. The debate between 1950 and 1965 centered less on the programmatic details of Medicare proposals than on whether the circumstances and claims of the aged warranted a central government as opposed to a private or a state remedy. The very name of the program — Medicare — misdescribed the limited hospitalization proposals that in fact constituted the legislative agenda in the late 1950s and early 1960s. What the public expected was much broader than what the Medicare legislative battle addressed. And when a broad Medicare program unexpectedly emerged from the bargaining of 1965, there was little public agreement about the program's purposes and the cost-control implications of the program's design. Likewise, the indexation of Social Security in 1972 — the result of congressional bargaining in an election year — produced long-run increases in Social Security payments without a glimmer of broad review.

Programmatic innovation thus proceeded without purposive clarity or agreement on strategies of implementation. The Vietnam War meant that expenditures for "guns" accompanied increases in the "butter" programs of the welfare state. The result was predictable, if lamentable. The United States faced the stagflation strains of the mid-1970s with the worst of all combinations: a large, rapidly growing system of social programs and a very incomplete comprehension of where we were coming from and what we were hoping to accomplish.

IMPLICATIONS FOR MEDICAL CARE

The concern of this paper is whether the cross-national evidence and the general policy directions illuminate current American medical policy trends as well as the policy directions not taken. What, in short, are the straightforward implications for medical care of the argument about welfare state developments introduced at the outset of this paper?

That argument, simply put, is that the broader politics of America's reaction to stagflation (and later the budget deficit) have dominated American health policy in the past fifteen years. For those who concentrate on disputes within the medical polity, attention has centered on the regulatory disappointments of the HMOs, the emergence of cost containment as a preoccupation (even obsession), and the much-noted disputes over the relative merits of regulatory versus so-called competitive strategies in reforming an expensive, troubled American medical world. These phenomena, undeniable at the surface of discussion, constitute for those purposes the consequences as much as the causes of American health developments.

Macroeconomic events—the inflation of the Vietnam years and the stagflation that worsened after the 1973–74 oil crisis—set the direction of social policy response but did not determine the particular shape. The economy required restraint; that restraint was achieved differently and to varying degrees in the welfare state economies of the OECD. The American political response to the economic strains was one of a widespread sense of crisis in social policy—the "overreaction" to which Klein and O'Higgins refer. The definition of the problem as one of crisis meant that as the low growth of the economy reduced revenues and the tax cuts of 1981 coupled with the arms buildup of the Carter-Reagan years produced very large deficits, new initiatives like national health insurance would become increasingly unthinkable. Deficits, a large defense budget, and the political unwillingness to raise taxes have put medical care policy in a paralytic vise. Only policy proposals that promise reductions in federal expenditure—like the heralded DRG innovation in Medicare hospital reimbursement (1983)—are on the agenda of active discussion. Otherwise social policy energy has concentrated on protecting current programs from further budget cutbacks. And the Gramm-Rudman-Hollings Act of 1985 has institutionalized the politics of constraint, making large-scale programmatic innovation practically unthinkable.

The crisis formulation of the 1970s put medical care on the defensive; the deficit politics of the 1980s have boxed discussion still more tightly. The United States is, by international comparison, well known as a big spender for medical care. The nearly 11 percent of GNP that is expended for medical care results from widespread third-party payments, public and private. This fragmented and expensive system leaves sizable proportions of the society under- or uninsured. Access problems are bound to worsen as state health programs, federal programs, and private employers compete to shift costs to other parties, driving as hard a bargain as they can with beleaguered providers and insurers. Within the federal Medicare program, the debate hovers between those intent on increasing the out-of-pocket expenses and those who favor stricter limits on what medical providers can charge. It is rare to find serious discussion of recasting the program as a whole so as to extract a better bargain for the $70 billion level of expenditures.

I have characterized the welfare state debate in the United States as the triumph of rhetoric over reality. For the world of medical care, that triumph was evident in two of the most common disputes of the past decade: regulation versus competition and the related cost-control debate. In both instances, the broader reaction to the welfare state's troubles conditioned the struggle within medicine.

The competition/regulation dichotomy makes little analytical sense. There is no form of competition that does not rest on rules that enforce price competition as the central way in which suppliers gain customers. Equally, there is no form of state regulation that obliterates competition among providers for customers, advance, favor, and honor. The dispute over competition and regulation is in fact over what form of competitive regulation is desirable and what its consequences would be for equity of access, fairness of finance, and quality of care. In developing this rhetorical dichotomy, American political discourse sets itself apart from the rest of the OECD world. But that divergence in turn resulted from the peculiar American interpretation of the welfare state strains of the stagflation era a crisis requiring retrenchment and precluding creative or flexible use of resources to meet changing needs.

The American form of cost-control disputes is equally distinctive. It is widely believed that governmental insurance triggered medical care inflation in the 1960s and that only the rigors of competition will restrain this failing industry. Again the broader context of cross-national findings makes one skeptical of the claim. In the rest of the OECD world, medical expenditures were the subject of considerable tinkering and restraint, but nowhere was there a major transformation of the postwar models of universal health coverage under public auspices. In these regions, increased expenditures in public medical programs are of great concern. And since the public programs are near-monopsonistic purchasers of care, the decision to reduce services affects all citizens directly. In the American case, the central state is but one payer (or purchaser). In recent years, it has become a participant in the scramble to spread the inflated costs of medical care to other budgets. In Medicare, for example, the cost-control effort is directed at reducing general deficits, permitting costs to spill onto other actors whether they are the elderly, the providers, or other payers.

The turbulent world of medical care in the 1980s is, in my view, not the product of forces internal to medicine. Having come late to the welfare state's expansion, and having done so in the context of economic abundance and ideological hesitancy, the American polity was exceedingly ill prepared for the strains of the 1970s. In the 1980s we have been living with the debris.

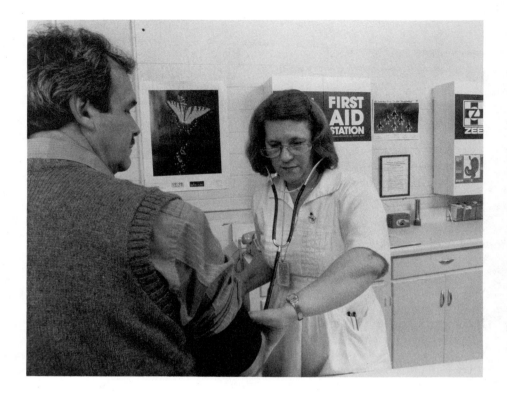

4

The Critical Role
of Nurses

N URSES OUTNUMBER DOCTORS, dentists, and every other single group of health professionals in the United States. They are responsible for a major proportion of patient care, and the issues that surround this profession have important implications for every health care delivery setting in the nation and for national health policy as well. In the past decade, nursing has undergone a major transition. Some call it a revolution. Enormous changes in modes of patient care have brought the nurse into direct application of complex health care technologies. Nursing responsibilities have also been affected by policy changes in the hospital setting that have led to a greater proportion of acutely and severely ill patients and of surgical patients in the hospital. The aging of the population, with a greater need for long-term care has also affected nursing. New nurse specialists have developed; primary among them is the nurse practitioner, who has obtained advanced clinical training for treating patients with common health problems in ambulatory settings. Other areas of expanded opportunities and responsibilities for nurses include long-term care nursing, nursing anesthesiology, and nurse midwifery. While some of these changes mean increased emotional and physical demands on nurses, they have also opened new doors.

Despite many positive developments, there is a darker side to current trends. Nurses' salaries have not kept pace with the increased skills required nor the added responsibilities. Also, working conditions are some of the most stressful anywhere, with long inconvenient hours, inflexibility of schedules,

and inadequate support staff. Nurses continue to experience a lack of autonomy, with many key decisions affecting their work made by doctors and
hospital administrators. Nurses have responded to these pressures in
different ways. Many are becoming active in the health policy arena, really
for the first time, and they are working to widen the scope of control over
work and career mobility.

A persistent problem related to the nursing work force is the issue of a
"nursing shortage." Despite the fact that there are more nurses today per
capita than ever before, the demand has risen steadily in relation to population.
There are two million registered nurses in the United States today; approximately 80 percent are employed at any one time. In 1987 there were about
20,100 nurse practitioners, 3,100 certified nurse midwives, and 23,000 nurse
anesthetists. Nurses salaries make up approximately one-third of a hospital's
expenses. Nursing schools, of which there are 1,451 in the nation, report
difficulty in attracting sufficient qualified applicants. Many nurses opt to leave
their profession for family reasons or because they want to seek higher paid
employment. Employers complain that the current pool of nurses is not
adequate for their needs, and the policy literature on the nursing profession
has continued to focus on this issue for the past 20 years.

In 1988, the Secretary of the Department of Health and Human Services,
Otis R. Bowen, released the Report of the Secretary's Commission on Nursing,
which was the result of a study undertaken to address issues related to the
nursing shortage. The executive summary of that report is presented here in its
entirety, which includes the commission's recommendations and conclusions.
In addition, the report suggests strategies for addressing the nursing shortage
as well as other problems in the profession.

In "The Nursing Shortage — Myth or Reality?" Linda Aiken and Connie
Mullinix examine the question of supply and demand, which the U.S. Department of Health and Human Services and the Institute of Medicine believe to
be in balance although statistics and the media indicate a severe shortage of
nurses. Since the number of vacant positions is up, there may be a change in
demand rather than a declining supply. On the down side, the number of hospital
beds and inpatient days are decreasing, and enrollment in nursing schools is
declining. The authors offer a perceptive analysis of the changing role of nurses
and recommendations for appropriate use of their special expertise.

Emphasizing the educational opportunities needed for nurses, Claire Fagin
details the effect on the profession of changes in health care delivery, both in
and out of hospitals in "The Visible Problems of an Invisible Profession."
Nursing practice is deeply affected by regulation and reimbursement policy as
well as by interprofessional tensions. She identifies the problems of image,
declining enrollment, and internal divisions as the chief issues that should be
addressed by the profession in order for nurses to take their rightful place in
the health care system.

U.S. Department of Health and Human Services

Secretary's Commission on Nursing, Executive Summary, Final Report

In late December 1987, in response to reports of widespread difficulties recruiting and retaining registered nurses (RNs), Health and Human Services' Secretary Otis R. Bowen, M.D., established the Secretary's Commission on Nursing. The charge given to this 25-member, public advisory panel was to: 1) advise the Secretary on problems related to the recruitment and retention of RNs; and 2) develop recommendations on how the public and private sectors can work together to address these problems and implement immediate and long-range solutions for enhancing the adequacy of the supply of RNs. The Commission was given the calendar year 1988 to accomplish these tasks.

The first five months of the Commission's tenure were devoted to an assessment of the magnitude, causes, consequences, and future implications of the nurse shortage. The results of this assessment were presented in the Commission's Interim Report, presented to the Secretary in July 1988. Based on this assessment, the Commission concluded:

- The reported shortage of RNs is real, widespread, and of significant magnitude. There is evidence to support the conclusion that the current shortage cuts across all health care delivery settings and all nursing practice areas. The shortage is most acute in urban hospitals, critical care and medical/surgical units, and nursing homes.
- The current shortage of RNs is primarily the result of an increase in demand as opposed to a contraction of supply. Although RN supply continues to grow, the number of new RN graduates has declined, and there are strong indications that RN supply has not kept pace with increased demand.
- The shortage of RNs is contributing to the deterioration of RNs' work environment and may also be having a negative impact on quality of patient care and access to health services.
- Projections for the future are not encouraging. In the short term, the quantity of care provided by the existing pool of RNs will be difficult to increase without significant intervention. In the long term, there is considerable evidence to suggest that the demand for RNs will continue to increase, and a continued imbalance with supply is anticipated.

Working from this assessment, the Commission then turned its attention to the task of developing action-oriented recommendations designed to alleviate the current shortage and assure a healthy nurse labor market in the future. Recommendation development was an iterative process that spanned five public meetings of the Commission and that led not only to the drafting of recommendations but also to the construction of a series of companion strategies designed to secure the successful implementation of each recommendation. The results of these long and thoughtful deliberations form the heart of this Final Report.

The Commission advances 16 specific recommendations and 81 directed strategies to achieve them. These are presented in groups, as they address the following issues:

- utilization of nursing resources:
- nurse compensation;
- health care financing;
- nurse decision making;
- development of nursing resources; and
- maintenance of nursing resources.

The specific recommendations are listed below, along with a brief statement explaining the rationale which supports each set of recommendations. Section 3 of this report contains all of the recommendations, more detailed rationales, and specific implementation strategies. These strategies provide guidance regarding the Commission's assessment of viable actions that can be undertaken to realize the objectives stated in the recommendations. Although not listed here in the Executive Summary, these implementation strategies are an integral component of the recommendation package and should be given careful consideration by all readers interested in the Commission's work.

UTILIZATION OF NURSING RESOURCES

As stated earlier, the Commission has concluded that the current nurse shortage is primarily the result of a rapidly increasing demand for RNs. Some of this increased demand for RNs is arising because health care delivery organizations are compensating for reductions in non-nursing staff—both clinical and non-clinical—as well as in other categories of nursing personnel. The four recommendations advanced in this area are intended to encourage nurse employers to use scarce RN resources in an efficient and effective manner, thereby enhancing the adequacy of the existing RN supply. These recommendations call for the provision of adequate support services for nurses, utilization of the most appropriate mix of nursing personnel, adoption of automated information and other labor-saving technologies in order to increase RNs' productivity, and improvement in the internal management of nurse resources within health care delivery organizations. The specific recommendations are as follows:

1. Health care delivery organizations should preserve the time of the nurse for the direct care of patients and families by providing adequate staffing levels for clinical and non-clinical support services.
2. Health care delivery organizations should adopt innovative nurse staffing patterns that recognize and appropriately utilize the different levels of education, competence and experience among registered nurses, as well as between registered nurses and other nursing personnel responsible to registered nurses, such as licensed practical nurses and ancillary nursing personnel.
3. The federal government should sponsor further research and encourage health care delivery organizations to develop and use automated information systems and other new labor-saving technologies as a means of better supporting nurses and other health professionals. Health care delivery organizations should work with researchers and manufacturers to ensure the applicability and cost-effectiveness of such information systems and technologies across all practice settings.
4. Health care delivery organizations, nursing associations, and government and private health insurers should collaborate to develop and implement methods for costing, budgeting, reporting and tracking nursing resource utilization, both to enhance the management of nursing services and to assess their economic contribution to their employing organization.

NURSE COMPENSATION

Evidence analyzed by the Commission indicates that nurse compensation is inadequate and that the severe wage compression over the span of a nurse's career is of particular concern. The Commission believes that inadequate compensation is one of the roots of the current nurse shortage. On the demand side, low RN compensation levels relative to those of other personnel for which RNs can substitute encourage employers' inappropriate utilization of RNs in carrying out non-RN functions. On the supply side, compensation levels lower than those of other professions requiring comparable educational preparation may encourage existing nurses to leave the profession, thus exacerbating the current shortage. In the longer-run, inadequate compensation is also likely to discourage potential nurses from entering the profession, contributing to a continuation of the shortage. The following compensation recommendation is advanced to address these concerns.

5. Health care delivery organizations should increase RN compensation and improve RN long-term career orientation by providing a one-time adjustment to increase RN relative wages targeted to geographic, institutional and career

differences. Additionally, they should pursue the development and implementation of innovative compensation options for nurses and expand pay ranges based on experience, performance, education and demonstrated leadership.

Health Care Financing

The Commission recognizes that many employers of nurses, especially those in the nursing home and home health sectors, may not have sufficient financial resources to support the compensation enhancement advocated in the preceding recommendation. Thus, the health care financing recommendation listed below and its accompanying implementation strategies given in Section 3 are put forth in the hopes of ensuring that the reimbursement levels and procedures do not constrain the efforts of efficiently organized health care delivery organizations to offer competitive compensation packages.

6. Government should reimburse at levels that are sufficient to allow efficiently organized health care delivery organizations to recruit and retain the number and mix of nurses necessary to provide adequate patient care.

NURSE DECISION MAKING

The Commission believes that failure on the part of health care delivery organizations, physicians, and health policy making bodies to fully recognize the decision making abilities of RNs has contributed to problems in recruiting and retaining nurses, hindered the development of a career orientation in professional nursing, and limited the efficiency and effectiveness of patient care delivery. With improved representation on policy-making, regulatory, and accreditation bodies, nurses can make unique, critical, and effective contributions to the health care delivery system. Furthermore, the technological, ethical, and managerial challenges facing health care delivery organizations dictate more collaboration among members of the health care team. The recommendations below address the active involvement of nurses in decision making at all levels.

7. Policy-making, regulatory, and accreditation bodies that have an impact on health care at the national, state, and local levels should foster greater representation and active participation of the nursing profession in their decision-making activities.
8. Employers of nurses should ensure active nurse participation in the governance, administration, and management of their organizations.
9. Employers of nurses, as well as the medical profession, should recognize the appropriate clinical decision making authority of nurses in relationship to other health care professionals, foster communication and collaboration

among the health care team, and ensure that the appropriate provider delivers the necessary care. Close cooperation and mutual respect between nursing and medicine is essential.

DEVELOPMENT OF NURSING RESOURCES

While nearly all evidence indicates that the current nurse shortage is demand-driven, the recent downturn in nursing school enrollments is cause for serious concern that the shortage will grow worse in the future. Additionally, the distribution of RNs across specialties and employment settings is currently problematic, and there is evidence that the formal education received by many new nurses leaves them inadequately prepared for the rigors of clinical practice in today's complex health care environment. Finally, the Commission believes that increased public awareness regarding the image of nursing can contribute to a reversal of recent enrollment trends. The recommendations contained within the development of nursing resources category are aimed at facilitating the education of nurses, and thereby increasing the supply of qualified RNs, through increased targeted financial support and improved program accessibility, updating the relevancy of nursing curricula, and promoting nursing as a career.

10. Financial assistance to undergraduate and graduate nursing students must be increased. The burden of providing this assistance should be equitably shared among the federal and state governments, employers of nurses, philanthropic and voluntary organizations. The preferred method of providing this support is the use of service-payback loans as well as scholarship funding for those in financial need.
11. State governments, nursing organizations, schools of nursing and employers of nurses should work together to minimize non-financial barriers to nursing education for individuals desiring to enter the profession as well as for nurses wishing to upgrade their education.
12. Schools of nursing, state boards of nursing, and employers of nurses should work together to ensure that the curricula are relevant to contemporary and future nursing practice, prepare nurses for employment in a variety of practice settings, and provide the foundation for continued professional development.
13. The nursing profession should take responsibility for providing immediate and sustained attention to the promotion of positive and accurate images of the profession and the work of nurses.

MAINTENANCE OF NURSING RESOURCES

Although certain in their assessment of the current status of the nurse labor market and confident that the recommendations put forth in this report embody the best approaches to resolving the current nurse shortage, the Commission believes that the federal government should spearhead a sustained effort devoted to: monitoring the nurse labor market; collecting improved data and conducting further research on the demand for nurses, as well as the supply and nursing practice; and following through on the implementation of the recommendations and strategies outlined in this report. The recommendations that follow are designed to accomplish these goals.

14. The Department of Health and Human Services should create a commission having a duration of at least five years that will monitor the implementation of the recommendations in this report as well as the development and maintenance of nursing resources. This commission should be constituted as an advisory body reporting directly to the Secretary.
15. The Department of Health and Human Services, private foundations, and employers of nurses should support and carry out research and demonstrations on the effects of nurse compensation, staffing patterns, decision-making authority, and career development on nurse supply and demand as well as health care cost and quality. Research should be sponsored on the relationship of health care financing and nursing practice.
16. The federal government should develop data sources needed to assess nursing resources as they relate to health planning and manpower.

The Commission does not view the development of these recommendations as the final step in addressing the nurse shortage. Rather, the more important and challenging task still lies ahead. The Commission strongly encourages the organizations addressed in this report to examine carefully the Commission's diagnosis of the problem, to assess honestly and carefully the relevance of each issue to their own particular organization, and to implement without hesitation the appropriate recommendations. The Commission recognizes that some of the identified problems transcend the interests of one particular organization and expects that, in these cases, the relevant institutions, organizations, associations, and individuals will make a good faith effort to collaborate in the implementation of the recommended solutions to the problem. It is the sincere belief of the Commission that the health of this nation will be at risk if the changes suggested in these recommendations do not occur.

In a recent study of hospitalized patients, those queried mentioned the following as nursing functions: taking doctors' orders, giving medications, serving meals, giving shots, and providing bedpans. The nurse's role has frequently been viewed as being analogous to that of the traditional wife and mother in a household.

J. L. MUYSKENS

Linda H. Aiken/Connie Flynt Mullinix

The Nurse Shortage: Myth or Reality?

The proportion of vacant positions for registered nurses in hospitals doubled between September 1985 and December 1986, reaching the levels of the last national nursing shortage of 1979. Current reports of vacancies are perplexing in the light of the size of the nation's supply of nurses. The output of nurses has doubled over the past 30 years, greatly exceeding the population growth, and licensed registered nurses now number 2.1 million. Between 1977 and 1984 alone, the number of employed nurses increased by 55 percent, as compared with an 8 percent growth in population. Intuitively, it would seem that an increased number of nurses would be the solution, but the problem persists nevertheless.

The reported shortage of hospital nurses exists in the midst of a substantial reduction in hospital inpatient capacity nationally. The demand for acute inpatient care in general hospitals has fallen, resulting in 50 million fewer inpatient days in 1986 than in 1981. Since 1983, hospitals have closed more than 40,000 beds, and average hospital occupancy rates dropped to 63.4 percent in 1986. Enrollments in nursing schools have also decreased markedly, raising the possibility that fewer nurses than anticipated will be available in the future.

There is now a contentious debate about whether a shortage of hospital nurses truly exists and about its causes. In 1981, the Institute of Medicine was commissioned by Congress to reconcile the evidence of an increased supply of nurses with continued reported shortages. The study concluded that the national supply of generalist nurses was adequate for the present and short-term future. Cyclical vacancies in positions for hospital nurses were attributed primarily to local labor-market conditions, although a shortage of nurses in certain specialties was noted. Recommendations were made to the hospital industry on the need to restructure nursing roles and develop improved financial rewards and opportunities for career advancement in clinical care. The National Commission on Nursing made remarkably similar recommendations in 1983. But in 1986, the American Hospital Association was again

Linda H. Aiken, R.N., Ph.D., is trustee professor of nursing and sociology and associate director of the Leonard Davis Institute of Health Economics, University of Pennsylvania, Philadelphia, Pennsylvania.

Connie Flynt Mullinix, R.N., M.P.H., M.B.A., is clinical assistant professor, School of Nursing, University of North Carolina, Chapel Hill, North Carolina.

reporting that high vacancy rates in positions for nurses were disrupting hospital care, whereas the U.S. Department of Health and Human Services again concluded that the national supply of nurses was in balance with the demand.

EMPLOYMENT PATTERNS OF NURSES

The shortage of nurses is measured by the hospital industry as vacant budgeted full-time-equivalent positions for registered nurses. Vacancy rates, however, are not an objective measure of the need for bedside nurses. Moreover, the number of budgeted positions for nurses reflects a number of factors, including budget constraints as well as local wage rates. Despite these limitations, we have chosen to analyze vacancy rates because they are used by the industry to reflect the changing supply of nurses.

There are several commonly held but erroneous beliefs about nurses' work patterns. One misconception is that nurses have left nursing in large numbers and are either inactive or working at jobs outside health care. In contrast, nurses have one of the highest rates of participation in the labor force among workers in predominantly female occupations. Almost 80 percent of registered nurses are actively employed either full-time or part-time, as compared with 54 percent of all American women. Not much is known about those who do not renew their licenses and, therefore, are not counted in the population of registered nurses. But less than 6 percent of registered nurses are employed in other occupations and are not seeking a position in nursing. Given the responsibilities of women for child rearing and other domestic concerns, an employment rate of 80 percent may be almost as high as can be expected. Thus, it is unlikely that unemployed nurses represent a large potential resource for hospital employment. However, nursing is somewhat unusual in that 27 percent of the total pool of registered nurses work part-time. Clearly, a change in the number of hours worked by more than 500,000 part-time registered nurses could substantially affect the supply of full-time-equivalent nurses.

Some observers have suggested that the shortage of nurses in hospitals may be due to the increased demand for nurses in ambulatory settings and new administrative positions in health care. However, hospitals' share of the ever-growing pool of nurses has not changed substantially since 1960. Sixty-eight percent of all employed nurses work in hospitals. Hospitals have dramatically increased the number of nurses they employ in the aggregate and in relation to numbers of patients, even when the recent increase in outpatient visits is taken into account. In fact, hospitals are employing more registered nurses than ever before and are even replacing non-nurses with nurses—just the opposite of what would be expected during an actual shortage of nurses.

In response to reduced numbers of inpatients, hospitals employed 133,376 fewer full-time-equivalent workers in 1986 than in 1983. In contrast, the number of full-time-equivalent nurses increased by 37,500 during the same period. A substantial increase in the ratio of nurses to patients resulted. In 1972, hospitals employed 30 nurses per 100 patients (average adjusted daily census); by 1986, the figure had increased to 91 nurses per 100—an 82 percent expansion (Fig. 1). Aides and licensed practical nurses were replaced by registered nurses. In 1968, registered nurses accounted for only 33 percent of hospitals' total nursing-service personnel; by 1986, registered nurses accounted for 58 percent.

THE CHANGING DEMAND FOR NURSES

The rapidity with which the current shortage developed suggests that increased vacancy rates must be due to a changing demand for nurses, not to a declining supply. There are three primary explanations for the recent increase in the demand for hospital nurses. First, hospitalized patients are sicker and require more care than in years past, on average, because of the reduction in discretionary admissions and the shorter average length of stay. However, there is no basis to suggest that the average condition of hospitalized patients changed dramatically enough between 1982 and 1986 to require a 26 percent increase in the ratio of registered nurses to patients. Although the changing case mix may provide a partial explanation for the increased demand for nurses, it cannot be the only explanation.

A second explanation for the recent increase in vacancy rates is related to changing budget constraints in hospitals. When vacancy rates were at an all-time low of 3.7 percent in 1984, the Medicare Prospective Payment System

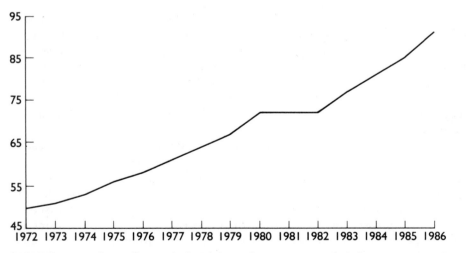

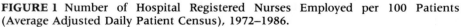

FIGURE 1 Number of Hospital Registered Nurses Employed per 100 Patients (Average Adjusted Daily Patient Census), 1972–1986.

was just being implemented and fears of severe hospital-budget limits were widespread. As a result, some budgeted positions were eliminated. Unexpectedly high operating margins, however, provided the opportunity for hospitals to budget for more nursing positions.

A third explanation is related to changes in nurses' relative wages. In most labor shortages, wages are adjusted and other incentives are developed to attract additional workers. These market adjustments fail to occur in nursing with the rapidity or magnitude seen in other labor markets. Labor economists have described nursing as a "captured" labor market. In any given community, a small number of hospitals employ most of the local nurses—a phenomenon known as oligopsony in labor economics. Employers offering nurses jobs with weekday hours usually have no trouble employing nurses and thus do not compete with other employers on the basis of salary. There is no demand for nurses outside the health care field that is sufficient to create competitive pressures on the hospital industry, as there is, for example, for computer programmers. Moreover, hospital administrators tend to assume that there is a finite number of nurses in any given community, and that wage competition among hospitals will be costly and will not resolve community shortages. The majority of nurses, if they want to work, must accept the terms offered by hospitals.

Registered nurses are versatile employees in a hospital context. They can provide all the services for which hospitals sometimes employ nurses' aides and licensed practical nurses, and they can also often perform a wide range of other functions, including those assigned at other times to secretarial and clerical personnel, laboratory technicians, pharmacists, physical therapists, and social workers. Nurses substitute for physicians under some circumstances, and commonly assume hospital management roles after regular work hours. Thus, when nurses' relative wages are low as compared with other workers', it is advantageous for hospitals to employ them in greater numbers and in lieu of other kinds of workers. Even if nurses' wages are 20 to 30 percent higher than those of licensed practical nurses or secretaries, it may still be more economical to hire nurses, because they require little supervision and can assume responsibility for a wide range of duties. The increased demand for nurses created by low relative wages can lead to shortages in some geographic locations, in specialty units, and on undesirable evening, night, and weekend hours.

The relative-wage theory is supported by data spanning several decades (Fig. 2). From 1946 to 1966, for example, the increases in nurses' wages lagged behind those in comparable women's occupations. Nurses' wages over the period increased by 53 percent, whereas teachers' salaries increased by 100 percent and female professional and technical workers' salaries increased by 73 percent. In the early 1960s, more than one in five budgeted positions for nurses was vacant. There was great concern at the time that the increased demand for hospital care accompanying the introduction of Medicare and Medicaid would exacerbate the shortage of nurses. But these new programs

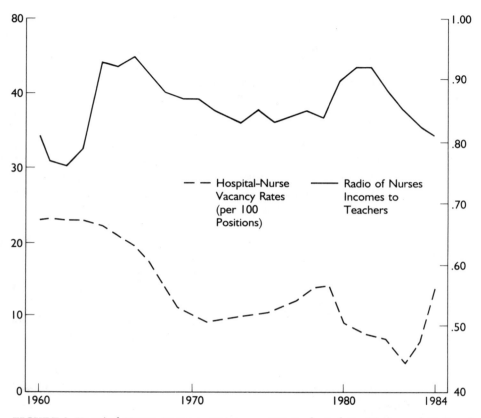

FIGURE 2 Hospital-Nurse Vacancy Rates per 100 Budgeted Positions and Ratio of Nurses' Incomes to Those of Teachers.

were accompanied by substantial wage increases for nurses. Employment rates among nurses increased substantially after these wage increases, as did enrollments in nursing schools. The proportion of vacant budgeted positions for nurses in hospitals dropped from 23 percent in 1961 to 9 percent by 1971. But, after hospital wage and price controls in 1971 and state rate setting and the voluntary hospital cost-containment effort a few years later, nurses' wages declined relative to other groups' and the proportion of vacant positions for nurses in hospitals increased again, leading to the shortage of 1979. There was a wage response to the 1979 shortage; nurses' wages rose an average of 13 percent annually in both 1980 and 1981. By 1984, the proportion of vacancies had reached a low of 3.7 percent.

The substantial wage increases received by nurses in 1980 and 1981 did not continue subsequently, and by the time the new Medicare prospective payment system was implemented, nurses' wages had been eroded. Hospital nurses have received only modest wage increases since 1982. By 1985, average salaries for teachers were 19 percent higher than those for nurses, and average salaries for all female professional and technical workers were 10 percent higher. Despite all the publicity about the shortage of hospital nurses, nurses' wages increased only 4 percent in 1986.

DECLINING NURSING SCHOOL ENROLLMENTS

Since 1983, enrollments in nursing schools have dropped by 20 percent. The number of new nurses graduating annually is predicted to fall from a high of 82,700 in 1985 to 68,700 or lower by 1995! All types of nursing programs have had declining enrollments; associate-degree programs have had a decline of 19 percent, and baccalaureate programs 12 percent. Enrollments in three-year hospital diploma programs have been declining for more than two decades and now account for only 14 percent of graduates annually (Fig. 3).

The country's demographic profile is partly responsible for declining enrollments because of the smaller size of 18-year-old cohorts in recent years. However, interest in nursing as a career has fallen precipitously among college freshmen in both community colleges and four-year institutions (Fig. 4).

There are many reasons for the declining interest in nursing. Whereas starting salaries of nurses are now comparable to those of other college graduates, the average maximum salary for nurses is only $7,000 higher than

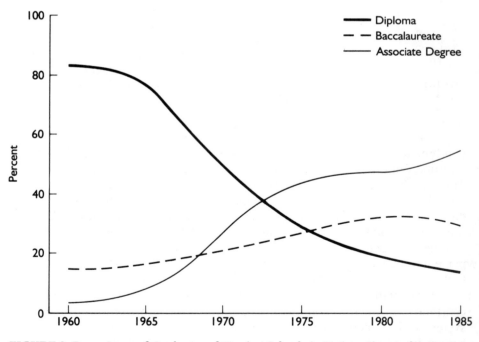

FIGURE 3 Percentages of Graduates of Nursing Schools in Various Types of Programs, 1960–1985.

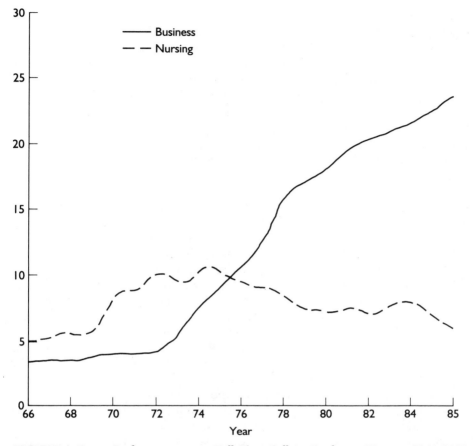

FIGURE 4 Career Preferences among Full-Time College Freshman Women, 1966–1985

the average starting salary. Since more women are choosing to work continuously in the labor force, the low raises discourage them from choosing a career
in nursing. Moreover, employers do not offer substantial differences in salary
in return for advanced education in nursing. Thus, the economic return on a
baccalaureate degree in nursing is poor as compared with the return in
alternative fields. Women today have many more career options than they had
in years past. Most other careers offer comparable or higher economic rewards and
do not require night and weekend work—a notable disadvantage of nursing.

RECOMMENDATIONS FOR CHANGE

A number of issues deserve careful reconsideration and experimentation. First,
public-policy makers must recognize that hospital rate setting can induce labor
shortages by artificially depressing wages in occupations like nursing, in

which hospitals are the dominant employers. In the short term, depressed wages will increase the demand for nurses, because they can substitute for other personnel, and result in acute spot shortages and high vacancy rates. Over the long term, recruitment to nursing will be seriously eroded by the absence of an adequate salary range that rewards skill and experience.

Second, one of the most unattractive aspects of nursing is the requirement of night and weekend work. With sicker patients, hospitals now need many more nurses on these unpopular shifts than they needed in the past, when it was not unusual to have a single nurse covering a unit at night. Most women want to work regular daytime hours and will even choose less interesting, less skilled, and worse-paying jobs to accomplish this. Preference for day work explains why vacancy rates are low in ambulatory care despite lower average salaries. Other industries that operate on a 24-hour basis offer substantial differences in wages for evening, night, and weekend work in order to attract sufficient voluntary staff coverage. Hospitals offer only small differences and try to make shift rotation a requirement of employment. Curiously, most of the innovations hospitals have adopted to reduce vacancies during unpopular shifts actually encourage nurses to work fewer hours. For example, some hospitals pay nurses a full-time salary to work two 12-hour weekend shifts (24 hours per week) but will not pay full-time nurses equivalent hourly rates for unpopular shifts. In view of all the expenses associated with continued high vacancy rates, increasing marginal wage rates to fill vacancies on unpopular assignments might not be as costly as is commonly assumed.

Third, the work requirements of nurses and other personnel in hospitals should be restructured. The ratio of support personnel to professionals is substantially lower in the hospital industry than in other industries. Given the complexities of operating busy hospital inpatient units, there is an astounding absence of secretaries, administrative assistants, and mid-level non-nurse managers. Moreover, the computerization of hospitals has lagged far behind that of other industries. Nurses are currently performing many nonclinical, administrative, and management functions in hospitals. Fewer better-paid and better-educated nurses in combination with an improved nonclinical support staff might yield better care without substantial increases in operating costs.

Fourth, hospital management should introduce incentives to encourage experienced nurses to remain in clinical care. A differentiated wage structure that recognizes experience and advanced education is critical. Employment benefits such as pensions, tuition support, and sabbaticals could be used much more effectively to develop "loyalty" and thus reduce costly staff turnover.

Fifth, physicians should take leadership roles in the development of more effective collaborative models of practice with nurses in hospitals. Much of the dissatisfaction of nurses with hospital practice is related to the absence of satisfying professional relationships with physicians. Many nurses choose administration over clinical practice in an effort to obtain greater status—in their interactions with physicians. More effective nurse-physician collaboration in clinical care activities would improve the professional satisfaction of both groups and contribute to improved patient outcomes as well.

CONCLUSIONS

The evidence suggests that under current market conditions in many local communities, the demand for nurses is greater than the supply. Regardless of the reasons for this imbalance, there is only a limited number of possible solutions. Expansion of nursing-school enrollments to increase the national supply of nurses might eventually solve the vacancy problem but is unlikely to occur, given demographic trends and the declining interest of young people in nursing careers. Recruiting inactive nurses into the work force is also not a promising solution because employment rates are already high among nurses and may have reached a ceiling. Expanding the number of nurses trained abroad is an expedient option but one that might create more problems, in terms of quality of care, than it would solve. The development of incentives to induce part-time nurses to work more hours is a promising option that should be pursued. Finally, if all the above methods to increase the supply of nurses still do not eliminate disruptive vacancies, restructuring hospitals to make more appropriate use of the special expertise of nurses is a difficult but obvious alternative.

None of these recommendations are new; they have been advocated consistently by every panel studying nursing shortages. Implementation, in contrast, has been slow, despite encouraging evidence from the few hospitals that are making the suggested changes. The fact is that nursing shortages are a consequence of complacent management and the reluctance of administrators to reexamine traditional practices. In the light of the attitudes of young women and their changing aspirations, what is now an artificially created shortage may become a critical problem in the future. Nurses are an essential resource for hospitals and the nation's health. Addressing their needs and aspirations realistically and examining their work conditions meaningfully are prerequisites for high-quality patient care now and in the future.

With a suddenness that surprised even long-time observers of cyclic shortages of nurses, the demand for registered nurses is outstripping the supply, and the factors that add up to this shortage suggest that there is no quick solution to the problem.

JOHN K. IGLEHART

Claire M. Fagin

The Visible Problems of an "Invisible" Profession: The Crisis and Challenge for Nursing

The opening article in the special fall 1986 issue of *Inquiry* discussed the large group of "disenfranchised citizens" lacking health insurance who are hidden from the public and for whom there is a lack of public and political outrage. How interesting that this simple phrase can also describe nurses and the paradoxical situation of the nursing profession in today's health care delivery system. That is, as patient needs become greater, requiring more and better-educated nurses, the invisibility of the nursing profession seems to increase in equal measure—until, of course, the specter of a "nursing shortage" looms, at which point all kinds of pundits, usually external to the profession, arise with instant and generally noxious solutions. Because we can expect a reenactment of this scenario shortly, now is the appropriate time to discuss the challenges and issues facing nursing and the health care field.

To do so requires some understanding of the present and of the way in which nursing has or has not met past challenges. The issues can be grouped in several ways, but no matter what the grouping, all must address the supply of nurses and the factors that influence supply, such as enrollment, entry-level requirements, and other educational issues; factors influencing demand, such as changes in health care delivery both in and out of hospitals; nursing practice and its regulation and reimbursement; and interprofessional factors.

THE SUPPLY OF NURSES

At this time the Department of Health and Human Services (DHHS) holds the view that the supply of nurses is in balance with demand as far as aggregate numbers are concerned. It admonishes the states, the private sector, and the health care industry to assume responsibility for assuring a continuing supply of entrants into the profession.

Claire M. Fagin, Ph.D., S.A.A.N., is professor and dean, School of Nursing, University of Pennsylvania, Philadelphia, Pennsylvania.

DHHS uses two models to forecast manpower needs: a historical model and a criterion-based model developed by a panel of experts. With regard to aggregate supply, both models project an oversupply of licensed practical nurses, who will face a growing shortage of jobs. The panel does, however, point to a shortage of nurses holding baccalaureate degrees (BSNs). The panel of experts differs from the historical model by taking into consideration such changes in the heath care delivery system as the recent reduction in hospital utilization and the increases in utilization of nursing homes and community health services.

Nursing homes and community settings require nurses who are prepared educationally for more independence in practice. The trend data show that by the year 2000 there will be roughly one-half as many BSN and higher-degree nurses, one and one-third times as many associate degree nurses, and one and one-half the LVNS/LPNS (licensed vocational nurses/licensed practical nurses) required to meet the conservatively estimated nursing personnel need. This represents a deficiency of 619,100 prepared at the baccalaureate and higher level; an excess of 296,900 prepared at the associate degree level; and an excess of 204,200 LVN/LPNs.

These conclusions are supported by the recent report of the American Hospital Association indicating that although full-time employment in hospitals has fallen, the employment of registered nurses increased significantly between 1981 and 1983 and was relatively stable between 1983 and 1984 (the latter period showing a .3% increase). Employment of LPNs fell 9.9% and ancillary nursing personnel declined 8.4% during that time. Hospital utilization declined sharply in 1984, and during 1985 more than 4,000 hospital employees lost their jobs. In the 1985 AHA survey, the number of physicians, dentists, and registered nurses increased, whereas there was an even larger drop in the number of LPNs working in hospitals.

The three-year National Commission on Nursing Implementation Project gives considerable weight to these data and their implications for the future. The project grew out of a study on nursing sponsored by the American Nurses Association, the American Hospital Association, and other national organizations. The governing body of the project represents nursing, medicine, hospitals, insurance, and consumers. The commission reviews data relating to projections of consumer needs, overall health care trends, and nursing supply and requirements for the years ahead. Its assumptions and conclusions in the first two areas are essentially the same as those of others and are familiar to all of us. Their predictions for nursing's immediate future, however, are perhaps less obvious:

- An increased number of nurses will be needed outside acute care organizations.
- Traditional settings will require a greater proportion of nurses with advanced preparation to manage the needs of clients.
- There will be an increased need for highly technically skilled nurses in acute care settings.

- Nurses will move with clients across settings.
- The nursing role will include managing and coordinating care, consulting with self-help groups, advocating, teaching and directing, and providing direct care and referral.
- The trend will continue toward higher levels of educational preparation.
- Organized nursing will seek practice changes and direct reimbursement through legislative action.
- There will be an organized effort to restrict the practice of nurses.
- There will be a shortage of baccalaureate degree nurses and an oversupply of associate degree nurses.
- Health care systems will increasingly secure nursing services by contracting with organized nursing services.
- Nursing costs and revenues will be explicitly identified in all health facilities.

There have been several articles in the lay and professional press decrying a nursing shortage of crisis proportions. In particular, hospitals appear to be experiencing a growing shortage of nurses educated and qualified to work in the extremely demanding areas of specialty practice such as critical care, intensive care, operating room, oncology, and other areas requiring extra experience and education.

All observers of the nursing marketplace know that there have been periodic nursing shortages since World War II. The most recent shortage ended in 1983 with the introduction of diagnosis related groups (DRGS) and the across-the-board staff cuts that subsequently occurred in some hospitals. Although the RN shortage rapidly became an RN oversupply in some areas, the rise in the acuteness of conditions of hospital patients, with the concomitant increase in critical care patients and the loss of reasonably healthy medical and surgical inpatients, appears to have laid the groundwork for another shortage.

There are close to 2 million registered nurses in the United States, and almost 80% of them are working in nursing. Of these working nurses, 66% are employed in hospitals. Thus, although there is a marked increase in opportunities for nurses in all types of health settings and related fields, the majority of nurses choose traditional hospital work for at least a part of their careers. That's the good news for hospital administrators and patients.

The bad news is that remarkably little progress has been made by hospital leaders to improve working conditions for nurses to ensure the future stability of their institutions and the care of the sickest segment of the health care marketplace. Numerous articles have been written dealing with compensation, autonomy, and various improvements in nurses' work environment, and I shall not discuss them here in detail. I will, however, elaborate on another problem that has widespread potential to adversely affect health care: the decrease in the number of highly qualified nursing students.

ENTRY-LEVEL REQUIREMENTS AND OTHER EDUCATIONAL ISSUES

Current information on the declining pool of young people choosing nursing as their future career is disquieting. During the early years of the women's movement, many of us, active feminists included, expressed concern about the possibility that this would happen during the 1970s. It did not then, but it now appears that many young women are acting out what Patricia Spack terms "women's new restrictions of opportunity," that is, are responding to pressure "to define themselves by participation in traditionally male professions, in the public rather than the private sphere."

The invisibility of nursing is integral to this dilemma. During the 1985 non-government sponsored World Forum for Women held in Kenya, speeches proclaimed the powerlessness of women in third world countries and the difficulty (if not impossibility) of finding women leaders. The speakers lamenting the lack of women leaders fell into the trap, described in the foregoing paragraph, that equates leadership potential with success in traditionally male professions.

I contend that the critical mass of women leaders in all countries, including those of the third world, can be found among women in traditional roles, including nurses in practice and education and in other health roles. It is interesting that the more than 3,000 nurse leaders who attended the convention of the International Council of Nurses held the same summer were virtually ignored at the Kenya meeting. Reports at this quadrennial meeting gave superb evidence of social reform and leadership in which all women could take pride and satisfaction. Yet the invisibility of the group in the media and at the Kenya forum must be viewed as symbolic of how the world, and the young people from whose ranks future nurses must come, view the profession.

During the early 1970s nursing, despite public derogation by leading feminist speakers, was showing a marked increase in popularity among a wide spectrum of college-educated and college-aspiring women and men. Students believed that the field offered opportunities for activists equal to or better than those achievable through the law and other professions. In this pre-yuppie generation the desire to help others was a primary legitimate motive for the socially minded young person.

Currently, however, nursing seems threatened by the new restrictions women are placing on themselves or are being influenced to place on themselves by society. Intelligent, achieving young women have often had a hard time selecting nursing as a career. Many have had to battle actively with families, guidance counselors, and teachers to matriculate at university schools of nursing. Yet enroll they did, and in my opinion the profession has the largest critical mass of women leaders in the world active in public life whose vantage point is that of a traditional profession which prides itself on skillfully using knowledge and compassion to care for sick people and to promote health.

The latest figures available from national testing services indicate a disastrous drop in interest in nursing among college-bound youngsters. Enrollment figures from hospital schools and associate degree programs show an even greater decline than do baccalaureate programs. The decline in associate degree and hospital-based programs should not be of concern, given the supply and need projections discussed earlier. The decline of applicant interest in baccalaureate nursing programs, however, presages a very dim picture indeed for the 1990s.

It might be hoped that "liberated" men would fill the breach. Although the opportunities for men (and, of course, women) in nursing are without bounds, there has not been an increase in men applicants to nursing programs. Men appear to be sticking with traditional, somewhat narrow career choices, just as many women appear to be limiting themselves to certain prestigious occupations in business and the professions traditionally held by men.

The narrowing of opportunity and choices for women and men should be of concern to all of us. Paradoxically, as the national pool of students interested in nursing has declined dramatically over the past five years, the opportunities for highly qualified applicants who do choose baccalaureate nursing programs have never been greater. If the downturn in student interest continues, we will see a nursing shortage of truly dangerous proportions in 10 years.

Are there solutions to this threat? Nursing has always suffered from short-term problems that have lent themselves to immediate solutions, which in turn have created long-term problems. Standards of education that have become norms in other fields have been recommended but never fully adopted by nursing educators and their institutional supporters. The proliferation and endurance of substandard nursing schools and programs created or maintained to address past nursing shortages are an example of a problem that contributes to the current dilemma. Discussions and pressures to maintain or even create new single-purpose training schools are occurring despite evidence that hospital schools are suffering an even greater decline in enrollment than other schools. This is no doubt largely because students and families view such schools as the norm for nursing but woefully outside of mainstream education.

Nursing must, once and for all, move its education programs squarely into the mainstream of higher education. This would require immediate planning for closure of all remaining hospital schools and for hospital participation in partnerships with colleges and universities to recruit and support students. Simultaneously, plans will have to be drafted to reduce prebaccalaureate programs and increase the number and strengths of college and university programs. These are steps the profession can and must take in collaboration with forward-looking members of other professions in the health and education arenas. Instead we are seeing too many fine schools closing or planning to close their baccalaureate programs for a variety of reasons, including "philosophical" and economic ones, enrollment problems, and difficulty maintaining faculty interest in teaching undergraduate students.

THE IMPACT ON THE NURSING PROFESSION OF CHANGES IN THE HEALTH CARE DELIVERY SYSTEM

Major changes in the health field have made the need for well-educated, caring nurses more urgent than at any time in the profession's history. High technology in and out of hospitals, the need for independent decision making, an appreciation of the financial ramifications of interventions in health care, and recognition of the special needs of an increasingly aged and chronically ill population all attest to this need.

In the early 1980s, Congress asked the Institute of Medicine (IOM) to study and report on future nursing supply and demand, especially with reference to such possibilities as the increased use of ambulatory care facilities and the enactment of legislation for national health insurance. The IOM's report, *Nursing and Nursing Education: Public Policy and Private Action,* was published in 1983.

The IOM made some estimates for 1990, believing that uncertainties in the future health care system would invalidate the projections for a longer-term period. The report indicated that by 1990, many more nurses would be needed to fill positions in administration and management of clinical services and health care institutions, in academic nursing, and in clinical specialty practices. It particularly highlighted the growing elderly population and the many services that nurses could provide to this population. It also focused on the need for graduate-level programs for geriatric nurse practitioners and other nurse practitioners, and urged that state laws limiting the autonomy of nurse practitioners and nurse-midwives be modified.

There is strong evidence that good nursing care has a positive effect on patient outcomes and that nursing services can contribute immeasurably to the goals of a competitive health care system. Because of this, some governmental and business officials strongly support the IOM's recommendations. The recent analyses of nurse practitioners (NPs) and other providers done by the Office of Technology Assessment indicate that NPs, physician assistants, and certified nurse-midwives (CNMs) provide care whose quality is equivalent to that of care provided by physicians and that NPs and CNMs are more adept than physicians at providing services that depend on communication with patients and preventive actions. The OTA report also recommends extending coverage for these workers and believes that in some settings this "could benefit the health status of . . . segments of the population currently not receiving appropriate care [and that among the] long-term effects could be a decrease in total costs."

Various legislative activities currently in motion could play a large part in altering the role of nurses in the 1990s. One important example is the bill introduced by Congressman Richard Gephardt in 1986 to establish community-based nursing organizations to provide Medicare Part B benefits on a prepaid, capitated basis to beneficiaries. This bill is likely to be enacted.

These organizations should be capable of demonstrating the cost effectiveness of direct nursing interventions in varied populations and under certain circumstances, such as the provision of preventive care. These organizations are expected to be structured like HMOs, with all care provided on a prepaid, capitated basis under the supervision of nurses, and with a major component of the care provided at home.

Although these "nursing HMOs" will care for multiple populations, they are expected to be particularly useful to the elderly by offering alternatives to nursing home care. Besides being of value to the community, they should enhance the image of nurses as direct providers of care who will receive direct payment for that care. The direct reimbursement of nurses is an important and sensitive issue—important because it increases the autonomy and attractiveness of the profession and sensitive because it can be a threat to physicians as well as payers. Nonetheless, Medicare, Medicaid, and other third-party payers often directly reimburse nurse practitioners, nurse-midwives, nurse-anesthetists, and psychiatric nurse therapists for their work with patients in a wide variety of specialty and generic roles.

Campaigns to persuade state legislatures to directly reimburse nurses can be expensive, since in almost all cases underfunded nursing organizations come up against well-funded, organized efforts of medical societies to prevent reimbursement changes. That nurses have been succeeding tells us as much about the way medicine is perceived currently as it does about recognition by legislators of the capability and potential of nurses.

In recent years there has been tremendous growth in opportunities for the direct and indirect involvement of nurses in nontraditional delivery systems. The number of nurses involved in entrepreneurial ventures continues to grow and is now of sufficient size for them to have formed a national interest group (the American Nurses Entrepreneurial Coalition). Opportunities for employment in managed care organizations, insurance companies, accounting companies, and myriad other organizations doing business in the health field have been described in newspapers and business journals. I believe we can expect continued growth in the number of nurses employed in nontraditional roles. Indeed, a recent article expressed concern that competition for nurses by these organizations will make hospital employment unattractive for nurses.

Accordingly, I suggest that hospitals recognize two facts. First, hospitals must learn to compete for nurses the way other organizations recruit and retain important workers. Second, because hospitals are the major employers of nurses and are the setting where nurses can make the most of their cost advantage, hospitals and the nursing profession should work together to find acceptable cost-accounting systems to track nursing productivity and manage cost and revenue directly. Currently there are efforts to create systems to document interventions and costs to provide data to third-party reimbursers of nursing care in any setting.

It has been predicted by one government official that hospitals in the 21st century will be huge intensive care units. In this connection, Knaus et al. studied treatment and outcome in 5,030 patients in intensive care units at 13 tertiary care hospitals. All hospitals had similar technical capabilities in their units but differed in organization, staffing, commitment to teaching, research and education. The authors examined whether these substantial differences in the structure and process of intensive care influenced effectiveness of care, as measured by hospital mortality rates. The hospital with the highest rank (69 deaths predicted, but 41 observed) had superior interactions between nurses and physicians and coordination of the intensive care unit staff. This hospital also had the most comprehensive support system. The clinical specialists with master's degrees and extensive experience in intensive care units had as their primary responsibilities the orientation and development of the nursing staff. This hospital "was the only institution which had a routine policy to cancel major elective surgery if adequate unit nursing staff were not available—a decision that could be made by the unit nurse in charge."

CHANGES IN EDUCATION

Master's-prepared nurse specialists are the pivotal professionals in these highly sophisticated clinical arenas. They work directly with clients and families with complex problems, but they also teach students and staff nurses, support and consult with primary nurses, and manage patient units.

In 1980, 5% of registered nurses had a master's degree. According to the IOM report, master's-prepared nurses are a scarce national resource. It can be expected that at least 10% of nurses will hold a master's degree in the early 21st century. Based on expected needs, the emphases in master's programs will continue to be on specialty clinical practice, with gerontology and community health nursing receiving considerable attention as specialties, and with courses in management and finance essential in all programs.

By the 1990s the rapidly moving trend linking university faculty and clinicians will be seen in one or another model throughout the U.S. nursing sector. There will also be flexible partnerships in nursing homes and community agencies. These models will surely increase nursing's visibility, improve interprofessional relationships, and alter nursing education. Indeed, these changes will pose significant challenges to curriculum developers to create programs to prepare nurses, including those for nursing leaders who will be pivotal in the major partnership roles.

Because many of the changes are likely to require graduate education, nursing programs that award the baccalaureate degree should be the standard. Because the practitioner of nursing in and out of hospitals is expected to play both a more independent and a more interactive role with patients, families, and colleagues, nursing education must be built on a broad liberal arts, scientific, and clinical foundation on which to base nursing judgments. As in other fields, basic nursing education must serve as a pipeline to leadership. Fundamental management skills should be included in most baccalaureate curricula so that graduates will have the requisite knowledge and skills needed to meet the challenges of producing primary health care in all environments. Technological literacy, of course, will be expected of all nurses.

As with other disciplines, the doctoral degree will be required for career faculty appointments in all universities and most colleges in the 1990s. This is already the case in academic health centers and other leading health care institutions. Many positions in nursing practice leadership will also require (or prefer) nurses with doctoral degrees. Various groups, including the National Academy of Sciences, link the future of the nursing profession to the quality and quantity of doctorally prepared nurses capable of conducting sophisticated research on nursing issues.

INTERPROFESSIONAL TENSIONS

Although physician-authored articles on health care provision often fail to note the competition and potential conflict between nurses and physicians, it is the subject of many formal discussions and informal conversations. The outcome of these interprofessional conflicts is extremely difficult to predict because it will be affected by many variables, each of which needs to be examined.

We do know that during the 1990s the United States will have a substantial physician surplus. Competition among physicians, and between physicians and hospitals, will be intense as physicians invade institutional services and hospitals invade ambulatory care. There are likely to be concomitant losses in physician autonomy.

These tensions are bound to provoke questions in the nursing profession. Will physicians, in an effort to protect their income, move into nursing? Will organized medicine increase its opposition to nursing's development, autonomy, and access to reimbursement? My answer is, "Yes, but. . . ." On the negative side, it has been noted that nurses neither control their labor supply nor hold a monopoly over any set of socially significant, or even insignificant, roles. Thus, nursing roles can be manipulated both within and outside the profession—a dangerous condition.

On the positive side, several factors lead me to believe that nursing will emerge in the 21st century as a distinctive profession essential to an effective and affordable health care system. First, the public interest in cost, accessibility, and quality is likely to result in greater support of nursing. This is already evident in consumer pressure for access to nurse-midwives and in its expressed willingness to utilize nurse practitioners. Second, the future health care delivery scene will shift its major focus from cure to care, and this shift will call for the skills which have formed the bases for nursing as long as nursing has been described. Third, there is now a critical mass of nurse leaders in positions of influence. Fourth, the acknowledgment of women's rights facilitates nursing's claims for its legitimate roles. Fifth, because more women are making lifetime commitments to their careers, nurses are more likely to act cohesively in support of their individual and common professional interests than they were in the past when so many nurses worked only episodically. Sixth, the quest for independence on the part of nurses and control on the part of physicians will decline before the end of this century. Instead, an interdependent, collaborative mode could emerge to resolve the critical issues of health care. Seventh, by the year 2000, the majority of nurses will have at least the baccalaureate degree. Their mainstream orientation and better communication and management skills are likely to serve well the profession as a whole and the patients it cares for.

The combination of physician oversupply and nursing shortage may put another cast on interprofessional issues. To extrapolate from the present situation, let us imagine that current nursing shortages will continue. If applicant pools diminish in both quality and quantity, will surplus physicians move into the nursing sphere? We are already hearing about physicians applying for management positions in nursing and of residents being asked to provide some services for which nurses have traditionally been responsible. The trend may continue to a point where physicians will assume mid- and upper-level positions in the nursing profession, particularly in positions of practice and administration.

We can also expect to see various other groups seeking these positions, including health administrators, persons with degrees in health policy, and other health professionals prepared in either generalized or specialized programs. Nursing has always tolerated a certain amount of incursion into its territory, but the tolerance level may decrease if nonnursing professionals preempt a critical mass of nursing positions, especially those at the higher levels.

SUMMARY AND CONCLUSIONS

In examining the future challenges and issues facing nursing in the coming years, I have discussed the supply of nurses, factors that influence supply and demand, and interprofessional tensions. Nursing is confronting problems of image, declining enrollment, and continued internal divisions. At the same time, the need and opportunities for nurses are growing with changes in health care practice, developing health care technology, and burgeoning health-related industries.

It is becoming clear that we are headed for a period of severe nursing shortage — the kind that leads to declining levels of quality care. Yet we are not seeing the creation of new strategies or even the implementation of previous recommendations for change which would mitigate current problems and prevent future ones.

Improving nursing's image to attract new entrants cannot be divorced from the realities of the confused education system and the work place. Nurses, with the crucial help of others in the health care industry, must address these problems now so that we keep our best people in the fulltime work force and attract the brightest young people to this caring profession.

Projections for our future health care system suggest enormous reliance on the skills and training of highly qualified nurses. Care delivered in the hospital setting to increasingly severely ill patients, as well as that delivered at home and other ambulatory settings, where some of the emphasis is likely to be on prevention and rehabilitation, will require nurses to have the greatest skills, knowledge, and intelligence as they deal with the increasingly complex health care system. The fit of nursing's abilities with the course of events most of us anticipate should, given appropriate strategic change, lead to the maturing of the profession and entry into the 21st century with strengthened skills, an accurate and positive image, and an assured future.

Nurses are by far the largest group of health care professionals. . . They are often the professionals with whom patients have the most sustained contact. And because of the profession's perceived tradition of holism and "care more than cure," nursing is often upheld as a hopeful paradigm for the future.

But the paradigm is changing.

GERALD R. WINSLOW

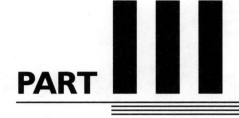

PART **III**

Critical Issues
for the 1990s

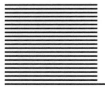

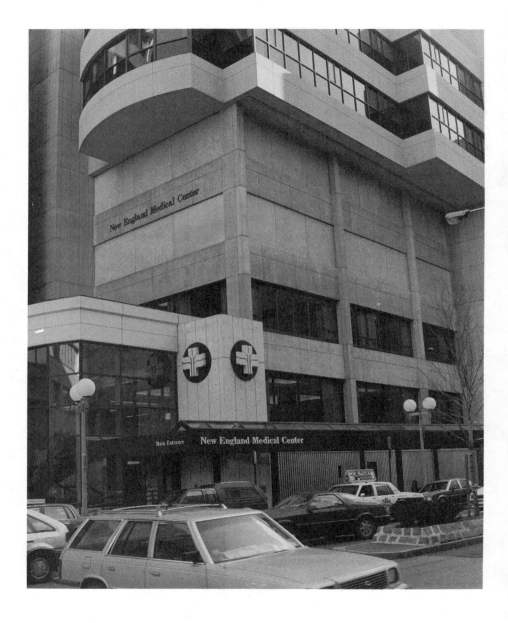
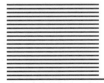

5

The Rising Costs
of Health Care

I SSUES RELATING to medical care costs are raised in each section of this book. They underlie all aspects of the health care system, and they influence all policy questions. It is not unreasonable for us to ask, "Why is it that the U.S. spends three times as much per person for health care as many other Western nations with little or nothing to show for this extra expense?"

There are three fundamental forces behind the tremendous upward spiral of health care expenditures: rising prices per unit of service, an increasing volume of services per capita, and growth in the population, particularly the growing number of elderly. The most obvious causes are related to inflation, including inflation in the price of medical services above the consumer price index; improved and costly techniques and technologies; an increase in the practice of defensive medicine by physicians to avoid malpractice suits; a greater number of people who use the services, which is partly a function of the nation's aging population; and the structure of the system itself, particularly the way we pay doctors and hospitals.

Medical care costs increased by over 51 percent between 1984 and 1989, nearly three times the period's rate of inflation. Health care expenses in 1988 were $541 billion, or more than 11 percent of the gross national product, compared to 8 percent in 1975 and 6 percent in 1965, when costs were over 500 percent lower for health services. At the same time, the percentage of health care costs paid by the government and by private insurance companies increased considerably. In 1987, Medicare, Medicaid and other government programs accounted for 41 percent of medical costs; private insurance paid for

[203]

32 percent, predominantly with employer contributions, and the remainder was paid by individuals out-of-pocket.

The results of these recent increases have been dramatic. The government has begun to tighten the health benefits covered by Medicare and Medicaid through hospital and physician payment reforms, and employers have developed strategies to reduce their costs by providing incentives for workers to contain their use of medical services or to change the type of plan they utilize. Insurance companies have in some cases begun to require prior approval for hospital admissions and concurrent review of lengths of stay, and there is a clear trend among insurers to avoid coverage of patients who are very sick, and therefore the poorest risks. Employers also have undertaken a variety of new approaches to underwriting benefits, including cost sharing and financial incentives.

The health care market no longer reflects the traditional dichotomy between fee-for-service and prepaid care. Pure fee-for-service plans that included first dollar coverage have declined from 90 percent in 1984 to 28 percent in 1989, as monthly premiums, deductibles, and co-payments increased for most plans and as a variety of managed care plans entered the picture. Health maintenance organizations and preferred provider organizations, which offer care with selected hospitals and doctors for a fixed price, have vastly increased in popularity with employers. Also, new alternative delivery systems have developed that utilize different reimbursement models, including risk sharing, case management, utilization review, and premium pricing. In addition to the great variety of HMOs and PPOS, some alternative delivery systems on the medical marketplace today include state-licensed prepaid plans, competitive medical plans, exclusive provider plans, and primary care networks.

The system is fluctuating rapidly. Costs continue to rise. At the same time government and corporate payers are reconsidering what levels of health coverage they will provide and in what structures care will be available. Clearly, they would like to see individuals use greater measures of prevention and exercise restraint in their utilization of services. They would also like to see physicians and hospitals contribute to efforts toward cost containment at the same time that patients begin to shoulder a greater portion of the cost burden.

Because these measures were not undertaken voluntarily, the federal government instituted systems of its own that have had a drastic effect on the manner in which care is administered and have compromised physician autonomy and patient choice in a manner heretofore considered unacceptable. In 1983, Medicare, which insures 30 million elderly and disabled people, instituted a prospective payment system for hospitals that fixed payments for admissions based on diagnosis-related groups (DRGs), to slow the rate of increase in hospital costs through decreasing admissions and lengths of stay. In 1984, Medicare applied a fee freeze for physicians' charges, and a number of other measures have been instituted since then to reduce the federal government's liability for the costs of health services, including a surcharge for specified benefits.

Those who pay medical care bills, principally the federal and state governments, insurance companies, and corporate employers, continue to seek reductions in their expenditures for health services or at least slow the rapid rate of increase in those expenditures. Although the government has been the leader in the move toward cost containment, private industry has also begun to play a major role, as providing employee health care coverage has become a major expense that cuts into profits. The target of the government's cost containment efforts have largely been the elderly and the poor, beneficiaries of Medicare and Medicaid; while private industry has taken aim at employed middle-income recipients. In both cases, people are discovering that their access to health care services has been altered, and through constraints imposed by payers, they feel the pressure to conform to new cost containment measures.

Cost containment strategies include a wide range of activities, some of which have already been employed by the government such as preadmission screening for hospital admission, placing a ceiling on hospital and physician charges, reducing waste in such areas as laboratory tests and unnecessary hospital admissions, raising the amount of out-of-pocket payment required, deductibles, co-payments, regionalization and centralization of selected major services, setting payments according to diagnostic categories, and decreasing the availability of health care services, especially to those who receive government coverage and those who have no coverage. Other measures are designed to get either the recipient or the provider to voluntarily submit to cost containment through such means as stressing behaviors to reduce the risk of disease. In some cases the approach has been to stimulate competitive markets and price competition, in others it has been through increased regulation of providers. The results of such measures thus far include a vast increase in the gap between the kind of services available to the poor and the rest of the population and a rise in dissatisfaction and even alarm among members of the middle class over the financial costs and quality of services available to them. The government has also threatened to tax both health insurance contributions and health insurance benefits.

The quality of the system that will grow out of these measures is uncertain. It is possible that the end result will be a hierarchical system in which health care will be available to people according to their ability to pay for coverage or services and thus the poor and the unemployed will receive minimal care, and they will sometimes find essential care unavailable; another small group will receive optimal care, and a large middle group will receive medium-level care unless they are willing to pay for expensive services that are not covered by most health insurance plans. This would be far from the kind of equitable, high-quality system that most Americans desire, and it would call on physicians to alter drastically their current practice philosophy.

This chapter includes an outline of patterns of spending for health services during 1986 and forecasts for spending through the year 2000 drawn up by the Division of National Cost Estimates, Office of the Actuary, Health Care Financing Administration. The authors underscore some deviations from historical trends, and they discuss the effects of the population's demographic composition on spending for health, taking the view that spending will increase in future years as a result of the evolution of that composition. They project that national health expenditures will leap from $458 billion in 1986 to $1.5 trillion by the year 2000—15 percent of the GNP.

The second article in this chapter on health care costs describes the 1988 Annual Report to Congress of the Physician Payment Review Commission. The commission, created by Congress in 1985 to look at methods of paying physicians for services provided to Medicare beneficiaries, conducts analyses and provides advice to Congress and the administration on physician payment issues, and it makes recommendations for policy reforms. In the following article, Philip R. Lee and colleagues on the commission staff present an overview of the commission's 1989 report to Congress.

In "A Hard Look at Cost Containment," Eli Ginzberg assesses the results of two decades of cost containment efforts and draws on the lessons we can learn from them to predict the future. He does not expect Americans to give up their attachment to quality health care services either for the large middle class or for the unemployed and poor. Instead he predicts that health care expenditures will continue to rise, and those who are struggling to contain costs will continue to seek new answers until we reach the upper limits of toleration on the proportion of the GNP we are willing to invest in health care.

Health economist Victor R. Fuchs in "Has Cost Containment Gone Too Far?" outlines a framework for looking at direct effects of three methods utilized in cost containment policies: (1) increasing production efficiency, (2) reducing prices, and (3) delivering fewer services. He differentiates between techniques that rely on physicians to contain costs and those that rely on patients, and he focuses on the effects of changes in the quantity of services.

Division of National Cost Estimates, Office of the
Actuary, Health Care Financing Administration,
Department of Health and Human Services

National Health Expenditures,
1986–2000

NATIONAL HEALTH EXPENDITURES IN 1986

Nationwide in 1986, a total of $458 billion was spent for health, an amount
equal to 10.9 percent of the gross national product (GNP). The growth of that
spending accelerated slightly in 1986 to a rate of 8.4 percent, following an 8.1
percent increase in 1985. Most of the acceleration is accounted for by higher
price inflation.

Spending for health rose more rapidly between 1985 and 1986 than did the
GNP, so that spending as a share of the GNP rose from 10.6 to 10.9 percent.
This increase is attributable less to acceleration of health spending than it is
to a sluggish performance by the economy as a whole. The 8.4 percent growth
in national health expenditures from 1985 to 1986 was the second lowest in
over two decades, but so was the 5.2 percent growth in nominal GNP.

Spending for health in the United States during 1986 amounted to an
allocation of resources equal to $1,837 per person. Roughly 60 percent of those
funds were channeled through private hands, either patients themselves or
private health insurers. The remaining 40 percent was channeled through
Federal, State, or local governments, mainly through the Medicare and Medicaid programs.

INDUSTRY SUMMARY

Before examining expenditure patterns, it may be useful to consider some of
the trends evinced by the health industry itself. These trends demonstrate
some interesting aspects of the demand for health care and shed some light on
patterns within the industry.

In terms of employment, the health services industry is still recovering from
a short-term dip in economy share. The trend in the private health services
industry share of total employment is quite pronounced: that share nearly
doubled from 1965 to 1983. However, the growing effects of cost containment
(including a large degree of uncertainty) served to depress employment growth
after 1983. Coupled with substantial industrial growth elsewhere in the economy in 1984, this produced a slight dip in the health industry share of total
nonfarm employment. There is reason to expect that that share will resume its
rise, but perhaps at a lower rate than has been seen historically. The growth of

hours worked and of payroll in the private health sector has followed a pattern similar to that of employment. Generally speaking, both have outpaced their economy-wide counterparts, frequently by substantial amounts. On the other hand, recent years have seen a different pattern. Following nearly identical growth rates in 1983, the total private nonfarm economy handily outperformed the health industry in 1984. Again in 1985, the two groups performed very similarly, and only in 1986 did the health industry re-emerge with faster growth. The effects of cost containment seem to have reduced the annual rate of growth, but it is too early to tell whether that shift is a shortrun or a longrun phenomenon.

Within the health industry, however, one very clear longrun trend is the increasing importance of providers outside of hospitals. In 1976, hospital employment (including government hospitals) accounted for almost two-thirds of all health service employment; a decade later, that share had fallen to 55 percent. There can be no doubt that cost containment has played a role in this trend. The rate of decline increased markedly after 1982, coincident with the beginning of the drop in hospital admissions.

The trends in health services employment, hours, and earnings are consistent with our understanding of the U.S. economy. Health care is principally a service, and service industries tend to grow more rapidly than do manufacturing or agriculture as an economy reaches the level of maturity currently evinced in the United States. Most of this growth stems from the longrun income elasticity of demand for services in general (and for health care in particular). Also, third-party financing obscured the true price of health care, leading consumers to use more of it than they otherwise would have done. In addition, health care increasingly had come to be treated not as just another commodity in the consumer's market basket, but rather as a socially ensured right of existence. Consequently, the market demand for health care took a life of its own, independent of price and income pressures. It was not until the early to mid-1980's that private industry, followed by government, began to challenge the social perception of health care as a right rather than as a part of a total consumption market basket. The ensuing interactions among consumers, providers, and financiers have modified the long-term trends in growth, at least for the short run.

Price inflation is another area in which the health industry differs from other parts of the U.S. economy. Prices paid by consumers for medical care rose 7.7 percent from December 1985 to December 1986, 1 percent faster than the 1984–85 change. Taken together, the 12 months of 1986 averaged 7.5 percent higher than the 12 months of 1985. This acceleration in health care price inflation came at a time when the rate of increase in the Consumer Price Index (CPI) for all items had slowed dramatically. The aggregate CPI change from 1985 to 1986 was only 1.9 percent, the lowest growth of the last two decades. Gasoline prices had dropped 22 percent and other energy prices had also fallen, although not nearly as much.

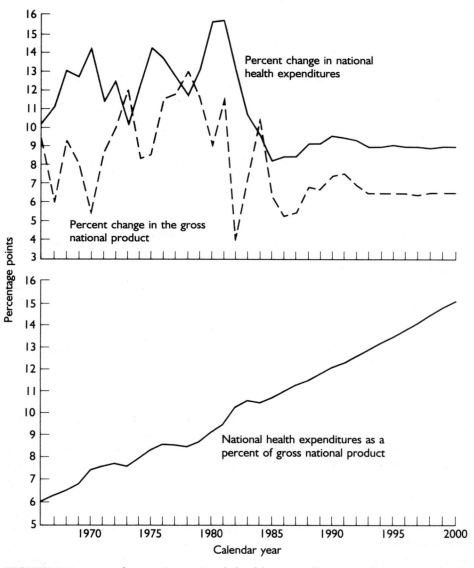

FIGURE 1 Percent change in national health expenditures and gross national product, and national health expenditures as a percent of gross national product: Calendar years 1966–86 and projections 1987–2000

Source: Health Care Financing Administration. Office of the Actuary: Data from the Division of National Cost Estimates

With an upturn in growth of national health expenditures last year, and a downturn in growth of the gross national product (GNP), health spending rose to 10.9 percent of the GNP in 1986. Barring unforeseen events and assuming that current laws and regulations continue into the future, health expenditures will continue to grow more rapidly than will the rest of the economy through the end of the century, by which time health spending will account for 15 percent of the GNP.

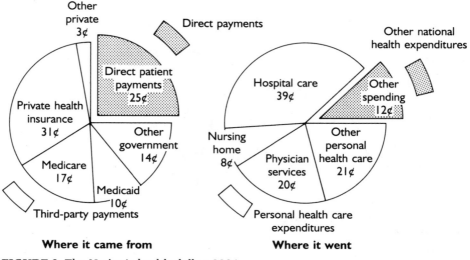

Where it came from   **Where it went**

FIGURE 2 The Nation's health dollar: 1986

Source: Health Care Financing Administration, Office of the Actuary: Data from the Division of National Cost Estimates.

Almost three-quarters of national health expenditures were channeled through third parties. Nearly two-thirds were channeled through private hands. The bulk of that expenditure was for patient care, and the remaining 12 percent was spent for research, construction, administration, and government public health activity.

However, it is not entirely appropriate to compare the CPI for medical care with the CPI for all items on their face values. First, the deep cuts in gasoline prices masked an underlying inflation rate of 3.9 percent in other categories of goods and services; the 13.2 percent deflation seen in energy prices did not translate into price cuts elsewhere. Second, service prices in general (including household utility prices) rose 5.0 percent from 1985 to 1986, compared with a drop of 1.0 percent in commodity prices. Service prices, in general, are likely to rise faster than commodity prices, because of lower productivity growth in the labor-intensive service sector. Thus, when evaluating health care prices, it is more appropriate to use service prices as a gauge than it is to use all prices. Third, the CPI for medical care contains a conceptual "price" of health insurance, which is not strictly a personal health care item. In the absence of this insurance component, the CPI for medical care would have risen 6.2 percent from 1985 to 1986. When looking at the relative growth of medical care prices, then, the best comparison may be between 6.2 percent and 5.0 percent. However, although less dramatic than the difference between the change in the CPI for medical care and the change in the CPI for all items, this margin is substantial in its own right. Within the medical care "market basket" priced for the CPI, the largest price increase — 8.6 percent — was for prescription drugs. Physician fees were up 7.2 percent and hospital prices increased 6.0 percent.

USE OF COMMUNITY HOSPITAL SERVICES

A substantial portion of the slowdown in growth of personal health care spending in recent years is attributable to changes in the use of community hospital services.

The effect of private sector initiatives to reduce hospital use appear to predate by about 2 years those of the more well known Medicare prospective payment system (PPS). Inpatient days for people under 65 years of age began to fall in mid-1981, as did admissions for that group. Days and admissions for the population 65 years of age or over began to fall in mid-1983, just into the first phase of PPS. Although some of the change in use by those under age 65 may be attributable to government programs such as Medicaid, the principal source of payment for that part of the population is private insurance. The latter group found itself under pressure from employers to reduce health care costs when insurance premiums became a major labor cost late in the 1970's.

Although total inpatient days have fallen since early in 1983, the opposite has occurred for outpatient visits. In fact, the trend of growth of visits began to accelerate early in 1985. Part of this phenomenon may be attributable to the changes in the sites that were once used for inpatient services. Many insurers encouraged patients to have preadmission testing done on an outpatient basis rather than an inpatient basis; other procedures, such as lens implantation, were moved from an inpatient to an outpatient setting in their entirety. Although the bulk of hospitals' revenue continues to come from inpatient services, outpatient visits began to outnumber inpatient days beginning in 1985, a change that appears to be permanent.

One other trend in community hospital use that may be worth examination is that of surgical procedures, because surgery tends to be associated with use of intensive (and expensive) hospital services. Beginning in 1981, the slope of the trend line flattened rather abruptly, and the number of operations remained roughly unchanged for 4 years. Beginning in 1985, however, the trend line resumed its former growth, a resumption that continued unabated through 1986.

The patterns of use of community hospital services demonstrate three things about that use. First, inpatient services have experienced a major reversal in trend. Admissions are at a 16-year low for patients under age 65 and at a 5-year low for patients 65 years of age or over; inpatient days are at an 18-year low. Second, hospitals have had some success in recovering those inpatient services in an outpatient setting. Third, surgical procedures in aggregate seem to be back on historical trendlines.

ELEMENTS OF NATIONAL HEALTH EXPENDITURES

Personal health care

Total spending for the direct provision of medical care goods and services—
personal health care expenditures—amounted to $404 billion in 1986, 8.8
percent more than in 1985. That is an amount equal to $1,620 per person and
represents 12 percent of U.S. personal income.

Compared with 1985 estimates, the data for 1986 indicate a slight increase
in the direct patient payment share of personal health care expenditures, 28.7
percent of the total, up from 28.4 percent. There are a number of partial
explanations of that increase. For example, almost one-fifth of it is attributable
to the Medicare program. Medicare coinsurance and deductible amounts were
increased in 1986, reaching an aggregate level of $12.7 billion. There is
anecdotal evidence of similar changes in private health insurance programs as
well. In addition, the 1986 national health expenditures estimates are preliminary, and subsequent data revisions may reduce or even reverse the change in
the direct payment share of total spending.

A substantial proportion of the increase in personal health care expenditures is attributable to price inflation, but the underlying trend in spending has
been essentially unchanged for the last decade. Price inflation—both
economy-wide and health-specific accounted for 54 percent of the personal
health care expenditures. Population growth accounted for another 11 percent,
and the remaining 35 percent is attributable to changes in consumption per
capita and in the "intensity" of consumption because of demographic change
of the population, changes in income levels and distribution, and so on.
Personal health care expenditures grew about 4 percent from 1985 to 1986 after
removing the effects of price inflation), close to the 10-year average growth in
"real" (price-deflated) spending.

Hospital care

Hospital revenues in 1986 amounted to $180 billion, 7.4 percent more than in
1985. Most of that money came from third parties. Private health insurers paid
36 percent of the total, Medicare and Medicaid paid 38 percent, and other
government programs paid 15 percent. However, the amount paid directly by
consumers increased disproportionately from 1985 to 1986, from 8.7 percent to
9.4 percent.

The increase in the direct payment portion of hospital revenues is attributable to changes in third-party financing and in coverage. Medicare beneficiaries were liable for increased deductible and coinsurance amounts in 1986,

because of changes in the cost per day of hospital care. Many privately insured employees and dependents faced similar changes in co-payment schedules, as employers sought to shift some of the cost of health care back to workers. In addition, there is evidence that the number of uninsured people in the United States is increasing, raising the amount of consumer liability.

Concomitant with the increased direct payment share of hospital spending, the Medicare share of spending dropped from 1985 to 1986, the first decrease since the early 1970's. This decline can be traced back to relatively low growth in Medicare payments per admission; the share of community hospital inpatient days and admissions accounted for by patients 65 years of age or over was unchanged from 1985 to 1986. New data from the American Hospital Association's annual survey of hospitals have resulted in revised estimates of hospital spending in 1994 and 1985. The new 1984 estimate is 0.6 percent higher than reported previously, and the 1985 estimate has been raised 0.3 percent.

Physician services

Spending for the services of physicians reached $92 billion in 1986, an increase of 11.1 percent from 1985.

Data on use of physician services show mixed growth. For example, both hospital admissions and inpatient days were lower in 1986 than in 1985, suggesting fewer physician contacts in an inpatient setting. On the other hand, emergency room visits grew 6.2 percent, implying increased outpatient contact. Further, the number of surgical procedures performed in community hospitals increased 2.2 percent, an indication that surgical income had increased as well.

Data on employment and hours suggest strong growth in physician activity in 1986. Total employment in offices of physicians and surgeons increased 6.6 percent, and hours worked by nonsupervisory employees increased 7.3 percent; both these figures were the highest in a decade. Nonsupervisory payroll was up 11.8 percent from 1985, again suggesting considerable strength in office business. The 1986 estimates of expenditure for physician services embody a shift of financing from private health insurance to direct payment. There is a substantial body of anecdotal evidence suggesting that privately insured people are paying higher proportions of their health bills in the form of copayments, which supports the shift observed in financing shares. Further, we estimate that "reasonable charge reductions" under Medicare Part B — the difference between what is billed and what the program recognizes as valid charges — will be shown to have increased some $200 million from 1985 to 1986; these reductions are the beneficiary's liability. On the other hand, the Medicare Part B deductible ($75 per year) was unchanged from 1985, effectively lowering the beneficiary share of total Part B allowed charges. The net effect of these occurrences is unclear.

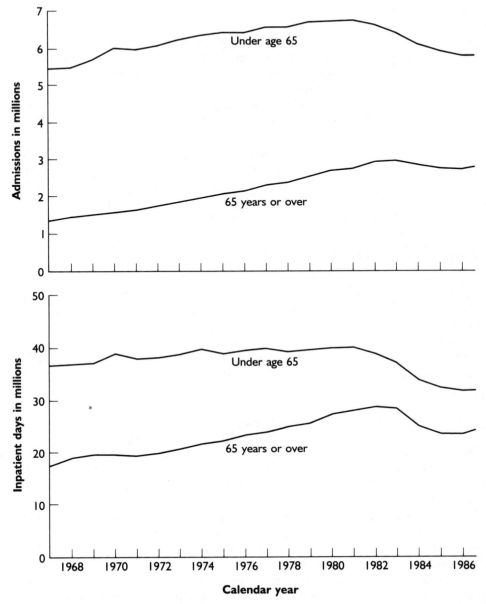

FIGURE 3 Number of community hospital admissions and inpatient days for populations under age 65 and 65 years of age or over: Calendar years 1967–86

Source: American Hospital Association: Data from the National Hospital Panel Survey, Chicago, 1987.

Since 1982, use of community hospital inpatient services has fallen, first for the population under age 65, and then for the population 65 years or over. Figure shows trends with seasonal, daily, and irregular variations removed.

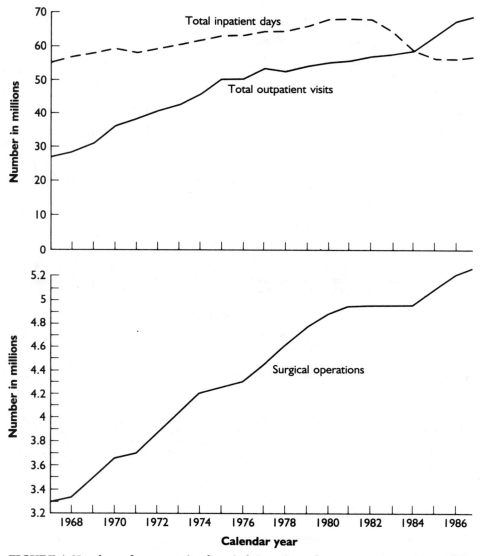

FIGURE 4 Number of community hospital inpatient days, outpatient visits, and surgical operations: 1967–86

Source: American Hospital Association: Data from the National Hospital Panel Survey, Chicago, 1987.

There has always been steady growth in use of community hospital outpatient services and of surgical operations performed in community hospitals. In fact, the same period in which the use of inpatient days declined witnessed an upswing in the trend of outpatient visits. The number of surgical operations accelerated after 1984. Figure shows trends with seasonal, daily, and irregular variations removed.

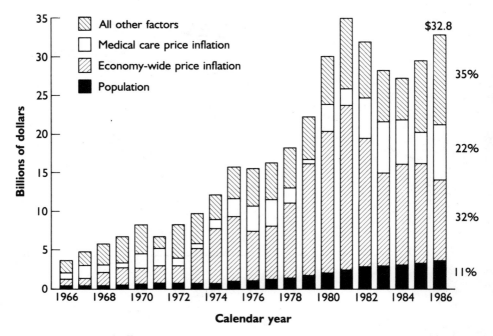

FIGURE 5 Factors affecting change in personal health care expenditures of billions of dollars: Calendar years 1966–86

Source: Health Care Financing Administration, Office of the Actuary: Data from the Division of National Cost Estimates

Price inflation has always accounted for a substantial part of the increase in personal health care expenditures. From 1985 to 1986, 32 percent of the $33 billion increase in that spending was attributable to economy-wide price inflation, and another 22 percent to medical care price inflation in excess of the general rate of price inflation. Population growth accounted for 11 percent of the change, and the remainder was attributed to other factors—changes in consumption per capita and in "intensity" as a result of rising income levels, aging of the population, and so on.

Nursing home care

We estimate the 1986 revenue of nursing homes to be $38 billion, up 9.1 percent from 1985.

In the estimates presented in this article, the Medicaid share of total expenditures has been falling. This may be attributable to State efforts at containment of total program costs. Medicaid certification has been tightened and nursing homes are giving priority to private pay patients. Recent General Accounting Office reports on access to care underscored this trend and added the observation that hospitals are encountering increasing difficulty in placing Medicare patients as well. Both of these phenomena may be reflected in the upward trend in the direct payment share of total nursing home expenditures.

Other personal health care

In addition to the three large expenditure categories mentioned previously, $94 billion was spent in 1986 for other personal health care. That amount — 9.2 percent more than in 1985 — was used to purchase dental care, drugs and drug sundries, eyeglasses and other medical commodities, home health and other professional services, and other medical goods and services.

Other national health expenditures

In addition to personal health care expenditures, $54 billion was spent in 1986 for other categories of health.

Government public health activity programs such as those at the Centers for Disease Control, which target diseases and conditions rather than beneficiary populations, cost $13 billion, increasing 9.2 percent — a rate consistent with historical experience.

The cost of administering public and private health programs, plus the net cost of private health programs, plus the net cost of private health insurance — the difference between earned premiums and incurred benefits — amounted to $24.5 billion.

New data on commercial insurance carrier experience in 1985 have led to a downward revision of previously published estimates for this category, resulting in a growth of 4.7 percent from 1984 to 1985, and of 3.8 percent from 1985 to 1986.

Noncommercial biomedical research consumed $8 billion in 1986, and another $8 billion was put in place as new hospital and institutional construction. The continued decline in construction is attributable to failing occupancy rates and to the uncertainty created by cost containment programs such as PPS regarding the future of inpatient care and capital reimbursement.

FINANCING HEALTH EXPENDITURES

The estimates of 1986 health spending shown in this report reflect the changes in financing of care that have been occurring over the last 4 years.

Medicare

Facing hospital insurance trust fund insolvency near the turn of the century, the Medicare administrators have actively sought ways to reduce spending while maintaining or improving the quality of care provided to more than 31 million aged and disabled program enrollees.

Medicare program benefits amounted to $76 billion in 1986, 7.8 percent more than in 1985. Because of the nature of the program, two-thirds of benefit payments were for hospital services; almost all of the remainder were for physician services. Nationwide, Medicare is the largest single purchaser of hospital care and physician services, accounting for 29 percent of all hospital revenue and for 21 percent of physician services.

Now in the third year of PPS, Medicare has actively sought to make hospitals more prudent providers of care. The decline in length of stay for the population age 65 or over, 98 percent of whom are eligible for Medicare hospital benefits, is attributable largely to the incentives created by PPS. The decline in admissions for the same group may be related to review activities carried out under the auspices of the program.

Medicaid

Originally intended to provide medical services to low-income women and children, Medicaid has evolved over time into the largest third-party financier of long-term care in the United States. Total Medicaid benefits (including both Federal and State shares) came to $44 billion in 1986, of which $16 billion were for nursing home care.

Counts of recipients demonstrate the extent to which Medicaid has become a long-term care vehicle. In fiscal year 1985, 21.8 million people received program benefits. Of that number, 2.5 percent received skilled nursing facility (SNF) care, and 3.8 percent received intermediate care facility (ICF) services (excluding ICF services for the mentally retarded). Yet, of fiscal year 1985 vendor payments, 13.5 percent were for SNF care and 17.4 percent were for ICF services. Nursing home recipients received an average of $9,300 in skilled nursing care and $7,900 in intermediate care in that year.

Private health insurance

As has been the case in recent years, growth in private health insurance was more rapid among self-insured policies than among the traditional carriers — the Blues and commercial carriers. Taken together, health insurance benefits rose 7.7 percent in 1985 (the reasonably complete data), to a total of $113 billion.

For insurers, 1985 was a profitable year, but less so than 1984. The difference between premiums and losses grew 3.2 percent from 1984 to 1985. Preliminary and projected data for 1986 indicate net underwriting losses for the industry, caused by very low growth in premiums (low by historical standards). Early 1987 data indicate that the situation will change dramatically: Some health policies are experiencing 20- to 30-percent increases in premium rates.

Direct patient payments

In 1986, $116 billion was spent for health care that was not covered by a third party. For the most part, this money came from patients or their families directly. Unlike total spending, less than one-third of direct patient payments were for institutional (hospital or nursing home) care. The largest amounts of direct payments were for physician services and drugs and sundries. Direct spending for nursing home care was only the third largest component.

During the last 4 years, the steadily downward trend in the share of personal health care expenditures paid directly by consumers has begun to waver. Part of this is attributable to changes in private and public health insurance co-payment schedules, and part of it is because of changes in the size and nature of the uninsured population.

EFFECTS OF DEMOGRAPHIC CHANGE

Population is often cited as an engine of demand for goods and services. Abrupt alterations in demographic structure—usually caused in modern times by rapid fertility changes—can create new needs or eliminate old ones. Because many industries require several years to adjust to demand changes, population shifts can result in dislocation of production.

But the biggest impacts are expected to occur in the next century because health care use rises rapidly after about age 65. The aged population is expected to continue growing rapidly until the mid-1990's. Then a temporary slowing will set in as the small birth cohort of the 1930's depression turns 65 years of age. By 2010 the postwar baby boom will reach retirement age and the rapid growth of the aged population will resume until the peak year birth cohort (about 1970) reaches age 65 in 2035.

Historically, the age and sex compositions of the population have contributed relatively little to growth of inpatient hospital care as a percent of GNP. The largest contribution (5.7 percent per year from 1965 to 1985) was from "intensity" of care—real goods and services provided per inpatient day. The second largest contribution to annual growth, 1.1 percent per year, was by hospital price inflation over and above general price inflation. Changes in the age and sex mix of the population, in contrast, added only 0.6 percent per year to expenditure growth.

At the same time that spending for inpatient care was growing, so was GNP—the resource base from which that spending was financed. In the historical period, hospital spending outpaced GNP growth by some 4.5 percent per year. Consequently, inpatient hospital expenditures rose as a share of the GNP, reaching 3.0 percent in 1985.

PROJECTIONS TO THE YEAR 2000

Based on historical trends and relationships and on recent experience, we project that national health expenditures will reach $1.5 trillion by the year 2000: 15.0 percent of the gross national product. Total spending per capita will rise from $1,837 in 1986 to $5,550 in 2000.

Assuming the continuation of current laws and regulations, we see little change in the distribution of services or of financing sources between now and the turn of the century. In fact, we project that hospital care will increase slightly as a share of total spending-cost containment notwithstanding (though we have recognized and extended the shift in composition between inpatient and outpatient care). Aging of the population will cause Medicare's share of total spending to rise a small amount as well, but the overall patterns of spending look remarkably similar over the 14-year span.

Still, growth in health spending is expected to moderate in the future. During the period 1965 through 1986, national health expenditures grew at an average annual rate of 12.1 percent. In contrast, the average growth from 1986 to 2000 is projected to be 9.0 percent. That historical growth in health spending will be more rapid than growth in our ability to pay, one factor prompting Congress, States, and private industry to initiate alternate ways to pay—for health care, alternatives such as health maintenance organizations, preferred provider organizations, and Medicare's prospective payment system.

The future being unknowable as it is, we have tried to steer a middle course in constructing our projections. We have focused on average annual rates of change, assuming no unanticipated events. Historical patterns in health spending were evaluated, with special emphasis given to the effects of Medicare's prospective payment system and to the recent impact of private sector initiatives on expenditure patterns. The resulting scenario serves as a baseline from which alternative estimates can be constructed to meet the needs of or to satisfy differing views of the reader.

CONCLUSIONS

In this article, we have presented historical estimates of national health expenditures by type of expenditure and source of funds through 1986, and we have projected those expenditures through the year 2000. We have assumed that historical trends and relationships will continue into the future, except as modified for the effects of public and private cost containment initiatives.

Health spending increases are projected to decelerate, primarily because of implementation of the Medicare PPS as it affects hospital inpatient expenditure growth, private sector initiatives to reduce the rate of increase of health costs, and lower projections of economy-wide inflation. However, spending is expected to continue to rise substantially faster than growth in the GNP.

Significant implications for the economy arise as the health sector continues to absorb large percentages of the GNP. The major implication is that, as more labor and capital are drawn into the health sector, relatively fewer resources are available for producing goods and services in other sectors.

We find little evidence that the incentives inherent in current cost-containment policies will reverse the ever-increasing share of GNP represented by total health spending. Substantial evidence does exist to indicate that current policies and initiatives will continue to cause changes in the mix of services provided. The increasing share of GNP used by health care may reflect, at least in part, a conscious choice by the nation for increased quantity and quality health care. Unfortunately, it may also reflect a piecemeal and disjointed approach to reimbursement reform by the public and private sectors. Thus far, it may be argued, a disproportionate share of reform has been focused on community hospital inpatient services. Concentrating in this one sector may have exacerbated cost-containment problems in other health care sectors.

The century of specialization has collected vast information about each and every organ of the body. The data available through modern research methods is beyond the wildest dreams of the medical scientist of even fifty years ago. But this information has been derived from, and applies to, isolated bits of human tissue. . . . This is, of course, the basic dilemma of the analytic method. In spite of the rich harvest of information we have reaped, the fact remains that people are still complaining of their aches, their pains and their inadequacies.

IDA ROLF

Physician Payment Review Commission

1988 Annual Report to Congress

SECTION I. BACKGROUND

The Commission was established because of the growing consensus among physicians, Medicare beneficiaries, and government officials about the need to reform physician payment in the Medicare program and the need to forge agreement on the elements of that reform. Pressure to reform physician payment under Medicare flows from many sources. Perhaps most prominent is the continued rate of increase in Medicare expenditures, but equally important are the erosion of financial protection for beneficiaries, fears that efforts to control expenditures will diminish access to services or reduce the quality of care, inequitable payment rates for physicians, and excessive program complexity.

The health sector has experienced rapid growth in medical technology, and in health facilities and personnel. With that growth has come a dramatic increase in health care expenditures. The burgeoning health sector has been successful in responding to the needs for biomedical research, hospital beds, physicians, and health care coverage over the past decades. However, the unrestrained increases in health care costs threaten to overshadow these accomplishments as the government, employers, and insurers find it increasingly difficult to pay the price.

Health care costs have continued to rise despite a variety of efforts to control them in the public and private sectors. In the 1980s, the rate of increase in national health care expenditures accelerated in relation to the GNP. In 1987, U.S. health expenditures reached an estimated 11.2 percent of GNP and are projected to reach 12 percent of GNP by 1990. Between 1975 and 1985, per capita health expenditures increased by over 11 percent a year in nominal terms, or 4.5 percent in real terms.

Medicare is the nation's largest payer of medical bills in an industry of over $450 billion. Enacted in 1965, it is a social insurance program that finances primarily acute health care services for 32 million aged and disabled persons. The program has two parts. Part A, the Hospital insurance (HI) program, provides inpatient hospital coverage and limited home care and skilled nursing facility benefits. Part B, the Supplementary Medical Insurance (SMI) program, covers the costs of physician services and such additional benefits as outpatient laboratory tests, durable medical equipment, and outpatient hospital care.

As in the private sector, the Medicare program has also experienced a rapid increase in expenditures. Federal outlays for Medicare amounted to nearly $83 billion in fiscal year 1987. This represented about 8 percent of the entire federal budget and almost 2 percent of the gross national product. Spending increases for Medicare have made the program a major target of policy reform and budget control efforts. Medicare outlays increased at 15.5 percent a year between 1975 and 1987.

In recent years, concern over rising health expenditures has focused on payment for physicians' services. Despite efforts in the public and private sector to control them, the costs of physician care have increased more rapidly than those for hospitals. In 1986 physician services accounted for about 75 percent of Part B expenditures, which amounted to 25 percent of all Medicare spending. In addition to the expenses associated with their own services, physicians may actually influence more than 70 percent of other medical services used by beneficiaries. Because of physicians' influence on health care utilization, any reforms in the current payment method for physicians need to be considered in light of their more general consequences for health delivery and spending.

After three years of moderate increases in Part B expenditures, which averaged about 12 percent annually, outlays rose 18 percent in 1986. This increase, coupled with the announcement that the beneficiary premium for Part B would increase by 38.5 percent in 1988, intensified concern about accelerating Medicare costs. The premium increase dramatized the impact of rising costs on beneficiary out-of-pocket spending. Although the Medicare program initially reduced the financial burden of health care costs on beneficiaries, beneficiaries are again spending at the pre-Medicare level of 15 percent of their income on medical care. While all beneficiaries experience the effects of increased out-of-pocket costs, the burden of rising premiums, coinsurance, and balance billing is unevenly distributed. The financially disadvantaged (disproportionately women and minorities), the very sick, and heavy users of noncovered services are at the greatest financial risk.

In part, increased Medicare expenditures have resulted from the current customary, prevailing, and reasonable (CPR) method of paying physicians, which generates a distorted and inequitable structure of prices. Payments vary by type of procedure, locality, specialty, and site of care. These payment differentials cannot be explained by documented differences in the underlying costs of providing services. Although these differentials have not arisen from deliberate decisions to favor certain styles of practice on grounds of cost, quality, or access, they may nevertheless affect practice patterns, because they often provide inappropriate financial incentives that influence such decisions as what services to employ in the care of patients, where to practice, and whether to specialize. These distortions can reduce access to care and quality of care as well as increase costs to beneficiaries and Medicare program expenditures. They have been criticized as being inequitable for both physicians and beneficiaries.

There has been a growing consensus among public and private payers that further controls on the price of physician services alone will be of only limited effectiveness in moderating the increase in expenditures. Nearly half of the increase in 1987 outlays for Part B was attributed to the increase in the volume of services. A fee schedule for Medicare can standardize payments and rationalize incentives that influence physicians' choices about practice location, specialty, and type or quantity of services. But changes in payment policy must be coupled with efforts to encourage more appropriate use of services. Only by increasing the efficiency of care can expenditure growth be constrained without reducing access or quality of care and without shifting financial burdens to beneficiaries. The Commission is developing an integrated strategy directed at these policy goals.

RECOMMENDATIONS IN THE 1987 REPORT

The recommendations contained in the Commission's first report dealt with both immediate and longer-term directions for reform. The key long-term recommendation was that Medicare move toward a fee schedule for paying physicians.

Fee Schedule

The Commission concluded that Medicare's existing customary, prevailing, and reasonable (CPR) method of paying physicians was sufficiently flawed and that it should be replaced by a fee schedule, rather than modified. The CPR method has

- encouraged fee inflation and excessive use of services;
- resulted in distorted prices that have led to inappropriate patterns of medical care and inequities among physicians; and
- become administratively complex and difficult for both physicians and beneficiaries to understand.

The Commission noted that a properly designed fee schedule would provide better incentives for appropriate medical care and reduce the complexity faced by program participants and managers.

Geographic Variation

The Commission expressed concern that geographic variation in payment may reduce beneficiary access in some rural and low-income urban areas, and be unfair to physicians practicing in those areas. It recommended a payment increment for primary care services provided in underserved areas and promised intensive attention to geographic variation in the coming year.

Inherent Reasonableness

The Commission endorsed the goals of the approach specified by Congress to make adjustments in existing payments for specific medical services based on assessments of their "inherent reasonableness." At the same time, it noted that the data requirements of the regulatory process specified by Congress for defining inherent reasonableness would limit the extent to which the process could be used to make such adjustments. So, the Commission proposed to evaluate the potential of using a consensus process for developing recommendations for changes in payment and, in the meantime, to respond to requests for advice during congressional budget deliberations by comparing Medicare relative payments with available relative value scales based on resource costs or the professional judgment of physicians.

Assignment and the Participating Physician Program

In recent years, Congress has acted to strengthen beneficiary access to physicians who accept Medicare allowed charges as payment in full. The Commission proposed a period of monitoring and evaluation to assess the results of these recent policy changes. Effective beneficiary education about the program and timely claims processing for participating physicians were indicated as matters for future Commission attention.

SPECIFIC ADVICE TO CONGRESS ON BUDGET RECONCILIATION

Soon after the 1987 report was released, the committees with jurisdiction over Medicare asked the Commission to advise them on how to meet the fiscal year 1988 budget objectives they expected to be set for the Medicare program as part of the congressional budget process. The Commission considered options that could be implemented quickly enough to reduce anticipated increases in physician payments during fiscal year 1988. After holding hearings on these options, it developed recommendations, guided by the principle that short-term policy changes should move the payment system in the direction of long-term reform.

The Commission recommended that some of the budget savings be derived from a reduction in the amount by which fees could be updated according to the Medicare Economic Index (MEI) that is used to limit annual increases in prevailing charges. To move the system toward a more rational pattern of relative payments and to protect beneficiary access to care, however, the commission proposed that primary care services be exempted from the reduction.

The Commission developed a methodology to identify procedures most overvalued by Medicare and recommended modest reductions in prevailing charges for them. The Commission noted that such reductions were likely to be consistent with the changes in relative payments that would occur under a fee schedule.

The methodology employed by the Commission compared relative payments by Medicare with relative value scales that had some of the attributes of the scale the Commission envisions for its fee schedule reform. The scales selected were those at least partially based on resource costs and those that were developed with a substantial amount of physician input.

The Commission initially identified eight procedures meeting the criterion that their relative values under Medicare be consistently higher than those in each of the other relative value scales, and substantially higher in most. When additional data became available, the Commission extended the analysis, upon congressional request, and identified five more procedures that met the criterion. For each of the overvalued procedures, the Commission cautioned that any reductions in prevailing charges should not apply in localities that already had relatively low charges, defined as those with prevailing charges below 75 percent of the national mean for the procedure.

The Commission reiterated its recommendation that Congress consider a payment increment for primary care services delivered in specified underserved areas and elaborated on a methodology for designating eligible areas.

Much of the Commission's advice was reflected in provisions of the Omnibus Budget Reconciliation Act of 1987. The Commission also began to advise Congress on approaches to controlling Part B expenditure growth in response to congressional concern over the increasing burden of Part B outlays on beneficiaries and taxpayers. The Commission expects to continue to work closely with Congress, to provide timely and relevant advice on physician payment policy.

SECTION II. SUMMARY OF 1988 REPORT

In its first report to Congress a year ago, the Physician Payment Review Commission (PPRC) established goals for Medicare physician payment policy and charted a direction for Medicare program reform. In that report, the Commission endorsed the concept of a fee schedule for Medicare. The Commission's 1988 report describes its subsequent work in shaping long-term options for reform and recommending short-term refinements in current policy consistent with those options.

During the past year, the Commission made progress in building the conceptual and technical framework necessary to develop a fee schedule proposal. It also examined options to promote the appropriate use of medical services, which could moderate expenditure growth without reducing Medicare beneficiaries' access to high quality care. As it develops policies for reform, the Commission gives particular consideration to the consequences for beneficiaries.

PROGRESS ON THE FEE SCHEDULE

In the past year the Commission has made significant progress in developing a proposal for a Medicare fee schedule. It has focused on the conceptual basis for a relative value scale (the relative rates of payment among different physician services), whether the payments for a service should vary by specialty, and how payments for services should vary by geographic area. It has also identified changes in the use of coding that would be required for a fee schedule to be implemented, and has planned a consensus process to develop the changes.

The Commission has considered several other issues related to the development of a fee schedule. Those issues include geographic variation in Medicare charges, policies related to assignment and balance or extra billing, and payment for diagnostic services with a substantial nonphysician component.

Basis for the Relative Value Scale

Two major bases for a relative value scale are feasible—historical charges and resource costs. The rationale for using what physicians have historically charged is that such charges reflect a market valuation of physicians' services. But the market for the insured services of physicians does not function well, and the resulting pattern of charges reflects serious distortions. Indeed, reducing these distortions is the principal reason the Commission is advocating a fee schedule. The Commission recommends basing a relative value scale primarily on resource costs.

A resource cost basis would reflect estimates of what relative values would be under a hypothetical market that functions perfectly. Under such a market, competition drives relative prices to reflect the relative costs of efficient producers.

The most difficult task in developing a relative value scale (RVS) based on resource costs is that roughly half the costs reflect physicians' time and effort. The usefulness of such an RVS depends on the accuracy with which the relative amount of physician time and effort for various services can be estimated.

Procedure Coding

Ambiguity in coding can complicate the development and use of a fee schedule. If a coding system is not interpreted uniformly by providers and payers, it is difficult to assign accurate relative values to codes and to ensure that assigned fees are applied to the intended services.

The Commission is working to make the interpretation of codes more uniform under the fee schedule. In cases such as global surgical services, this can be accomplished by standardizing carrier interpretation and implementation of current codes. The Commission has developed a process for this reform that uses an interspecialty consensus panel to develop a generic description of global services and groups of physician experts to identify the specific components of individual global services.

In the case of visit services, ambiguity in coding may persist after carrier standardization. The Commission is recommending that current visit codes be evaluated to ascertain their specificity, reliability, and correlation with resource costs. If the current system cannot provide a sound basis for valuing, reporting, and paying for visit services, more specific definitions of visit codes will have to be developed. The Commission is investigating potential options for this type of reform.

Setting the Conversion Factor

A conversion factor transforms a relative value scale into a fee schedule. The level of the conversion factor will determine projected expenditures for physician services, given an expected volume of services. The Congress could set the initial conversion factor to be budget neutral—that is, so that the projected level of expenditures under the fee schedule was equal to the amount that would have been spent under the old payment system—or to increase or decrease projected expenditures. Though the implications for the federal budget are likely to be the principal determinant of the initial conversion factor when the fee schedule is implemented, the effect on beneficiary access and financial liabilities must also be considered.

Updating the Fee Schedule

Once the fee schedule is implemented, the RVS and adjustments such as geographic multipliers and the conversion factor will need to be updated. Processes must be developed to make these modifications.
The Commission is examining several alternative processes such as:

- a formula approach linking the conversion factor to an index to yield a predetermined increase in Medicare expenditures;
- using the existing regulatory rulemaking process of the Department of Health and Human Services (HHS);
- recommendations to the Secretary of HHS or to Congress by an independent board or commission; and
- negotiation between physicians and representatives of the federal government.

Geographic Variation in Charges and Interim Policy Changes

The Commission has conducted extensive data analysis on current patterns of geographic variation in Medicare prevailing charges. Geographic variation, while significant, is less extensive than anecdotal evidence might suggest. Variation is generally greatest for visit services and least for diagnostic procedures. Areas with charges that were relatively high for one procedure did not necessarily have relatively high charges for other procedures. Charges are usually higher in urban areas, but there remains substantial variation among urban areas and among rural areas.

Adjusting for costs of practice reduced some of the geographic variation in charges, but much of it remained. Differences between urban and rural areas decreased substantially, so that on an adjusted basis, urban charges were, on average, only slightly higher than rural charges.

The Commission examined a series of interim options to address excessive geographic variation in charges. Placing a floor and ceiling on the prevailing charges for each procedure would increase equity among physicians but could cause some charges to move in directions opposite of those likely under a fee schedule. In particular, a ceiling on prevailing charges might lower fees that later would be raised under a relative value scale. In addition, some of the reductions might be large and might be handled better in the context of comprehensive reform.

The Commission recommends that a floor equal to a fixed percentage of the national mean be placed under primary care services (office visits, nursing home visits, home visits, and emergency room visits). For example, after adjustment for costs of practice, no prevailing charge would be less than 80 percent of the national mean for the service. This would tend to increase beneficiaries' access to primary care services in some areas and might reduce their out-of-pocket costs since reductions in extra bills for unassigned claims could exceed the additional coinsurance from the higher prevailing charges. Equity among physicians would be increased. The budgetary cost of a geographic floor could be offset by a variety of policy options, including a geographic ceiling for specialized procedures.

Assignment and Participation: Current Status and Policy Options

Since its inception, Medicare has permitted physicians to decide on a claim-by-claim basis whether to accept assignment (to bill Medicare and accept Medicare's allowed charge as payment in full) or to charge the patient directly, leaving the patient responsible for the full charge even if it exceeds what Medicare will pay. The amount in excess of Medicare's allowed charge is known as the balance bill or extra bill.

Physicians currently accept assignment for almost three-fourths of Medicare claims, yet the cost to beneficiaries of the extra billing on nonassigned claims was nearly $2.5 billion in 1987. The Commission is concerned about both beneficiary financial liability under Part B—including liability under extra billing—and Medicare's long-standing policy to give physicians a choice whether to accept assignment. It is therefore examining evidence on the effects of current balance billing policy and reviewing options for change so that it can improve current approaches and determine what policies would be appropriate to accompany a fee schedule.

Recent changes in Medicare policy have focused on increasing incentives for physicians to accept assignment or to participate (that is, to agree to accept assignment on all charges for a year), on helping beneficiaries find physicians who will provide them care without extra billing, and on constraining extra billing while preserving some freedom for physicians to extra bill. These changes included creating the Participating Physician Program, providing beneficiaries with directories of participating physicians, and placing constraints on the billed charges of physicians who choose not to participate.

These changes have contributed to large increases in overall assignment rates and in the percent of total services provided by participating physicians. However, significant variation in assignment rates by geographic location, specialty, type of service, and site of service persists. Such variation differentially affects the ability of beneficiaries to avoid balance bills. It also suggests that physicians' de facto opportunity and inclination to balance bill varies. Analyses of the factors affecting physicians' assignment and participation decisions show that both economic and noneconomic factors are important. Increases in Medicare payment levels would increase assignment and participation, but with large financial implications for the Part B trust fund, beneficiaries, and physicians. Philosophical attitudes also have a major effect and are less amenable to alteration through policy changes.

Possible improvements within the framework of current policy, such as providing more information to physicians or expanding efforts to inform beneficiaries about participating physicians, are likely to have only a small effect on beneficiaries' ability to avoid balance bills.

More far-reaching reforms could be shaped by decisions on three policy issues: the scope of services and the population to which concerns about extra billing should apply; the relative importance of eliminating extra billing versus limiting it; and the mix of policies between the use of financial incentives and the use of limits on extra billing.

The Commission recognizes that a fee schedule has major implications for balance billing policy. A fee schedule, if budget neutral, is likely to have relatively modest effects on overall national assignment and participation rates, but much larger effects on individual beneficiaries and physicians. Decisions about setting payment levels under the fee schedule and about possible limitations on charges must take into account their potential impact on the ability of beneficiaries to obtain needed services.

Given that diagnostic tests have historically subsidized office visits, particularly among primary care practitioners, the Commission recognizes that major changes in payment for those tests should not proceed reform of payment for visits.

UTILIZATION, COST, AND QUALITY

Though the growth of Medicare expenditures for hospital services has slowed in recent years, expenditures for physicians' services have grown particularly rapidly, averaging 17 percent a year for the past decade. This rapid growth in expenditures has required increases in the program's support from general revenues and in the premiums that beneficiaries must pay.

While a number of factors have contributed to the growth of expenditures, the primary factor now driving the increases for physicians' services under fee-for-service is the increasing volume of services. Although increases in charges for each service have been tightly constrained for the past five years, this does not appear to have substantially slowed expenditure growth. The focus must now shift to limiting the rate of growth of the volume of services.

While most services provided to Medicare beneficiaries are of substantial benefit, some are unnecessary and others provide only a very small benefit despite substantial costs. The challenge for controlling the rate of growth in expenditures is to identify and selectively reduce the services of least benefit.

The primary concern about any effort to control growth in expenditures is the possible threat to access and quality of care. The Commission is very much aware of this as it considers alternative policies. It also plans to examine thoroughly Medicare's ability to assess and assure quality of care during the next year.

A Strategy to Moderate the Rate of Growth of Expenditures

Medicare needs an effective strategy to moderate the rate of growth of expenditures without threatening the quality of care. A successful strategy will require three elements: the will to reduce not only clearly unnecessary services but also services that provide only marginal benefit at disproportionately high cost; effective mechanisms to give patients and their physicians the means and incentive to reduce those services; and better knowledge of which services provide little or no benefit, so that reductions can in fact be targeted to them.

The responsibility to reduce services of least benefit must be shared by patients and their families, physicians, and the general public. Co-payments are intended to make beneficiaries aware of the costs of services, and to forgo services of little or no benefit. However, policymakers have been reluctant to rely on increased beneficiary copayments to control expenditures for fear they will reduce quality and access, particularly for the poor and the seriously ill.

Since physicians make or influence most of the decisions to use medical services, much of the responsibility for reducing services of minimal benefit will fall to them. They will be accountable to the public, as well as to their patients, for using services appropriately. Practice guidelines and feedback of utilization information will help them identify services of least benefit. Finally, the public must recognize that unless we forgo costly services that provide little or no benefit, expenditures will continue to grow rapidly.

Utilization Review

Medicare now relies on utilization review by Part B carriers and Peer Review Organizations (PROs) as its primary method of reducing unnecessary services. Despite improvements, however, problems remain. The clinical soundness of the review criteria used by PROs and carriers has not been systematically assessed, although these criteria vary considerably in specificity and scope. Little has been invested in research to improve the efficiency and effectiveness of utilization review, and the measurement of current program results is sketchy. Beneficiaries and providers frequently have problems getting prompt and understandable answers to questions, and communication with physicians about local utilization review processes and problems is very limited. In general, the administration of utilization review and related functions is compromised by funding limitations and the addition of new responsibilities without concomitant funding increases. The results are poor service and higher outlays for unnecessary services.

The Commission suggests several actions that may help increase the effectiveness of utilization review to reduce unnecessary services and to better limit the reductions to services that do not benefit the patient. In the short-term, the Health Care Financing Administration should comprehensively assess the clinical reasonableness, effectiveness, and administrative burdens of current criteria and processes for utilization review. Over the longer term, a focused research strategy is needed to strengthen the clinical foundation for review and to improve the effectiveness and efficiency of review techniques. Results should feed into ongoing program oversight and fundamental program design.

In addition, Medicare should consider broader use of preadmission and preservice review, management of high-cost cases, and intensified review of care outside the hospital. High-cost case management programs target probable high-cost patients for intensive attention and efforts to arrange less costly alternatives to inpatient care; the Commission will evaluate the potential of these programs for Medicare.

Finally, carriers and PROs must be provided adequate and predictable funding to carry out their current and future responsibilities. They should be allowed greater flexibility in using contracted funds to achieve their objectives.

Practice Guidelines and Feedback of Utilization Information

Uncertainty about the benefits of services to patients makes it difficult to identify and reduce services of least benefit. The Commission has begun to examine several methods to give physicians and their patients the information they need to determine which services are indeed of little benefit and the means to reduce them. Two methods are described in this report: practice guidelines to provide recommendations for clinical practice and feedback of comparative utilization information.

Practice guidelines are developed through consensus of expert physicians, building on the available information in the medical literature. They are intended to embody the best available knowledge of appropriate use of services in a form physicians can easily use. Sound and clinically credible practice guidelines would help physicians — and their patients — determine how much a particular service is likely to benefit the patient with a particular clinical presentation. Guidelines can also provide a sound clinical basis for utilization review.

If guidelines are to fulfill this promise, they must be clinically sound and credible. Both the process through which guidelines are developed and the ways they are applied must recognize the unavoidable uncertainty in medical knowledge and the essential role the attending physician's clinical judgment must play in medical practice. The Commission has begun to evaluate existing guidelines, alternative processes for developing sound guidelines, and how guidelines could be used in Medicare.

Providing physicians with information on their use of services compared with that of their peers can lead them to examine their practices and to reduce unnecessary services. This method is now being used in several projects. Evaluation of its effect on quality and costs will allow determination of its potential for use in Medicare.

Expenditure Targets

The Commission is examining the potential of expenditure targets to help moderate the rate of growth in the volume of services. Expenditure targets constitute a way of adjusting updates of physicians' fees in an area based on how total expenditures compare with a predetermined target. If physicians collectively control the volume of services, they can achieve a larger increase in fees. The intent of expenditure targets is to make clear to the physician community its responsibility to employ medical resources wisely. They offer the medical profession enhanced clinical autonomy and freedom from intrusion into medical decisions in return for its accepting this responsibility. Expenditure targets also could begin to address the disparities found among geographic areas in their per capita Medicare spending.

For expenditure targets to limit growth in expenditures and reduce geographic disparities, the physician community must translate their collective financial incentive into changes in what individual physicians do when caring for Medicare patients. The Commission will explore whether and how this can occur.

CAPITATION

Medicare payment for medical services through capitation arrangements currently offers an alternative to the fee-for-service system for a relatively small segment of Medicare beneficiaries. With the growth in capitated plans and increases in enrollment among the general population, the number of Medicare enrollees in such plans also can be expected to grow.

In the past year the Commission has focused its efforts on selected issues pertaining to the quality of care in HMOs and certain aspects of the payment mechanism that may contribute to problems in accessibility.

Quality of Care in HMOs

Key issues regarding the quality of care in HMOs include possible inappropriate use of services, particularly the underuse of services, as a result of improper use of financial risk arrangements at the level of individual physicians, and the adequacy of Medicare's current quality assurance activities. The Commission recommends that all HMOs participating in the Medicare risk contracting program be subject to a periodic accreditation process that focuses particularly on internal quality assurance programs and physician compensation arrangements. Also, regulations should be developed to require HMOs with risk-sharing contracts to provide physicians with detailed information regarding financial risk arrangements and beneficiaries with educational material regarding characteristics of HMOs that may influence patient care either positively or negatively.

Payments to HMOs

The prospective payment mechanism employed by HCFA to pay risk-sharing plans fails to provide appropriate, equitable levels of payment to certain HMOS. The best short-term solution to payment problems stemming from differences in patient mix is the incorporation of a health status adjustment (for example, diagnostic cost groups) into the current per capita payment mechanism. While some additional research is needed to refine the adjustment, a lengthy demonstration is unnecessary. Incorporating a health status adjustment should be done in concert with improvements in the actuarial process used to calculate Medicare per capita payments to HMOs, since this process currently has the potential to seriously distort payment levels.

Geographic variability in payments has probably discouraged some HMOs from entering into Medicare risk-sharing contracts, thus reducing beneficiary access to HMOs in certain geographic areas. A floor or lower limit should be established for county-specific payments. The Commission will assess the impact of alternative methods of establishing such a floor in the coming year.

MEDICARE DATA

Some changes in the Medicare Part B data system will be necessary to support both the continued development of current program management and implementation of alternative payment mechanisms. Adoption of a fee schedule may involve changes in the definition of certain types of data currently collected or the collection of new types of data. If implemented, a program of expenditure targets would probably require the designation of certain geographic boundaries and the collection of data specific to these geographic units.

The ability of the Health Care Financing Administration, carriers, providers, and beneficiaries to respond to changing data requirements is an important consideration in assessing the feasibility of any alternative payment mechanism and establishing a schedule for implementation. Changes involving the submission of additional data, the redefinition of currently submitted data, or systems modifications may require several years or more to implement and may involve substantial expenditures. Consequently, thorough advance planning and realistic goals are prerequisites.

During the coming year, the Commission will conduct a planning process to identify the specific changes in the Medicare Part B data system required to support the various physician payment mechanisms under consideration.

Tonsils, vermiform, appendices, uvulas, even ovaries are sacrificed because it is the fashion to get them cut out, and because the operations are highly profitable.

GEORGE BERNARD SHAW

Philip R. Lee/Paul B. Ginsburg
Lauren B. LeRoy/ Glenn T. Hammons

The Physician Payment Review Commission Report to Congress—1989

The Physician Payment Review Commission has developed proposals to rationalize the pattern of payments to physicians by Medicare and to slow the rate of increase in program costs so that they are affordable to beneficiaries and taxpayers. It outlines these proposals in its 1989 report, submitted to Congress April 28, 1989.

The Commission was created in 1986 to advise Congress on reform of the methods used by Medicare to pay physicians. The Congress expanded its charge in 1988 to include consideration of policies designed to slow the rates of increase in expenditures and utilization of physicians' services. Medicare is the nation's largest payer of medical bills in an industry that now accounts for more than 11% of the gross national product. Its expenditures have grown rapidly over the years, with spending for physician services being the fastest growing portion, rising an average of 15% a year. Taxpayers and beneficiaries pay for these services, and there is general consensus that the increases of the past cannot continue. While concern about expenditure growth is the most prominent factor behind efforts to reform Medicare payment policy, equally important are concerns about the erosion of financial protection and access to quality medical care for beneficiaries, inequitable payment rates for physicians, and excessive administrative complexity under current Medicare policies.

To rationalize the pattern of payments by Medicare, the Commission proposes a Medicare Fee Schedule based primarily on resource costs. To limit beneficiary financial liability, it recommends limits on balance billing. To control growth in expenditures, the Commission proposes the use of expenditure targets, increased research on effectiveness of medical services, and development of practice guidelines.

Philip R. Lee, M.D., is professor of social medicine and director of the Institute for Health Policy Studies, School of Medicine, University of California, San Francisco. He is also chair of the Physician Payment Review Commission.
Paul B. Ginsburg is executive director and Lauren B. LeRoy and Glenn T. Hammons are deputy directors of the Physician Payment Review Commission.

MEDICARE FEE SCHEDULE

The Commission recommends that Congress enact legislation this year that would replace Medicare's current "customary, prevailing, and reasonable" method of paying physicians with a fee schedule based primarily on resource costs. The Commission believes that the fee schedule should be implemented gradually, beginning with a transition fee schedule that would take effect 6 months after enactment and would move the payment system in a series of steps toward full implementation of the Medicare Fee Schedule in 1992. The Commission also recommends that the Medicare Fee Schedule cover all specialties, including radiology and anesthesiology, for which separate fee schedules now exist for Medicare payment.

A fee schedule consists of:

- a *relative value scale* (RVS), which indicates the value of each service or procedure relative to others;
- a *conversion factor*, which translates the RVS into a fee for each service; and
- a *geographic multiplier*, which indicates how payment for a service is to vary from one geographic area to another.

Relative Volume Scale

The Commission has reached a number of conclusions about the design of the RVS for the Medicare Fee Schedule. The Commission recommends that the RVS comprise two cost elements: relative physician work and practice costs.

Relative Physician Work.   The Commission has carefully evaluated the work by William Hsiao and his colleagues at Harvard University to develop a Resource-Based Relative Value Scale. It has found the methodology for estimating relative physician work to be fundamentally sound and has drawn heavily on it in developing its RVS for the Medicare Fee Schedule. The Commission's evaluation calls for additional research to be undertaken by Dr. Hsiao and the Commission staff to strengthen the results of the study. Most of these tasks are already under way.

A national fee schedule requires that the codes for physician services be interpreted uniformly by all physicians and carriers. Only then can accurate relative values be assigned to each service so that fees reflect the resource costs associated with providing that service. The Commission's recommendations call for changes related to coding in two important areas: surgical global fees and evaluation and management services.

Codes for Surgical Global Services.   With the unanimous agreement of a consensus panel made up of surgeons and carrier representatives, the Commission has developed a policy to determine which services associated with an operation should be included in the global payment for surgery and which ones should be paid separately. Using data from the Hsiao study, the Commission has calculated the relative values for each operation accordingly.

Codes for Evaluation and Management Services. Physicians cannot accurately use the current codes for evaluation and management services, commonly referred to as *visit codes*, to reflect their time and work, because the levels of service (e.g., brief, intermediate, comprehensive) are not precisely defined. Based on analysis by the Commission and by Dr. Hsiao, the Commission concludes that the time spent by a physician for each type of visit is a good predictor of the amount of work involved. The Commission therefore recommends that time be incorporated in the definitions for visit codes.

This reform would make the codes more accurate for several purposes: helping physicians to use them properly, assigning relative values to evaluation and management services, and assisting carriers in determining whether physicians are billing correctly for these services.

Practice Costs. The Commission has developed a formula that it recommends using to incorporate practice costs into the RVS. The Commission's formula for incorporating practice in the RVS allows for overhead to be calculated independently of physician work.

Updating the RVS. The RVS would need to be updated annually to take into account changes resulting from new technology, refinements in the coding system, and evolving clinical practice. The Commission recommends that the process used to develop the Medicare Fee Schedule, in which the Commission provides the Congress with the information and advice it needs to make policy decisions, be used for updating the RVS. This process gives Congress the technical information and advice it needs, and it gives organizations representing those affected by the legislation—physicians, beneficiaries, and others—a chance to participate in the decision-making process.

Physicians, in particular, have a major role to play in revising the RVS. The Commission will continue to work closely with the AMA and the specialty societies. It has begun to explore ways of structuring the process through which the medical profession would advise it that would be acceptable to all groups.

Conversion Factor

The conversion factor transforms the RVS into a schedule of dollar payments for each service. The Commission recommends that the initial conversion factor be set so that outlays for physicians' services projected under the fee schedule are the same as those projected under the current payment system.

The conversion factor should be updated annually. The formula used to determine the update should have as one element the difference between targeted and actual expenditures, as described later herein in the discussion of expenditure targets.

Geographic Multipliers

The Commission recommends that the geographic multiplier reflect only variation in overhead costs of practice. The amount physicians receive for their time and effort, after subtracting overhead costs, should not vary by locality. Therefore, if physicians in two parts of the country provide the same quantity and mix of services to Medicare beneficiaries, they would receive the same net income from Medicare. This policy would reduce substantially the magnitude of geographic variation in fees.

Specialty Differentials

The Commission believes that when a service provided by physicians in different specialties is essentially the same, the payment should be the same. It therefore recommends that specialty differentials — differences in payment to physicians of different specialties for the same procedure code — be eliminated under the fee schedule.

In some cases, physicians in different specialties provide different services under the same code and yet receive the same payment, because distinct codes that would accurately capture these differences do not exist. New codes should be established in such cases to reflect legitimate differences that are substantiated. Identification of such coding changes would be part of the process for updating the RVS.

Assignment and Balance Billing

The Medicare Fee Schedule must be accompanied by policies to limit beneficiaries' financial responsibility for charges in excess of what Medicare allows. The Commission does not recommend mandatory assignment but proposes these policies to increase protection for beneficiaries as follows:

- Limiting charges for unassigned claims to a fixed percentage of the fee schedule amount. These charge limits would replace current Medicare maximum allowable actual charge limits. Precedents for this approach exist in recent federal legislation phasing in limits of 125% of the Medicare allowed amount for overpriced procedures and 115% of the allowed amount for the radiology fee schedule.
- Eliminating balance billing for qualified Medicare beneficiaries. This step would involve clarifying the provision in the Medicare Catastrophic Coverage Act of 1988 (Public Law 100-360) that requires state Medicaid programs

to pay Medicare cost sharing for beneficiaries who are not otherwise eligible for Medicaid, but who have incomes below the federal poverty level. The current legislation covers Medicaid payment of deductibles, premiums, and coinsurance, but does not require physicians to accept the Medicare allowed charge as payment in full, as they do for other Medicare beneficiaries covered by Medicaid.

- Continuing the Participating Provider Program and its payment differential that provides higher fees to participating physicians.

The Commission has concluded that limitations on balance billing are needed because the market for physicians' services does not function well enough to protect Medicare beneficiaries. Limited balance billing would also provide a safety valve concerning errors in setting fee schedule amounts and an opportunity for those physicians who are especially highly regarded by patients or who systematically take on the most difficult cases to be paid more than the fee schedule amount.

Impact on Physicians and Beneficiaries

The Commission has constructed simulation models to project the impact of the Medicare Fee Schedule on categories of physicians and beneficiaries. Table 1 shows the changes in Medicare payments for selected services. Fees for evaluation and management services, such as office visits and hospital visits, would increase, and fees for many surgical procedures would decrease. Table 2 shows the impact on major specialties included in the first phase of the Hsiao study. Medicare payments would increase for family physicians and internists and decrease for thoracic surgeons, ophthalmologists, and radiologists.

The Medicare Fee Schedule would change the distribution of payments among geographic areas (Table 3). The geographic multiplier, reflecting overhead costs only, would result in higher payments to physicians in rural areas and lower payments to physicians in very large metropolitan areas.

Beneficiaries in general would experience a moderate reduction in out-of-pocket payment of coinsurance and balance bills, most of which would result from the limit on balance billing. The magnitude of these reductions is relatively uniform across different categories of beneficiaries (e.g., by age, sex, income).

Transition

The Commission recommends a transition that would adjust payments in the direction of the Medicare Fee Schedule to give physicians and beneficiaries time to adjust, allow for midcourse corrections, and increase the chances that private payers will implement similar changes.

The Commission's plan would call for a transitional stage that would retain customary and prevailing charge screens. It would base changes in prevailing

TABLE 1 National Mean Allowed Charges in 1988 for Selected Procedures by the Medicare Fee Schedule and Customary, Prevailing, and Reasonable (CPR) Charge System*

	Procedure	Medicare Fee Schedule, $	CPR, $	Change, %
Evaluation and management				
90050	Limited office visit	29	23	24
90060	Intermediate Office visit	35	28	26
90250	Limited hospital visit	33	26	29
90260	Intermediate hospital visit	40	30	35
90620	Comprehensive consultation	104	93	13
92014	Eye examination and treatment	39	42	−6
Surgery				
27130	Total hip replacement	1955	2404	−19
27244	Repair femur fracture	1188	1299	−9
33512	Coronary artery bypass	2816	3894	−28
35301	Rechannel of artery	1154	1573	−27
44140	Partial removal of colon	1065	1256	−15
49505	Repair inguinal hernia	405	588	−31
52601	Prostatectomy (transurethral resection)	920	1128	−18
Diagnostic				
52000	Cystoscopy	111	105	6
70470	Contrast computed tomographic scans of head	78	113	−31
71010	Roentgenographic examination of chest (one view)	10	12	−20
93000	Electrocardiogram, complete	25	35	−30

*Fees are for procedures performed by the most common specialty in the most common place of service.

screens on the difference between current payments and those projected for the Medicare Fee Schedule. Comparable geographic adjustments to prevailing charges would also be included.

Implementation of the Transitional Fee Schedule would begin about 6 months after enactment of the legislation. After 2 years of experience, the full Medicare Fee Schedule would be implemented, along with coding reforms and changes in locality boundaries. In addition, prevailing and customary charge screens would be eliminated, so that all services would be paid at the fee schedule amount.

POLICIES TO SLOW INCREASES IN EXPENDITURES

Reducing inappropriate and unnecessary services is the best way to contain costs while not sacrificing access and quality of care.

TABLE 2 Percent Change in Medicare Allowed Amounts by Specialty under Medicare Fee Schedule Compared with Customary, Prevailing, and Reasonable (CPR) Charge System

Specialty	% Change*
Medical	21
Internal medicine	18
Family practice	40
Dermatology	1
Surgical	− 11
Ophthalmology	− 16
General surgery	− 10
Orthopedic surgery	− 8
Urology	− 4
Thoracic surgery	− 19
Otolaryngology	7
Obstetrics/gynecology	1
Hospital based	NA
Radiology	− 25
Pathology	− 24
Anesthesia	NA
Other physicians†	

*NA indicates not applicable.

†Other physicians includes important Medicare physician specialties not evaluated in the Hsiao study: cardiovascular disease, clinic, general practice, gastroenterology, nephrology, neurology, neurosurgery, plastic surgery, psychiatry, pulmonary disease, and miscellaneous.

TABLE 3 Percent Change in 1988 Medicare Allowed Amounts by Area under Medicare Fee Schedule Compared with Customary, Prevailing, and Reasonable (CPR) Charge System

Area*	Specialty Group	% Change
Very large metropolitan		
	Medical	− 1
	Surgical	− 26
	All physicians	− 14
Large metropolitan		
	Medical	17
	Surgical	− 12
	All physicians	− 3
Small metropolitan		
	Medical	26
	Surgical	− 7
	All physicians	3
Large rural		
	Medical	31
	Surgical	− 5
	All physicians	13
Small rural		
	Medical	38
	Surgical	− 7
	All physicians	15

*Very large metropolitan areas include counties in metropolitan statistical areas of 5 million or more populations, large metropolitan includes counties in metropolitan statistical areas of 1 million to 5 million populations, and small metropolitan are all other metropolitan counties. These areas accounted for 14%, 37%, and 33%, respectively, of Medicare allowed charges in 1988. Large rural (nonmetropolitan) counties have populations of 25,000 or more, small rural includes all other nonmetropolitan counties. These areas accounted for 9% and 7%, respectively, of Medicare allowed charges in 1988.

The Commission recommends three approaches to slowing expenditure growth as follows:

- giving physicians collective incentives to contain costs through expenditure targets,
- increasing research on effectiveness of care and expanding the development and dissemination of practice guidelines, and
- improving utilization management by carriers and peer review organizations.

Expenditure Targets

The Commission recommends that a national expenditure target for physicians' services under Part B be used to determine annual conversion factor updates under the fee schedule. The target would reflect increases in practice costs, growth in the number of enrollees, and a decision concerning the appropriate rate of increase in volume of services per enrollee. The last factor would reflect trade-offs between beneficiary needs, technological advances, and affordability.

If actual expenditures during a year are equal to targeted expenditures, then the conversion factor update for the following year would be equal to the increase in practice costs. Whether the update would be higher or lower than the increase in practice costs would depend on differences between actual and targeted expenditures.

As an example, assume that practice costs are increasing by 4%, enrollment is growing 2%, and volume of services is projected to increase by 7% per enrollee. This would lead to a 13% increase in expenditures. Now assume that the target is set at 11%, thus permitting a volume increase of 5% instead of the projected 7%. If actual expenditures rise 13%, the conversion factor update for the following year would be 2% (a 4% increase in practice costs minus the 2% by which the target was exceeded). If actual expenditures rise only 9%, the conversion factor update would be 6% (a 4% increase in practice costs plus the 2% by which expenditures were below the target).

The Commission recommends beginning with a single expenditure target at the national level, but anticipates that the policy will evolve to one with multiple targets. For example, targets could be established for states or carrier areas or for categories of services.

Expenditure targets are designed to stimulate efforts by the medical community to work with the Medicare program to increase knowledge of the effectiveness of services, to use this knowledge to increase the appropriateness of care, and to participate more actively in medical review. Encouragement would come from tying the annual update in the Medicare Fee Schedule conversion factor to the difference between the actual rate of increase in expenditures for physicians' services and the target rate of increase. Expenditure targets would not alter the financial incentives for individual physicians and their patients. Rather, the incentives would fall to the physician community, which could respond through education and support of the existing infrastructure of medical review. For example, the AMA and national specialty societies could develop practice guidelines and disseminate them. They could provide technical assistance to carriers and peer review organizations in the development of criteria for review and political support for sanctions of physicians who persisted in providing care that was inappropriate and did not meet standards of quality. To allow time for these efforts to develop, the

Commission recommends that target rates of increase for the first few years not depart substantially from baseline rates of increase.

Effectiveness Research and Practice Guidelines

The Commission recommends a substantial increase in federal support for building our knowledge of the effectiveness and appropriateness of medical practices and getting that knowledge to practicing physicians and their patients. We need to know more about which of our diagnostic tools work and which patients would benefit from particular therapy. This knowledge is essential if we are to reduce unnecessary and inappropriate services.

To increase this knowledge, we need more research to determine the medical outcomes and the costs of alternative medical practices and procedures, and to determine the best ways to organize and provide care. This work would include clinical trials, epidemiologic studies of data generated by clinical practice, analyses of the cost-effectiveness of alternative ways to organize care, and assessment of techniques used in managed care to influence physicians' clinical decisions.

The knowledge we have about effectiveness and appropriateness must be made available to physicians and their patients. Practice guidelines synthesize the best that we know from research and the judgments of practicing physicians into a form that can be readily used. The Commission recommends that the federal government actively encourage the development and dissemination of practice guidelines so that they are incorporated into physicians' practices, made available to patients, and used as the basis for coverage, payment, and medical review criteria developed by hospital medical staffs, carriers, and peer review organizations.

The Commission calls for the federal government to support practice guidelines through funding, coordination, and evaluation. Funds should be used to support and build on existing private sector activities by the medical profession and others. Federal oversight should focus on ensuring the integrity of the process, including the quality of the methods used and of the resulting guidelines, and facilitating efforts to share information, identify issues, and set priorities. The federal government also has a role as administrator of Medicare. The Health Care Financing Administration should reinforce the importance of basing medical review on sound criteria by assisting peer review organizations and carriers in selecting and using review criteria that are consistent with practice guidelines.

Utilization Review

The Commission supports the current efforts by the Health Care Financing Administration to move toward a more comprehensive approach to medical review and calls for further actions to strengthen the review process. If utilization and quality review are to be effective tools both to improve the quality and efficiency of care and to control the growth in Medicare expenditures, the Medicare program will have to create a comprehensive medical review system that looks beyond individual services to complete episodes of care. This requires systematic integration of information drawn from claims data, analysis of practice variations, and peer review of physician practice.

To take on these responsibilities, carriers and peer review organizations will need additional resources and time, more administrative flexibility, and the cooperation of the medical community. The Commission makes a number of recommendations in its report concerning the transition from the current system that has emphasized claims payment to one of comprehensive review.

INFRASTRUCTURE FOR PAYMENT REFORM

Successful implementation of the payment reforms described herein will require investments in the administrative infrastructure of Medicare. We applaud recent efforts by the Health Care Financing Administration to introduce a unique physician identifier, to incorporate diagnostic information on claims forms, and to develop a common working file including data from both Part A (hospital) and Part B (physician) of Medicare.

The Commission recommends two further changes to strengthen the ability to implement these payment reforms. First, Medicare should require providers to submit all claims, whether or not assignment is accepted. Second, the Health Care Financing Administration should take steps to accelerate the trend toward electronic claims submission. In addition, the ability of the carriers to implement a fee schedule and expand their medical review activities is dependent on funding that is adequate and predictable. If there are to be major reforms in this program, the administrative resources to carry them out must be ensured.

CONCLUSION

Three years ago, Congress created this Commissison with a mandate to suggest policies to rationalize the payment for physicians' services by the Medicare program and to slow the rate of growth of expenditures for these services. We believe that a Medicare Fee Schedule will serve to rationalize payments by tying them to resource costs. It will be simpler and easier to understand for both physicians and beneficiaries. It will promote better care and provide additional financial protection for beneficiaries. Expenditure targets will help slow the increase in Medicare expenditures so that we as a society can meet other pressing social needs. And increased effectiveness research and practice guidelines will provide us with the knowledge and means to manage available health care resources more wisely. With these changes, we believe that Medicare can continue to meet the medical needs of our elderly and disabled citizens.

Eli Ginzberg

A Hard Look
at Cost Containment

By the end of 1987, health care expenditures in the United States will have passed the half-trillion-dollar mark. According to forecasts by the U.S. Department of Commerce and the Congressional Budget Office, the estimated expenditure of $511 billion will account for 11.4 percent of the gross national product (GNP)—another record high. In 1980 national health expenditures accounted for 9.1 percent of the GNP, just a decade after President Richard Nixon had warned that the nation was facing a health care crisis because its expenditures totaled $75 billion, or 7.5 percent of the GNP.

Nixon's warning was preceded and followed by a number of efforts by the federal government, often in association with the states and the medical establishment, to contain steeply rising health care expenditures. These efforts included the elimination of the 2 percent override in Medicare's reimbursements to hospitals, the introduction of professional standards review organizations to prevent excessive days of hospitalization, federal support for the establishment of health maintenance organizations (HMOs), a federal-state-area system of health care planning to control new hospital construction and the purchase of expensive equipment, and the reduction of federal support for the education of health professionals. With the election of Ronald Reagan to the presidency, the federal government redoubled its efforts to limit its health care outlays; its efforts were paralleled by those of many of the states and the corporate sector, seeking the same objective.

This article addresses three interrelated questions: What does the record reveal about the success of two decades of efforts at cost containment? What lessons can be extracted from this experience? What is the outlook for cost containment in the middle and longer term?

THE RECORD

Table 1 presents total and per capita national health care expenditures, in current and constant dollars, for selected years since 1960. Because the United

Eli Ginzberg, Ph.D., is director of Conservation of Human Resources in the Graduate School of Business, Columbia University, New York, New York.

TABLE 1 National Health Care Expenditures, 1960 through 1986.*

Year	In Current Dollars			In Constant Dollars†	
	Billions of dollars	% of GNP	Average % change from previous year shown	Billions of dollars	Dollars per capita
1960	26.9	5.3	—	34.0	185
1965	41.9	5.9	9.3	46.8	229
1970	75.0	7.4	12.3	62.2	292
1975	132.7	8.3	12.1	78.5	349
1980	248.1	9.1	13.3	93.3	397
1981	287.0	9.4	15.7	97.5	410
1982	323.6	10.2	12.8	98.5	410
1983	357.2	10.5	10.4	100.0	412
1984	390.2	10.3	9.2	102.8	420
1985	425.0	10.7	8.9	105.4	427
1986	465.4	10.8	9.5	107.4	431
1987‡	511.9	11.4	10.0	—	—

*Data are for selected calendar years and are from the U.S. Department of Commerce and the Health Care Financing Administration (Office of the Actuary, Division of National Cost Estimates).

†The Medical Care Price Index has been used to convert current to constant dollars.
‡Projected.

States population grew rapidly over this quarter century and the economy was buffeted by inflationary pressures, the best single index of expenditures is the per capita outlay in constant dollars, which shows a gain of 133 percent.

Table 1 also indicates the percentage of the GNP contributed by health care expenditures during the same years. This statistic reveals whether the increased expenditures for health care were matched by the growth of the economy and gains in productivity or required the transfer of resources from other areas of the economy. What the rising percentage demonstrates is that economic growth supplied only part of the additional resources that were needed to cover increases in health care costs.

The data underscore several facts: health expenditures in the United States have been increasing rapidly; they have accounted for a steadily rising share of the GNP; and the steepest rate of increase (in constant dollars) occurred in the five years after the introduction of Medicare and Medicaid.

LESSONS ABOUT COST CONTAINMENT

Throughout the 1970s, the federal government and many of the states sought to contain health care costs through planning, regulation, and controls on hospital costs. In the waning days of the Carter administration, however,

Congress balked at continuing on the regulatory route and rejected the President's proposal to impose an annual ceiling on capital expenditures for new hospital construction.

The Reagan administration entered office with a strong antiregulation bias and looked to enlarging the scope of the market and price competition to control health care costs. New competitive forces and a broadened role for price competition have increasingly come to characterize health care, however. Four specific developments are viewed as the foundations of cost containment: the introduction of prospective financing for Medicare beneficiaries who require hospitalization, the proliferation of new forms of prepaid health care delivery, the increasing supply of physicians, and the growth of for-profit health care enterprises.

In assessing the success or failure of cost-containment efforts, it is essential to consider the total use of resources in relation to total useful output, measured by quality as well as quantity. Cost containment should not be confused with cost shifting or with cost reductions in one area, such as inpatient care, without taking into account cost increases in another, such as ambulatory treatment. True cost containment depends on controlling the costs of the health care system as a whole, without impairing quality.

Hospital admissions and days of care peaked before the introduction of diagnosis-related groups in 1983; nevertheless, the federal government's shift to prospective reimbursement for hospital care for Medicare patients unquestionably accelerated the trend toward reducing the number of inpatient hospital days. Since expenditures on hospital care account for 40 percent of total health care outlays, many have interpreted the recent trends toward fewer admissions and shorter stays as major contributions to cost containment, especially because the growth of managed care systems and the expanding scope of ambulatory treatment are seen as further opportunities to reduce overall hospital days.

William B. Schwartz has recently challenged this optimistic view. He has pointed out that the current reductions reflect a one-time gain that results from removing the "fat" in the hospital system and that the underlying factors — continuing advances in technology, population growth, and rising prices (particularly more expensive labor) will reverse the initial decline in the rate of growth of health care costs and maintain an increase in costs of about 7 percent a year. I agree with the thrust of his analysis. Moreover, the cost per hospital admission has continued to increase, even as some of the fat has been removed; despite severe reductions in occupancy, down-scaling and closings of hospitals have been proceeding at a snail's pace, and most calculations of cost containment in inpatient treatment fail to take into account new expenditures for ambulatory care, nursing home services, and home care.

The rapid growth of enrollments in HMOs and preferred-provider organizations (PPOs) is perceived as the necessary precursor of effective cost containment. Admittedly, HMO enrollees have a much lower rate of hospitalization than patients under traditional fee-for-service. But several important countervailing factors need to be considered. HMO and fee-for-service costs have been found to grow at the same rate. Despite the recent rapid growth of prepaid plans, not more than one in six Americans was covered by an HMO or a PPO at the beginning of 1987. The current assumption that at least two of every five insured persons will be enrolled in a prepaid plan by 1990 is probably too optimistic in the face of the steeply growing costs of marketing, the absence of large savings to employers, the difficulties of structuring and managing large prepaid plans, and the growing insistence of employers and consumers on quality controls. The continuing, if somewhat slower, growth of prepaid health plans can be expected to exercise some restraint on cost increases, but it will not be sufficient to reverse their upward trend.

Between 1970 and 1986, the number of physicians per 100,000 population increased from 148 to 220. During the same years, the net pretax income of physicians, in constant dollars, averaged $35,942 (1970) and $35,133 (1985). Applying supply-and-demand analysis to physician services, most mainline economists have looked favorably on increases in the supply of physicians in the expectation that this increase would lower physicians' fee schedules and earnings. The income data just mentioned provide little support for such a conclusion. In most market areas and in most fields of specialization, established physicians are able to influence both the demand for their services (by encouraging return visits by their patients) and their incomes (by raising their fees).

Further increases in the supply of physicians are inevitable because of the large numbers of students already being trained. Even if a further increase of 20 percent in the supply of physicians would depress physicians' earnings by 20 percent, total health care costs would be much more likely to increase than to decline. Since physicians' earnings account for about 20 percent of total health care costs, the savings realized from a reduction in physicians' incomes would be 4 percent. Physicians are said, however, to be responsible for 70 percent of total health care outlays. Hence, a 20 percent increase in their number would generate an increased outlay of 14 percent, or a net increase in health care costs of 10 percent. Because most of the physical facilities of the health care system are now in place, it would be reasonable to reduce this estimate of the additional costs of the new supply of physicians by half—that is, from 10 to 5 percent. But with expenditures now in excess of $500 billion, even the incremental costs of the additional physicians would be substantial, adding $25 billion annually.

The emergence and rapid growth of for-profit hospital chains in the 1970s and the more recent incursion of for-profit enterprises into other areas of health care are viewed by many as the harbingers of greater cost effectiveness resulting from economies of scale, equity financing, and professional management. Some advocates have gone so far as to prophesy that a dozen or so large for-profit health care companies will soon come to dominate the entire health care sector.

Recently, Wall Street has become much less bullish on the for-profit hospital chains; several of the chains have moved from a policy of acquisition to selling off some hospitals that do not fit their new strategies, and their occupancy rates are many points below those of the nonprofit hospitals – a fact that does not augur well for their balance sheets in the future. Only a true believer in private enterprise and the competitive market will look to the for-profit chains for the solution to the problem of the nation's rising health care expenditures.

These are the lessons about cost containment that we can extract from the foregoing analysis: the declining use of hospitals will sooner or later level off, and the growing intensity of treatment will keep hospital costs increasing; prepaid plans are likely to grow more slowly than has been forecast, and the cost differences between such plans and fee-for-service care are likely to narrow; the expanding supply of physicians will lead to an increase, not a decrease, in total health care expenditures; and there is no basis for believing that the for-profit hospital chains will prove more cost effective than the nonprofit hospitals.

Moreover, the boundaries of medicine are continually being expanded, as demonstrated by the new programs for sports medicine, cosmetic surgery, wellness, substance control, and health education – not to mention the uncertainties that attach to the spread of the acquired immunodeficiency syndrome. Although hospital capacity may eventually be considerably reduced, alternative forms of care are likely to proliferate. And the number of physicians – the key determiners of the use of health care resources – will increase. All the above factors point to cost increases, not cost containment.

THE MIDDLE- AND LONGER-TERM OUTLOOK

On the basis of the best estimates of the federal government, total expenditures for health care will be in the range of $640 billion in 1990, with a GNP of around $5.5 trillion. If these forecasts prove to be more or less on target, health care expenditures as a proportion of the GNP will reach a new high of 11.6 percent in 1990. Should there be a recession before then, health care expenditures are likely to exceed 12 percent of the GNP. Nonetheless, in the period from 1985 to 1990, whether or not there is a recession, health care expenditures will increase by 8.4 percent, the lowest increase in any five-year period since the effort at cost containment was first launched.

Two questions remain: Why does the cost spiral continue? And what forces might sooner or later interrupt or possibly even reverse it?

The first question is relatively easy to answer. We have an "open system" with numerous sources of funding for health care. Even the federal government, the largest payer, covers only about one third of the total bill. Corporations, through their benefit plans, cover something over one quarter. The remaining major payers are consumers (who pay out of pocket), states, and other levels of government. With more than 23 million of the nation's elderly persons holding paid membership in the American Association of Retired

Persons, Congress will find it difficult, if not impossible, in the absence of an overriding financial crisis, to cut back substantially on Medicare benefits. In fact, Congress is about to consider the addition of coverage for catastrophic illness under Medicare and may even consider coverage for long-term care at some later time.

State governments are wrestling with the urgent need to improve their Medicaid programs and are exploring alternative ways to protect the uninsured through subsidized insurance or a mechanism for reimbursing providers who care for the insured. Many corporations have been successful in recent years in renegotiating health care benefits for their employees, with the result that employees now have less first-day coverage and pay more out of pocket for health care in the form of deductibles and coinsurance. Further large-scale give-backs by employees can probably be secured only at the risk of costly strikes, which most employers will seek to avoid.

The answer to why costs continue to rise, then, lies in our open system of health care payment in the United States, which depends on the decisions of the federal and state legislatures, large and medium-sized corporations, and consumers. The American people have indicated repeatedly, in response to surveys, that they want more and better health care services. And many nonprofit, for-profit, and government health care providers are able to continue to enter the capital markets and obtain new funding to meet these increased demands.

What about the longer term? Clearly, there is an upper limit on the proportion of the GNP that the American people will be willing to spend on health care—possibly 15 percent, perhaps as much as 20 percent. But before we reach that theoretical upper limit, other forces may come into play. We could face a major crisis in the federal budget, which could lead to the transformation of Medicare into a means-tested program. We could fail to provide essential care to increasing numbers of uninsured persons, thereby creating renewed political momentum for national health insurance. The competitive position of American business could become so endangered that a growing number of large, medium-sized, and small corporations would have no alternative but to cut back on employees' health care benefits. One can think of other pressures and responses, including limiting the introduction of high-cost technology and explicit attempts to ration high-cost treatments.

A society such as ours—which places a high value on pluralism, which is enthralled by technology, which resists domination by the federal government, which accepts the prevailing inequality of income and wealth, and which promotes the sovereignty of consumers—is not likely to opt for serious constraints on biomedical research and development or to favor the explicit rationing of proved health care services to the public. Its concerns are more likely to be focused on ensuring access for the entire population to an effective level of care and on finding a way of covering the health care costs of those who cannot pay their own way. Until we approach the upper limit of acceptable health care expenditures—an eventuality that may be far in the future—cost containment is likely to remain the elusive hare that the hounds pursue but never overtake.

Our message is simple and it's straightforward. The hospital field in the United States today is in fragile condition. . . . Congress can no longer balance the budget with cuts in the public Medicare and Medicaid expenditures without damage to all who rely on a sound health care delivery system.

CAROL MCCARTHY
President
American Hospital Association

Victor R. Fuchs

Has Cost Containment Gone Too Far?

Cost-containment strategies are sweeping through the health care system like fire through parched underbrush. Medicare's prospective payment system based on diagnosis related groups is leading the way, with health maintenance organizations, preferred provider organizations, state regulatory agencies, and deductibles and coinsurance close behind. The reasons for the changes in health care financing and organizations are well understood. But what about their effects? We know that there was a dramatic decline in the rate of growth of health care expenditures in 1984, but other than that it is too soon to expect systematic, definitive assessments.

Over the long run, the current reimbursement revolution is likely to change every aspect of the health care system: medical practice, medical education, medical research. Moreover, the effects are likely to vary greatly among patients by age, income, and employment status, and among hospitals and physicians by type, location, and specialty. The debate over whether cost containment has gone too far has already begun. This article does not attempt to resolve that debate or to discuss all of the eventual ramifications of cost containment. It does offer a framework for thinking about the direct effects of current policies on *health and social welfare*, and it shows why reasonable observers may differ in their evaluation of cost containment.

HOW COST CONTAINMENT WORKS

Regardless of whether cost containment is sought through competition or regulation or a combination of both, reductions in spending on health care can be achieved in only three ways. First, the producers of health care may be forced to increase *production efficiency*, i.e., to deliver the same amount of services with fewer inputs. Such gains in efficiency are always possible in every organization, but it is unlikely that they will prove to be a major source of cost reduction. Even under the old payment systems there was no reward for the

Victor R. Fuchs, Ph.D., is research associate, National Bureau of Economic Research, and Henry J. Kaiser, Jr., Professor, Department of Economics and Department of Health Research and Policy, Stanford University, Stanford, California.

inefficiency associated with using more resources for a given amount of services. The inefficiencies that critics pointed to had more to do with what care was delivered than *how* it was produced.

Second, even with the amount of services and production efficiency unchanged, health care spending can be reduced by *reducing the prices* paid for inputs. As with efficiency, it is always possible to squeeze input prices a little to trim nurses' wages and physicians' fees and drug industry profits. But it is highly unlikely that this will be the major source of cost reduction, especially over the long run. In the short run, supplies of inputs may be relatively inelastic and, therefore, their prices can be squeezed. In the long run, however, nurses, physicians, drug companies, and other inputs into health care must receive competitive compensation or the supplies will not be forthcoming.

The third, and by far the most important way to contain costs is to deliver fewer services. At the most fundamental level, cost containment must mean fewer hospital admissions, shorter lengths of stay, fewer tests and X-rays, and similar reductions across the spectrum of care. Thus, the question about the effects of cost containment can be restated: How will health and social welfare be affected by a reduction in the amount of health services? This question can be illuminated with the help of a few diagrams.

MAXIMIZING HEALTH AND SOCIAL WELFARE

Figure 1a presents a stylized description of the relation between health benefit and amount of services, defined to include all possible dimensions. For instance, an increase in the amount of care can be thought of as an increase in length of stay in the hospital (holding services per day constant), or as an increase in the number of tests per day, or as any combination of changes in days and tests that results in more services. For each patient the health benefit typically increases as the amount of services increases, but at a decreasing rate. Eventually a point is reached, Q_2, where the health benefit is at a maximum, and additional services do more harm than good. To be sure, health benefits also depend on the timeliness and appropriateness of services, but it is useful to focus on the effects of changes in the quantity of services, holding constant the levels of timeliness and appropriateness.

Figure 1a also records how cost changes as the amount of services increases. To simplify the presentation without undue violence to reality, it is assumed that cost rises at a constant rate, i.e., each additional unit of service adds as much to cost as does the preceding unit. If all the benefits of care are reflected in the health curve, the amount of services that maximizes social welfare is Q_1. If any less care is provided, the benefit would decrease more than the cost; if any amount greater than Q_1, is provided, cost would increase more than the benefit.

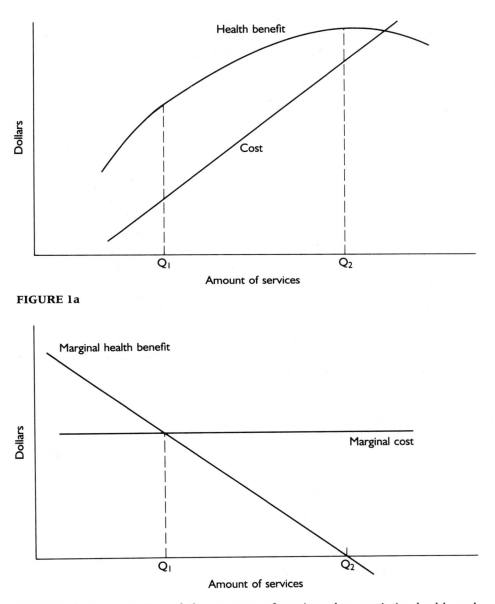

FIGURE 1a

FIGURE 1b Determination of the amounts of services that maximize health and social welfare.

The basis for defining the amounts of services that maximize health and maximize social welfare can perhaps be seen more clearly in figure 1b, which shows the marginal (i.e., additional) benefit and marginal cost curves derived from the total benefit and total cost curves of figure la. The exact shape of the marginal benefit curve will vary from disease to disease and from patient to patient, but the marginal benefit, on average, surely declines as the amount of services increases, and eventually becomes negative. Overall, the linear approximation may not be far off, and greatly simplifies the analysis.

THE EFFECTS OF LESS CARE

What happens as cost-containment strategies reduce the amount of services? The answer clearly depends on how much is being provided. Any reductions that occur to the right of Q_2 will result in an improvement in health; reductions to the left of Q_2 will decrease health. For social welfare, Q_1 is the critical point. Reductions in the amount of services to the right of Q_1 increase social welfare (because they reduce cost more than benefit); reductions to the left decrease social welfare (because they reduce benefit more than cost). Thus, the effect of cost containment on health may differ from the effect on social welfare; any reductions between Q_1 and Q_2 would simultaneously decrease health and increase social welfare. Both effects, however, depend on the initial distribution of patients by amount of services and on the change in services.

It is reasonable to assume that prior to cost containment different patients are receiving different amounts of services (relative to potential benefit); a stylized description of such a frequency distribution is presented in figure 2. Some patients are receiving the amount that maximizes the health benefit, Q_2; some are receiving more, and some less. Some patients may not even be receiving as much as Q_1. *This distribution and the size and pattern of the reduction in services determine the changes in health and social welfare.* Consider the following hypothetical scenarios:

1. Equal absolute reductions.

If cost containment results in a uniform absolute reduction, *a*, in the amount of services received by each patient, the average effects on health and social welfare will be determined entirely by the size of the reduction, *a*, and the *mean* ($\overline{Q}$) of the distribution prior to the change. For instance, suppose the reduction in services takes the form of two days less hospitalization for every patient. The effect on health will be favorable if (prior to cost containment) the mean length of stay was more than one day to the right of Q_2. If the mean was less than one day in excess of Q_2, the effect on health will be unfavorable; the further to the left the mean was, the more unfavorable the effect. In the same way, the effect on social welfare will be favorable if the mean was to the right of Q_1 by more than one-half *a* and unfavorable if it was not.

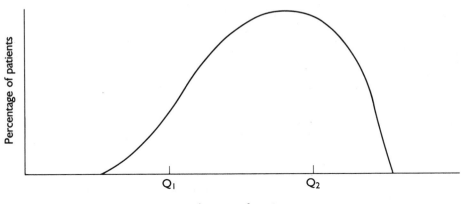

FIGURE 2 Hypothetical distribution of patients.

2. Equal percentage reductions.

Suppose that cost containment results in a uniform percentage reduction, α, in the amount of services received by each patient. For instance, suppose each length of stay is reduced by αQ where Q is the original amount. In that case, the effects on health and social welfare will depend on the size of α, the mean of the distribution, $\overline{Q}$, and the variance (σ^2) of the distribution. The larger is the variance, the smaller can be $\overline{Q}$ consistent with a favorable effect on health or social welfare.

Although the relation between the change in health and α, $\overline{Q}$, and σ^2 is complicated, the reason why the variance matters is not. If the variance is very small, as in figure 3a, an equal percentage reduction for each patient is almost the same as an equal absolute reduction, but if the variance is large (figure 3b), those patients who were receiving the greatest amount of services will receive much larger absolute reductions. This will result in more favorable (or less unfavorable) effects on health and social welfare than if every patient received the same absolute reduction.

Thus, equal percentage reductions will not decrease health even if $\overline{Q}$ is less than Q_2, provided the variance is sufficiently large and α is not tremendously large. For instance, if $\overline{Q} = Q_2$ prior to cost containment and the reduction in care was 30 percent ($\alpha = .3$) there would be a favorable effect on health if the variance exceeded .176. All these results are identical for social welfare if Q_1 is substituted for Q_2.

3. Unequal percentage reductions.

If the reductions are selective, i.e., if the patients receiving more services (relative to potential benefit) experience larger than average percentage reductions, the effects on health and social welfare will be more favorable than those

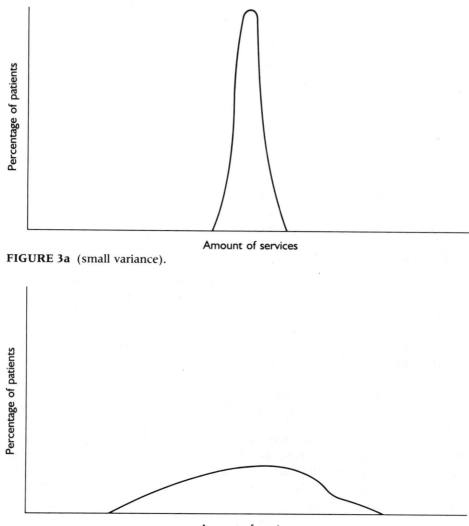

FIGURE 3a (small variance).

FIGURE 3b (large variance).

in case 2 for any given values of $\overline{Q}$ and σ^2. Of course, if the reductions are perversely selective, i.e., if those patients receiving fewer services (relative to potential benefit) experience larger than average percentage reductions, the effects will be less favorable than in case 2.

THE POLICY DEBATES

The foregoing analytical discussion should help to clarify key aspects of the current debate about whether cost containment has gone too far.

Disagreement over the criterion for judging "too far." Which side a person takes in this debate may depend on whether health or social welfare is the criterion. It is certainly possible (many experts would say probable) that reductions in the amount of services will simultaneously decrease health but increase social welfare because the value of the decreases in health will be smaller than the value of the resources freed for other uses.

Disagreement over the distribution prior to cost containment. Even individuals who agree that health should be the criterion may disagree about the distribution of patients with respect to Q_2 prior to cost containment. If $\overline{Q}$ is substantially to the right of Q_2 (a large amount of services that harm health), then equal absolute reductions in care will not reduce health on average. Some patients will be hurt by the reductions but others will benefit. Even if $\overline{Q}$ is to the left of Q_2 it is still possible for equal percentage reductions to be benign if the prior distribution has considerable variance.

Disagreement over how selective the reductions will be. Even individuals who agree about the criterion and about the prior distribution may disagree about how the reductions will be applied. If reductions are selectively concentrated on those patients who were receiving too much care, the effect will be very different than if the reductions are experienced by all patients.

In the absence of hard data it is not surprising that experts differ in their estimates of the prior distribution and of the probability that reductions will be selective. Those who believe that many patients receive excessive care and that the variance is large can point to the uneven incidence of surgery across geographical areas. They may also cite the findings of the Rand Health Insurance Experiment that although cost sharing resulted insubstantial reductions in the amount of care received by some families, no major effects on health were observed for either adults or children.

On the other hand, a study of the effects of Medicare and Medicaid on utilization of surgical operations casts doubt on the ability of patients to reduce care selectively when faced with less insurance coverage. Urban nonwhites experienced an increase of 50 percent in their utilization of 11 selected surgical procedures after the government insurance programs went into effect, but the average level of urgency or necessity of the procedures performed on these patients was the same as it was prior to Medicare and Medicaid. If any selectivity had been present during the period of limited or no insurance, the average level of urgency and necessity should have fallen as the amount of services increased. There is no doubt that deductibles and coinsurance can induce consumers to demand less medical care, but given the complexity of many medical decisions, it is questionable whether consumers know which services to cut back on and which to retain.

Selectivity will become increasingly important as the reductions in amount of care (relative to potential benefit) grow larger. The more selective the reductions, the greater can be the decrease in cost for any given change in health or social welfare. This suggests that the question "Is cost containment being pursued in the best possible way?" may be as important as how far it is pursued. Those strategies such as prepaid group practice that rely on physicians to contain costs are likely to result in more selective reductions than those relying on patients' responses to cost sharing: physicians have more understanding of the potential effects on health of alternative protocols. Moreover, the improvement and expansion of research and education programs designed to increase that understanding will be essential in the long run in order to contain costs in the best possible way.

The question is to decide whether health or economic growth should have priority in determining the type of environment in which we live.

RENE DUBOS

6

Competition vs. Regulation

Aʟᴛʜᴏᴜɢʜ ᴀᴛ ᴏɴᴇ ᴛɪᴍᴇ Americans believed that theirs was the best
health care system in the world, this is no longer true. In fact, a 1989
Louis Harris and Associates survey reported that Americans are more dissatisfied with their health system than either Canadians or Britons, despite our
higher levels of health care spending. The poll reported that 89 percent of U.S.
residents called for fundamental changes in the delivery of health services, and
61 percent would be pleased to trade the U.S. system for a model like that in
Canada. This new climate of public opinion reflects dissatisfaction with a
number of aspects of the current system, including limitations on access to
services, high costs, complex technologies, fragmentation of services, uneven
quality, and many others.

Some say this is but another expression of the basic American wish to have
our cake and eat it too. We want miracle cures, but we don't want prices to go
up, and we don't want to pay spiraling costs for the aged and the indigent
through our public health insurance programs — Medicare and Medicaid.

Although the system is meeting the personal needs of many people,
collectively there are failures. These failures reflect the tradeoffs that are
necessary under the current payment system. For example, over 25 million
low-income people have no insurance coverage and thus no means of payment
for health care, and these are often the people who most desperately need care.
In addition, the great expense and scarcity of many advanced technologies
force health care providers to weigh individual circumstances of patients

against economic constraints in making therapeutic decisions. Thus, providers find they must limit resources and keep treatment from patients who could benefit from the care. A recent report that infant mortality was higher in the United States than in Singapore and that the U.S. ranked only eighteenth in infant mortality worldwide raised many questions about the unavailability of prenatal care to certain groups in this country, which experts say could prevent needless deaths.

Currently, there is a hot debate about changes in financing and organization that may or may not rectify the problems faced by the health care industry and may or may not address some sources of dissatisfaction reflected in the Harris poll. In the 1980s, the trend toward for-profit medicine emerged in the form of privately owned proprietary hospitals and nursing homes, laboratories, emergency service centers, alcoholism and drug treatment programs, psychiatric hospitals, and other health services. This has been coupled with an increase in centralized ownership and investor-owned national chains, which tend to seek out the affluent markets. The policies under President Reagan during the 1980s favored employment of market principles in allocating health resources thus progressing toward greater competition in health care and away from strict regulation of the industry and universal coverage.

This chapter opens with a statement by health economist Victor R. Fuchs, who is perhaps best known for his 1974 book entitled *Who Shall Live?* wherein he outlined the difficult dilemma faced by the U.S. in deciding what kind of a health care system it can and will support. He pointed out that Americans cannot have it all, but indeed they can address the significant problems of cost and access in a manner that will result in major improvements in the health care system and in the health of the population. In this article Dr. Fuchs begins by asking the question whether the current movement toward competition is really even competition at all and in any event what the results have been. He then discusses the reasons for failure of the cost-containment efforts of the 1980s and closes with some projections for the future of the health care market.

Bruce C. Vladeck, currently president of the United Hospital Fund in New York, presents "The Case for Regulation." Although he concludes that it doesn't make sense to talk generically about regulation, he outlines the measures by which regulation can and should be a means to an end. For that matter, he points out, competition should also be viewed in this context. The conflict is not over competition vs. regulation, he says, but rather it is between two value systems — one that would emphasize the quality of available services and one that would emphasize the importance of access to services as a right of everyone in our society.

Alain C. Enthoven's article "Health Care Costs: Why Regulation Fails, Why Competition Works, How to Get There From Here," reflects the author's early espousal of the cause of competition in the health care marketplace. He takes an optimistic view of fair competition as a means to address the underlying causes of uncontrolled cost increases. He outlines the principles of a system of fair competition, which he says would result in the survival of health plans that offer good value to their customers, and he recommends that the government eliminate the barriers to this type of market system.

The question is to decide whether health or economic growth should have priority in determining the type of environment in which we live.

RENE DUBOS

Victor R. Fuchs

The "Competition Revolution" in Health Care

Any attempt to assess the effects of a revolution that is less than a decade old and still in progress is fraught with danger. The relevant data appear only with a lag and are subject to revision. Some of the most important effects necessarily occur slowly, and at this point any evaluation of recent changes in health care must contain large elements of forecast as well as measurement after the fact. My assignment poses an additional problem because the health care revolution has been widely advertised as one of "increasing competition." Is this characterization correct? To what extent have recent changes in organization and finance increased competition among health care providers? To answer these questions we first must consider what economists mean by competition and appraise the factors that limit competition in health care. The major portion of this article deals with the effects of the revolution regardless of whether related to competition or not. We will see that the cost-containment efforts of the 1980s did not result in a slowing of expenditures for health care. The reasons for this apparent failure and the implications for the future are discussed.

HEALTH CARE COMPETITION IN CONTEXT

Health care is, in many respects, similar to other goods and services. It is produced with resources that are scarce relative to human wants. Thus every society must have control mechanisms for determining how much health care to produce, how to produce it, and how to distribute it among the population. In principle, only three types of mechanisms are available: the market, central direction, and traditional norms. Kenneth Boulding has characterized these alternatives as the exchange system, the threat system, and the integrative system. All modern societies use a combination of the three, but the proportions vary greatly from country to country and from time to time within the same country.

Victor R. Fuchs, Ph.D., is research associate, National Bureau of Economic Research, and Henry J. Kaiser, Jr., Professor, Department of Economics and Department of Health Research and Policy, Stanford University, Stanford, California.

For the market approach to succeed, competition must be present. Without competition, sellers with monopoly power or buyers with monopsony power can take advantage of their customers or their suppliers with results that are neither efficient nor equitable. Most health care markets depart substantially from competitive conditions, sometimes inevitably and sometimes as a result of deliberate public or private policy. One question of interest is the extent to which the changes in finance and reimbursement of recent years have moved health care markets toward a more competitive structure. Another, to be discussed at the end of the article, is whether the competitive market approach is the goal toward which health policy should strive.

The term competition has a long and complex history in economics. To Adam Smith it was a powerful, beneficent instrument of change that would liberate the economy from the deadening influence of mercantilist restrictions. With extraordinary vision, he saw that if the anticompetitive influence of government were eliminated, the market system literally could create the "wealth of nations." He also warned against private attempts to limit competition, especially the propensity of people of the same trade to meet together "even for merriment and diversion, but the conversation ends in a conspiracy against the public."

Following the prescriptions of Smith, Ricardo, and other classical economists, nineteenth-century England developed the competitive market approach in full force, and the British economy prospered. Many noneconomists, however, railed against the evils of competition, and the term began to acquire an odious connotation.

In modern times, economic theorists have defined competition (and its many variants) with greater precision. *Perfect* competition means that the individual seller or buyer is so small relative to the total market that the actions of that seller or buyer have no effect on the market price. Each producer's output is indistinguishable from competitors', and there is perfect information on both sides of the market. Given certain assumptions about preferences, income distribution, and economies of scale, perfect competition constitutes an ideal in the sense that if it prevailed in every market, resources would be allocated in a socially optimal way.

A more practical approach to the question of competition emphasizes the following conditions: (1) A large number of buyers and sellers, no one of whom is so big as to have a significant influence on the market price; (2) no collusion among the buyers or sellers to fix prices or quantities; (3) relatively free and easy entry into the market by new buyers or sellers; (4) no governmentally imposed restraints on prices or quantities; and (5) reasonably good information about price and quality known to buyers and sellers.

In short, the structure of the market (number of firms and their size distribution), barriers to entry, and privately initiated or government-sanctioned collusion generally determine the extent of competition. In health care markets there is another consideration: Are the buyers of health care sensitive to costs?

If they are not, the question of competition among suppliers is less relevant. One consequence of competition, in health care as well as other markets, is a reduction in profits.

Let us look at each sector of the health care industry and ask whether recent changes have moved the sector in a more competitive direction. Health insurance has always been competitive, with hundreds of firms seeking business in most large markets. Nationally, over 1,200 firms sell health insurance, and the number has not changed materially in the 1980s. In some markets, Blue Cross and Blue Shield (the "Blues") have a dominant share, and they have been accused of competing "unfairly" by getting discounts from hospitals. Health insurance company profits are not known precisely and fluctuate markedly from year to year. The conventional wisdom is that they were low in the early 1980s, rose sharply in 1984 and 1985, and have been falling since then. Much of the recent pressure on profits comes from insurance company ventures in health maintenance organizations (HMOs) and preferred provider organizations (PPOs).

The number of hospitals certainly has not increased in the 1980s; indeed, it has decreased slightly, and this decrease has been widely applauded. Many hospitals have no close competitors because they are located in areas with small populations. Hospitals located close to one another have always competed, but in the past the target was usually physicians, and the bait was better equipment, bigger support staff, and the like. Now the target is more likely to be patients, who are wooed with amenities and services on the one hand, or with price discounts (to large buyers) on the other. If the total amount of competition among hospitals increased in the 1980s, profits should have fallen; however, there is no evidence of that through 1985. In that year, profits from the prospective payment system (PPS) were estimated at $5.1 billion or a profit/revenue rate of 15.3 percent. In 1986, however, profits probably did fall as the large buyers of care, both public and private, began to press harder on price and utilization.

The number of physicians has increased in the 1980s, but the rate of increase has been no more rapid than in the 1970s, when competition was rarely mentioned. Moreover, during the 1980s, there has been an effort to get medical schools to reduce enrollment or to close altogether, and the number of independent physicians has declined as a result of a trend toward larger groups and organized practices.

There has been a large increase in the number of organized health plans and a big increase in competition in that sector. Thus, an organization such as Kaiser Permanente, which frequently was the only plan in an area, undoubtedly has perceived a big increase in competition. At one time Kaiser was the only organization offering managed care in many markets, and their low costs relative to conventional insurance plans insulated them from competitive pressures. All that has changed. Furthermore, the increased emphasis on self-insurance by large firms and on experience rating by health insurers threatens the survival of Kaiser's community-rating approach. With respect to collusion, there probably has been some reduction through the elimination of laws that prohibited selective contracting.

Price discounting is more widespread now than in the past, although until we have information on utilization and quality of care we will not know whether discounts truly lower the cost of care. It is ironic that selective price discounting by hospitals and physicians now is hailed as evidence of competition, when one of the most frequently cited articles in health economics, Reuben Kessel's "Price Discrimination in Medicine," concluded that the existence of sliding fees proved that physicians had monopoly power.

Most of the barriers to entry into health care markets — licensure, accreditation, and certification — are about the same today as in 1980. The growth of for-profit firms, however, with their access to equity capital, may have encouraged entry in some areas. There certainly has not been any reduction in governmentally imposed prices; at the state level, especially, the trend has been toward more government intervention.

Finally, with respect to information available to buyers, there has been a small increase in the form of health plan evaluations and some primitive quality-of-care measures for hospitals. Yet, the fundamental problem remains: patients frequently have great difficulty determining how much and what kind of medical care they need, and they probably always will.

In short, except for the growth of organized health plans, I would not characterize the 1980s as a period of substantial increases in health care competition. I say this even though most physicians, hospital administrators, and other health professionals feel that they are under increased pressure, which they attribute to competition. Most of this pressure, however, really comes from another source, namely, more activist policies by the buyers of health care. The large buyers have decided to exert "countervailing power" against the sellers. This may be socially desirable, but it is not the same as competition. However, a shift away from open-ended, cost-unconscious third-party reimbursement is resulting in more emphasis on price as opposed to nonprice competition. Also, a shift from inpatient to ambulatory care has forced many hospitals to seek new sources of revenue.

WHAT REALLY HAPPENED?

In the three decades preceding 1980, demand for health care increased enormously, beginning with the rapid diffusion of private health insurance. The number of persons with hospital insurance jumped from 32 million at the end of World War II to 122 million by 1960, and coverage for physicians' services soared from fewer than 5 million to over 83 million. Then, when the spread of private insurance ran out of steam, tens of millions of additional Americans obtained health insurance coverage through the Medicare and Medicaid legislation of 1965.

Changes on the demand side were accompanied by substantial shifts in supply. Between 1950 and 1980, the number of short-term hospital beds per 1,000 population rose from 3.3 to 4.4, hospital personnel per patient soared from 1.8 to 3.8, and physicians per 1,000 population jumped from 1.5 to 2.1. Generous funding from the National Institutes of Health (NIH), as well as heavy investment by drug companies and other private firms, contributed to a scientific and technologic transformation of medical practice.

For three decades, "highest-quality care for all" dominated the health policy agenda. Not surprisingly, spending for health care jumped from 4.6 percent to 9.1 percent of the gross national product (GNP). As 1980 approached, however, concern shifted from increasing access and raising quality to curbing the skyrocketing cost of health care.

In assessing the possible mechanisms to achieve cost containment, policy-makers ruled out self-regulation by physicians and hospitals as ineffective. A so-called voluntary approach had been tried in the 1970s and been found wanting. Direct regulation by the federal government, as implied in the Carter-Califano proposals, also was rejected as inconsistent with the political-economic temper of the times. With air transportation, trucking, banking, and other industries being thrown open to the rigors of the unregulated market-place, there was little support in Washington for close regulation of health care. A few states, however, did adopt a regulatory approach through hospital commissions charged with setting rates and controlling utilization.

Prospective payment.   Probably the most important change in the 1980s was the introduction by the federal government of a prospective payment system (PPS) for Medicare beneficiaries, based on diagnosis related groups (DRGs). Although this change has helped to slow the rate of growth of hospital expenditures, it has little to do with competition. To see this, imagine that all hospitals were owned by one giant corporation, HMA (Hospital Monopoly of America). The switch from a system of cost reimbursement to a prospectively set fixed fee could result in a slowing of expenditures and put great pressure on HMA even though its monopoly position was unchanged.

The impact of PPS on hospital length-of-stay has been substantial. Hospitals reimbursed under PPS had much smaller increases in costs per case than those still covered by the previous Tax Equity and Fiscal Responsibility Act (TEFRA) system (+7.6 percent versus +18.1 percent between 1982 and 1984). The most important factor was a more rapid decline in average length-of-stay in the hospitals paid by PPS (−14.6 percent versus −7.9 percent).

The role of competition in this decline is unclear. A recent study of California hospitals by Melnick and Zwanziger concluded that those located in highly competitive markets were more responsive to cost containment in 1983–1985 than were hospitals in areas with very little competition. In 1983, however, the hospitals in the highly competitive markets had almost 50 percent higher expenses per admission, so it is not surprising that they would be affected more by PPS and similar cost-containment efforts. In a national study, Robinson and Luft reported that costs actually are higher in hospitals located in competitive markets than in hospitals that have no close competitors (controlling for wage rates, patient case-mix, state regulatory programs, and teaching status of hospitals). In the past, competition between hospitals typically took cost-increasing, nonprice forms such as meeting physicians' requests for new technologies. Currently, there probably is more emphasis on price competition, but extensive expenditures for advertising, community relations, and outreach programs show that nonprice competition is still significant. The new nonprice competition is focused more on patients and less on physicians.

Another aspect of cost containment in the 1980s is a reversal of the egalitarian ethos of the 1960s and 1970s. In recent years, we have seen reductions in health care programs for the poor, elimination of cross-subsidies by tying premiums more closely to experience, and attempts to reduce utilization via deductibles and copayment. Regardless of whether these changes are good or bad, they should not be mistaken for changes in competition among suppliers.

Consider the RAND health insurance experiment, which conclusively demonstrated that the "general law of demand" applies to medical care as well as to wheat and widgets. In a prospective, carefully controlled study, families with full insurance coverage used more care than those with cost sharing. Although this result often is cited in support of the competition argument, no such inference is warranted. Both the free-care families and the cost-sharing families received their care in the same markets, and the cost-sharing effect on utilization was as large in a site that had fewer than two dozen physicians as in a site that had several thousand.

From a theoretical perspective, it is not clear that more competition would enhance the cost-saving effects of deductibles and coinsurance. Given the inevitability of imperfect information, rival health plans faced with decreasing demand might increase marketing expenditures more than a monopoly would. At least some of these expenditures would be a dead-weight loss from the point of view of consumer welfare.

How effective was cost containment? The question of competition aside, did cost containment reduce the rate of growth of health care expenditures? The answer is that it did not, at least so far. The overall growth of real expenditures per capita was more rapid after 1980 than in the previous decade. Disaggregation reveals that expenditures for hospital care did slow appreciably after 1983, but expenditures for physicians' services accelerated rapidly throughout the 1980s. Indeed, spending for physicians grew at a faster rate from 1980 to 1986 than in the euphoric period following the introduction of Medicare and Medicaid in the late 1960s. Spending for dental care, other professional services, drugs and sundries, other personal care, and "program administration and net cost of private insurance" also accelerated in the 1980s. The increase in the last item was so great that one may suspect some accounting artifact. The growth of nursing home expenditures slowed somewhat after 1980, and government public health expenditures also grew less rapidly. The latter change reflects government policy and bears no relation to market structure.

FAILURE TO DECREASE SPENDING

To gain insights regarding the failure of the health care revolution to slow spending in the 1980s, it is useful to begin with a cost-containment identity:

$$\text{Expenditures} \equiv \begin{bmatrix} \text{quantity of inputs per} \\ \text{unit of service} \end{bmatrix} \begin{bmatrix} \text{prices of} \\ \text{inputs} \end{bmatrix} \begin{bmatrix} \text{quantity of} \\ \text{services} \end{bmatrix}$$

By definition, expenditures depend upon the reciprocal of productivity (the first term) multiplied by the prices of the factors of production (including profits) multiplied by the quantity of services (including quality as one dimension of quantity). For cost containment to have had an effect, it would have had to have worked through one or more of these three terms.

Productivity.   The first term, the reciprocal of productivity, is extremely difficult to measure, but in my judgment there was not much improvement. Moreover, the potential for change is not large. This term measures *production efficiency* in the narrow sense of the quantity of services delivered to patients, regardless of the value of those services. It does not purport to measure efficiency in the broad sense of changes in health outcomes or other aspects of patient satisfaction.

In my view, there is only limited potential for increasing the quantity of services produced with a given quantity of resources or for producing the existing quantity of services with fewer resources. No doubt every organization runs with some slack, and most individuals could work harder than they do. However, the notion that there is large potential for cost containment through increases in production efficiency is misguided. To put the matter in simplest terms, how much additional nursing services can be obtained from a fixed number of nurses? In the short run, nurses probably can be pressed to work harder, but, in the long run, they will quit or demand higher pay for the harder work. One obvious way to increase productive efficiency would be to reduce the number of physicians in specialties with large excess capacity, but such reductions will come slowly, if at all.

The limited measures of productivity that are readily available, such as the number of hospital personnel per patient or number of physicians per 1,000 patient visits, show no improvement since 1980, and perhaps a deterioration. To be sure, the quantity of services per patient day and per visit probably increased, but we do not know by how much. We do know that after 1980 there was a considerable increase in resources going into marketing, advertising, new computer systems, management consulting, and the like. Whether these additional inputs resulted in an equivalent increase in services to patients is unclear. Also unclear is whether the additional inputs required by hospitals and physicians to adapt to the changes in health care finance are "one-time" or whether they will continue. For the period 1980–1986, 1 would not be surprised if subsequent research shows that the productivity term made a negative contribution to cost containment.

Input prices.   The second term on the right-hand side of the cost-containment identity refers to the prices of inputs (of given quality), including inputs of capital and entrepreneurial skill. Thus this term includes profit as a price. The most important input to health care is labor, and fortunately we have good data on wages in health and other industries. These data show that hourly earnings of health care workers grew faster than the earnings of other American workers between 1979 and 1985.

The gap of over one percentage point per year cannot be explained by differences in employment growth. It is true that employment grew much more rapidly in health than in the goods sector (mining, manufacturing, and the like), but employment in other services (banking, finance, retail trade, personal services, education, and so on) grew almost as rapidly as in health.

Whatever else cost containment did, it did not noticeably depress the price of labor—the most important input. This is not surprising. The health industry must offer competitive wages if it is to be able to attract the quantity and quality of labor it needs.

Quantity of services.   If changes in productivity and input prices did not (and in my opinion cannot) contribute much to a slowing of health care expenditures, that leaves the third term, quantity of services, as the only significant mechanism through which costs can be contained. Sooner or later the only way to cut health care spending significantly is to reduce the quantity of services delivered to patients.

Recent cost-containment efforts did have a major impact on the quantity of hospital care delivered to Medicare beneficiaries. The number of bills (a good index of number of admissions) declined in the 1980s instead of rising rapidly as in the late 1970s; average length-of-stay decreased more dramatically than before; and the number of days of care stopped rising and then fell rapidly. If the average rate of decline of 5.5 percent per year were to continue for eight more years, the number of days of care would fall to one-half the 1980 level!

Total charges (deflated) continued to rise, but at a much lower rate than before 1980. The rate of increase in charges per bill was relatively unchanged, but reimbursement per bill rose 1 percent per year faster after 1980, contributing to better profit rates for hospitals under PPS.

With respect to the population under age sixty-five, the growth of participation in HMOs from 5 percent to 12 percent of the population (1980–1986) also must have had an appreciable effect on hospital use. HMO members typically use only about two-thirds as much hospital care as the rest of the population; thus the shift in proportions would explain a decrease in hospitalization of 0.4 percent per year even if everything else remained constant.

It seems clear that the cost-containment efforts did have an impact on hospital services, not only for the Medicare population but for patients under sixty-five as well.

Cost containment has yet to make an impact on physicians' services. The number of bills for Medicare beneficiaries grew somewhat more slowly after 1980 than in the 1970s, but the growth rate for allowed charges continued at almost 8 percent per year, deflated.

For the population as a whole, there is uncertainty about the trend in number of visits to physicians. At this point, the most reasonable conclusion is that number of visits probably did not change much one way or the other; the intensity of each visit probably increased.

OTHER EXPLANATIONS

The failure of cost-containment efforts in the 1980s to have much effect on expenditures does not come as much of a surprise to those who emphasize supply factors — hospitals, physicians, and technology — as major influences on costs. In 1980, a huge hospital capacity was already in place, and fewer patient days do not translate into equivalent reductions in costs until hospitals actually close. Hospital closure comes slowly, but the pace is increasing: eighty-three in 1986 compared with sixty-one in 1985 and an average of fifty-four per year in 1980–1984.

Physician supply.   A large physician supply also was in place in 1980, and continued to increase after that date. It takes at least a decade for changes in demand to affect the flow of new physicians into the market, and even longer for changes in the flow to have a significant effect on the size of the total stock and its distribution among specialties.

Fees for specialty care and the number of specialists have, as yet, been relatively untouched. The failure of fees to fall to a level that would eliminate the excess capacity while still providing a fair return to physicians with reasonably full workloads indicates that this market is far from the one envisaged by economists when they talk about competition.

Technologic change.   In addition to numbers of physicians, a major factor affecting costs is the pace and character of technologic change. In our pluralistic, heavily insured, malpractice-sensitive system, once a new technology is in place it tends to be used. Over the long run, technology, more than anything else, drives the cost of care. The technologic innovations that were introduced during the first half of the 1980s were mostly developed prior to the cost-containment efforts. It takes a long time to slow the pace of innovation. Unless this happens, however, other cost-containment efforts tend to have only a one-time effect. In the long run, changes in the rate, or at least the character, of technologic innovation must play a critical role in slowing the rate of growth of health care expenditures.

. Technologic change depends in part on new scientific knowledge, but it also is affected by demand. The old cost-based reimbursement system tended to encourage any innovation that promised to improve the quality of care, regardless of cost. Manufacturers of drugs, equipment, and supplies contemplating investment in the development of such innovations did not have to worry about whether the prospective improvement was worth the increase in cost. Under the prospective, closed-ended reimbursement that has been growing since 1980, developers of new technology are concerned much more with prospective benefit/cost ratios. This pressure probably will slow the overall rate of innovation and will shift the emphasis away from improving quality regardless of cost to innovations that are valued primarily for their cost-saving potential.

Thus, it was unreasonable to expect the cost-containment efforts of the 1980s to have any marked effect on health care spending within just a few years. To slow spending, it is necessary to slow the rate of growth of services; there is little possibility for big savings either in productivity gains (in the narrow sense) or in depressing the prices of inputs. The demand for services by patients can be affected by deductibles and coinsurance, but it seems unlikely that third-party payment will not always predominate. The major constraints on services, therefore, must come from the supply side: the number of physicians, their specialty distribution, their training, the incentives they face, and, most importantly, the facilities and technology at their disposal. Changes in these factors can come only with a long lag, but they probably will come if the large buyers of health care maintain and extend their cost-conscious behavior.

DISTRIBUTIONAL EFFECTS

The cost-containment efforts did not slow the overall rate of growth of spending for health care but probably did affect the distribution of care. Between 1981 and 1986, the days of hospital care per 1,000 population declined more rapidly for the poor than for the nonpoor in both absolute and percentage terms. Similar disparities occurred in trends for blacks compared to whites, and females compared to males. The Johnson Foundation's national access surveys in 1982 and 1986 showed that access and utilization measures for the poor and minorities deteriorated relative to the nonpoor and whites. This reversed the trend of the 1960s and 1970s, when differentials were narrowing. National Health Interview Survey data show the percentage of persons without any health insurance coverage rising from 11 percent in 1978 to 13.3 percent in 1986. The trend in the late 1960s and early 1970s was toward increased coverage.

These distributional shifts should not be regarded as "unintended" effects of cost containment. They are inevitable if one seeks to eliminate cross-subsidization and to make patients more cost-conscious in their use of care. In the absence of third-party payment, each patient would make his or her own calculations of marginal benefit (versus marginal cost). The result would be different standards of care for different people because, other things equal, the trade-offs would depend on income. In the absence of cross-subsidies for insurance, the poor and the sick will decrease their purchases of insurance and use of medical care.

Critics of a single standard of care are correct in asserting that some people get more care than they want (in the sense that they would rather use the resources for something else) while some get less than they would want. However, the egalitarian approach can be justified for its symbolic value, or because it contributes to political stability, or because the wealthy do not want to redistribute money to the poor for them to use as they choose but are willing if the money is used for health care.

THE FUTURE OF THE HEALTH CARE MARKET

Dissatisfaction with the cost-containment effort is mounting. Critics say that it is not stemming the growth of expenditures, it is leaving more individuals with little or no insurance, and it is making life difficult and uncertain for the manufacturers of drugs, equipment, and other health care supplies. Some critics allege a decline in the quality of care, but the evidence offered is largely anecdotal.

Physicians blame cost containment for forcing them into new modes of practice and for their loss of power to managers and administrators. Some reorganization and loss of power was inevitable, but where physicians have taken the leadership in efforts to control costs (as in the prepaid group practices) there is greater potential to retain professional satisfaction than when controls on utilization are imposed from the outside.

A counterrevolution in health care finance is brewing, based on dissatisfaction and fear among many different elements. At some point, a coalition of business interests, consumer advocates, and providers is likely to unite in a call for more federal involvement in health insurance and health care, although they will disagree on the form of that involvement.

Efforts to improve the current situation should be encouraged, but they should be based on realistic assessments of what has happened and what is possible. The failure of health spending to slow in the 1980s probably reflects the recency of the cost-containment efforts more than inherent ineffectiveness. Indeed, there has been a demonstrable impact on hospital utilization, which was the primary target.

Most importantly, any attempt to build a better system for providing health insurance and controlling health care must recognize certain fundamental problems. On the demand side, most people do not want to risk having to pay very large bills, so they seek health insurance, either privately or through government programs. Once individuals have insurance, however, they want to consume more medical care than they would consume without it — and more than is socially optimal.

Another difficult policy problem is deciding when the premiums people pay for health insurance should be based on their expected utilization and when they should not. Most Americans seem to feel comfortable about having cigarette smokers pay higher premiums than nonsmokers, but even enthusiastic advocates of experience rating are uneasy about requiring individuals born with genetic defects to pay above-normal premiums. Where to draw the line? Is alcoholism, for instance, to be regarded as similar to cigarette smoking, or is it more analogous to a genetic disease?

There also are fundamental problems on the supply side of health care. Competition often is impossible or undesirable because of economies of scale. For instance, how many hospitals are needed to serve a population of 100,000 efficiently? Probably only one; at most two. Similar constraints apply to competition in physicians' specialty care, especially if the physicians work full-time at their specialties. It is doubtful that a population of one million is large enough to justify enough independent maternity services or open-heart surgery teams to approximate competitive conditions. Thus, it is wrong to think that competition can serve as the only control mechanism for health care.

Even in markets large enough to sustain large numbers of hospitals and physicians, it is not clear that the public interest is best served by insisting that health professionals maintain rigorous arm's-length competition with one another. Patients can benefit from cooperation among physicians and hospitals, in both reduced costs and better service.

This article began by noting the similarity between health care and other goods and services. The differences also are important. The patient/physician relationship often is highly personal and intimate, similar in many ways to relationships within families or between teachers and pupils or ministers and congregants. It is, in part, what Boulding calls an integrative relationship, one that depends on mutual recognition and acceptance of rights and responsibilities enforced by traditional norms as well as market pressures and government regulations.

The production function for health is a peculiar one; it usually requires patients and health professionals to work cooperatively rather than as adversarial buyers and sellers. Mutual trust and confidence contribute greatly to the efficiency of production. Thus the model of atomistic competition usually set as the ideal in economics textbooks often is not the right goal for health.

The necessity for dealing with dying and death also reveals the problematic nature of standard solutions based on fully informed consumers and competitive suppliers. There are, of course, many advantages to providing more information to the consumers of health care, but there also are potential disadvantages. If there is cost sharing, fully informed consumers will be forced to make painful decisions concerning limitations on care for loved ones, decisions that can leave a lifelong residue of guilt and regret. Not infrequently, families and society as a whole would prefer to have physicians take responsibility for these difficult decisions, keeping implicit rather than explicit the inevitable trade-offs between life and goods and services. If there is no cost sharing, patients and their families usually will want any care that could possibly help, regardless of cost. The rationing will have to come from the supply side, and full disclosure is unworkable.

The market is a subtle and powerful instrument of control, and competition is an important component in making markets work well. But Alain Enthoven has concluded that competition in health care must be managed, and that government must be one of the principal managers. Moreover, I believe we err in thinking that the only options are markets or government regulation. There is room for, indeed need for, a revitalization of professional norms as a third instrument of control in health care. As long as physicians continue to perform priestly functions, as long as they are our ambassadors to death, as long as they control the introduction of new technology, they must be endowed with certain privileges and held to certain standards of behavior different from those assumed by the market or regulation models.

In my view, we will never be able to introduce enough direct patient payment into the system to make that a significant instrument of cost containment. Thus, we inevitably will have to rely on physicians and other health professionals to do much of the rationing. How equitably and how efficiently they do that, along with constraints on supply and on the quantity and character of technologic change, will determine the success of cost containment in the long run.

Health, as a vast social enterprise, is too important to be solely the concern of the providers of services.

WILLIAM L. KISSICK

Bruce C. Vladeck

The Market vs. Regulation:
The Case for Regulation

The current hostility toward regulation (and the converse promotion of competition) owes little to dispassionate intellectual analysis. Rather, it arises from a conjunction of short- and long-term political forces with the tendency of health policy makers to adopt new fads every two or three years. The case for regulation is not often made, for political reasons; but, as an unrepentant regulator, I would like to argue the case by listing, with brief discussion, ten characteristics of the health care system and the regulatory process which seem to me to make health care regulation desirable.

The focus is on the regulation of health care, including health care facilities, health care providers, and health insurance mechanisms — my remarks are not meant to apply to regulation more generally, although some of them do. One of the major shortcomings of the current debate over regulation and deregulation is the often willful failure to identify the extent to which regulation in one area may differ from regulation in another. There is no plausible defense for the Interstate Commerce Commission's protection of truckers or railroads at the expense of shippers and consumers, but few of us would be prepared to dispense entirely with the police. There has been considerable discussion of "public utility model" regulation of health facilities; but, as an economic entity, the typical labor-intensive, publicly supported, nonprofit hospital is profoundly unlike Con Ed or Pacific Gas and Electric.

THE NATURE OF MEDICAL CARE CONSUMPTION

The most important consideration in a discussion of regulation and competition in health care is that, no matter how much devotees of the market might wish it were otherwise, medical care consumption decisions are simply atypical: most citizens in their consumption of medical care services do not behave like the theoretical construct of a rational consumer on which most of Western economics is based. Indeed, if one stops to think about it, where health care

Bruce C. Vladeck, Ph.D., is president of The United Hospital Fund of New York.

matters are concerned, it may not even be desirable to encourage people to behave more like rational "economic man." The science of medicine still relies on the patient's nonrational acceptance of the physician's role as healer.

The current argument for greater competition in the health care sector is based on the initial assumption that health care markets are distorted because of the wide prevalence of insurance, specifically including first-dollar insurance, which induces consumers to over-consume. When insurance — especially insurance purchased through employment relationships in which the individual consumer is never directly involved in the decision-making on benefit packages — makes the out-of-pocket, immediate cost of health services zero, consumers at the margin will be more likely to incur health care expenses than they would be if they experienced an out-of-pocket liability. Remove the moral hazard created by insurance practices, goes the argument, and the greater price sensitivity of consumers will begin to create market discipline on providers.

This argument is perfectly sound so far as it goes, and there is no question that in many instances the phenomenon of moral hazard works just as it is supposed to in the economics textbooks. But the advocates of increased competition seldom go the further step: to inquire just why it is that there is so much health insurance around, particularly insurance that is so comprehensive in its coverage of relatively small discretionary expenditures. One can agree that low-probability, high-risk events, such as hospitalizations for severe illnesses, are precisely the sorts of things against which rational consumers will insure, accepting some degree of copayment as a rational pricing mechanism; but no one is arguing that the problem of medical care costs has been created by insurance for such episodes. It is first-dollar coverage for relatively more discretionary services or marginal elective surgery and things of that sort that has everyone so excited — even though, in the actuarial sense, insurance for something like routine physician visits is not really insurance at all, since there is relatively little risk in the pure sense and the incurring of a loss is entirely at the discretion of the insured.

While advocates of competition, substituting static elementary economics for any knowledge of history, attribute current health insurance practices to relatively insubstantial tax subsidies, the basic fact is that medical care expenses are the most insured-against hazard in this society. The proportion of people with health insurance is substantially greater than the proportion of automobile owners with liability insurance, even in those states with compulsory automobile insurance laws. Something is going on here; consumers are trying to tell us something that professional social scientists have sought to ignore. People have walked picket lines and taken bitter strikes not only to get health insurance per se but also to protect first-dollar coverage. As one goes up the socio-economic ladder, one finds ever-richer benefit packages with diminishing copayment. People want health insurance, and they want it without deductibles or coinsurance.

Consumers have sought the kinds of health insurance they have, not because they wish to act irrationally in the aggregate economic sense, but precisely because they don't wish to be forced to make rational trade-offs when they are confronted with medical care consumption decisions. No matter how we draw our curves or shape our abstract arguments, the elemental fact is that medical care is about living and dying, something considered by many to be of a rather different character from the purchase of tomatoes. The primary characteristic of most consumers of medical care most of the time is that they are scared. They are scared of dying, or disfigurement, or permanent disability; and these are serious matters. It is hardly fair to expect any of us to make rational decisions about matters of such import. As a society, we may be prepared to pay a substantial economic premium to insulate people from having to make such decisions.

This argument is flawed, the proponents of a greater role for markets will say, because most encounters between individual consumers and health care providers do not involve life and death situations; indeed, most physician visits and even most hospitalizations involve conditions that will go away on their own in the absence of medical intervention. That is probably true, but it is also probably irrelevant. The real question is not, as Schelling would have it, what we are prepared to spend to reduce in the fourth decimal place the extremely low probability of a very highly disvalued event. Rather, it is a question of how much we are prepared to spend to be able to seek reassurance of a variety of kinds in a variety of circumstances—when we are scared, or anxious, or lonely, when we are not dying. It is one thing for social scientists to tell us that freeing people from marginal trade-offs between out-of-pocket expenditures and the intangible benefits of health care is very expensive. It is quite another thing for them to then tell us that doing so is illegitimate and must be abolished by legislative fiat—talk about government interference in private decision-making!

EQUITY

Whether or not the content of medical care is effective from the perspective of narrowly drawn cost-benefit analyses, it is something we value highly. Indeed, it is something we value so highly that as a society we are committed to providing it to all, even if some can't afford to pay for it from their own pockets. As a matter of social policy, we certainly do treat health care very differently from housing, or clothing, or any other set of commodities other than food. We have taken the basic position that all citizens are entitled to receive it. Those who can't afford to pay for it themselves should receive it at public expense. To be sure, we may penalize them in many ways for their impecuniousness. Not least are what Uwe Reinhardt terms "hassle factors." But this probably has more to do with a disapproval of poor people than with a disavowal of the basic responsibility for providing care.

Everyone learns in the first week of Economics I that the one thing markets don't do very well is insure equity. Equity considerations are thus always the major arguments for public intervention in a market economy. What is often ignored, however, is that the very same equity concerns often require some degree of regulation in the form of government intervention. It is not enough, as marker advocates would contend, simply to redistribute income. To begin with, as a society we are prepared to distribute access to services, not to redistribute cash income. More to the point, narrow economic incentives will not satisfactorily distribute even services.

One of the most important characteristics of poor people, but one economists tend to ignore when they so blindly consign questions of equity to the outer fringes of nonmarket areas, is that almost by definition poor people fare less well in markets of any kind, even when they are given purchasing power. Most people receiving direct government subsidies for medical care have limited access to that care not merely because of low incomes per se but rather because of low income arising from certain kinds of social or ethnic status. Even when incomes are relatively more equal, these socioethnic disparities make access to health care difficult. The poor in the United States are characteristically old, or black, or hispanic, or young members of families with a single parent. At all income levels, people in these categories have special problems with health care services.

People are poor for a reason; and the same things that make them poor frequently make it less attractive to sellers to provide them with services, as well as making it more difficult for the poor to rationally consume services. If you are the head of a supermarket chain, or indeed of a chain of for-profit hospitals, the last place you are going to locate your next expansion is in the midst of a poor community, even in this day of food stamps and Medicaid. You want to go where the economic growth and the young, affluent markets are; and, by long historical practice in this and most other countries, that is generally where poor people aren't. For hospital services, after all, Medicaid is a kind of voucher; but inner-city hospitals continue to close; and, even if physicians could earn the same incomes in Harlem, they'd probably prefer to practice in Scarsdale.

As committed as I am to the necessity for regulation in the health care sector, I am confident that the healthier, more affluent three-quarters of the population would do just as well in their receipt of health care services in the absence of any major regulatory activity at all. It is that other one-quarter that I worry about, and that provides the major justification for what it is we in government do.

PUBLIC PURSE

Given our predispositions in this country away from public ownership (or direct public provision) of services and toward market solutions whenever they are thought to be available, the primary way in which Americans have sought to ensure access to health services for old and poor people is through subsidies in the form of Medicare and Medicaid. But that approach creates the most important political rationale for extensive regulation of the health care sector. Put most simply, the dollars we are talking about controlling are tax dollars; and the public tends to be rather protective of how its tax dollars are spent.

At the most elemental level, any industry that receives more than 40 percent of its revenue from government should simply accept at the outset that it is going to have to undergo a substantial loss of autonomy. Put more positively, we have an obligation to be at least as careful in our expenditure of tax dollars for health care as we are in our expenditure of tax dollars for highways, welfare, or sanitation. Whatever their cause, excessive hospital costs waste tax dollars as efficiently as more obviously unnecessary projects. We outlaw excess profits for defense contractors, but not for Medicare providers.

The historical record seems very clear to me. Extensive regulation of health care providers is the price we pay for not having national health insurance. Given a political stalemate in society which precludes development of a health insurance system like that in every other modern society, we have chosen to subsidize particular groups while consciously refusing to make major structural changes in the health care industry. Fee-for-service health care and reasonable cost, however, lead to inordinate public expense—unless there is substantial and effective regulation of fees and services. Equal access for the poor and elderly will feed cost inflation unless costs are directly controlled.

A somewhat more subtle, but equally critical, point links these concepts of equity and protection of the public purse. Government is always the provider or insurer of last resort. To the extent that our society is unwilling to deny life-saving or disability-preventing medical care to those without other resources, there is a role for government in arranging for their care. The more competitive the private insurance market, the more such people there will be—because insurers avoid bad risks and have a marketing strategy of selling low-cost, low-benefit programs to those with the lowest income (but the greatest probability of needing services)—and thus the greater the burden on public funds. There is, for example, essentially no private market for nursing home insurance; so, government pays for more than two-thirds of nursing home days.

SLAYING DRAGONS

In evaluating the competing claims for regulation and competition in health care, there is also the small matter of empirical evidence. The standard to which regulation is generally compared, that of the "efficient" performance of perfect theoretical markets, is almost purely a theoretical construct. Apart from a few markets for agricultural commodities, there are almost no true markets left in modern society; and one can even raise historical questions about how many ever really existed. It was Adam Smith, after all, who warned of the inevitable tendencies to monopoly, mercantilism, and other exercises of economic power. As a regulator, I'm growing tired of being beaten over the head by defunct economists.

Dispute rages over the fine points, but there is no question that state-operated hospital cost-containment programs work and, while my counterparts in New York may have overdone it, there is no verifiable evidence of seriously dysfunctional outcomes in any state with strong regulation, even New York. Well-managed HMOs do reduce costs, but it's hard to develop them, and harder still to get lots of people to voluntarily enroll in them. At the other pole of the debate, I think close examination of most of the currently trumpeted procompetitive plans would reveal how much regulatory content of their own they would require. In these plans, the focus of regulation is shifted from providers to insurers, but a powerful, external guiding hand remains. In order to make reality look more like the textbook theories, we would need lots of regulation anyway.

DESTRUCTIVE COMPETITION

One of the curious facts about the argument for increased competition in the health care sector is that there has been so much competition for so long, although of a kind that is less than perfectly desirable. Specifically, note the classic patterns of competition among hospitals, which are widely thought to have resulted in substantial excess capacity and enormous overinvestment in dubiously useful technology. In a market structure in which consumers do not make basic consumption decisions about hospital services themselves, in which they are forced to rely on the preferences and decisions of physicians, competition among institutions for physicians' favor is bound to be inordinately expensive and destructive. One could argue that the sorts of destructive competition we have seen among hospitals result from the nature of health insurance coverage. But that argument ignores the way in which people and physicians actually perceive and care about the hospitals with which they do business. The so-called technological imperative in medical practice may not be a technological or professional/scientific phenomenon at all, but rather a competitive one.

Competition among health insurers is, in fact, a major source of the expansion of comprehensive first-dollar health insurance. Moreover, as Diana Chapman Walsh has recently illuminated so superbly, the structure of the real health insurance market strongly discourages cost containment. Forcing insurers to sell packages that would make consumers more price sensitive would require extensive new regulation.

IDLE PROFITS

Closely related to this kind of competitive behaviors is the fact that the most expensive and most pervasive institutions in health care, those where the greatest expenses are incurred, are overwhelmingly run on a not-for-profit basis. Even in the absence of a fully satisfactory theory of the nonprofit firm, it is clear that the behavior of nonprofit firms varies in significant and critical ways from the classic theory of the for-profit firm.

THE GOLDEN MEAN

Traditionally, the possible social arrangements for the control of certain kinds of essential services have been defined as markers on the one hand and public ownership or direct public provision on the other. The sorts of regulatory phenomena we see in health care, or utilities, or other segments of American life are uniquely American, a sort of compromise between the two historical ideological poles. Moderation of this kind, suggested Aristotle, is a principal characteristic of effective democracy.

I do not imply that regulation is a "golden" mean between markets and public ownership, but I would suggest that there may be something of value inherent in the regulatory process itself that has been sought and then preserved by those who have made public policy. In contrast to the functioning of an ideal market, regulation is extraordinarily cumbersome, time consuming, and inefficient; but it has the virtues of its weaknesses. The most important of these virtues are due process, stability, and accountability.

DUE PROCESS

Whatever else one may or may not say about the regulatory process as it is practiced in most jurisdictions, it is certainly characterized by a high degree of formal due process. Given the interests involved, that may very well be a desirable attribute. In a pure market, individual physicians or individual nursing homes, for example, might well be badly battered by the forces of market competition in a way that was unfair from the perspective of anything but economic efficiency. Formal fairness is a value of some significance in and of itself, and I do think the regulatory process compares quite favorably to most competitive processes in its ability to provide for it.

STABILITY

Another thing which regulatory processes are good at providing, and which they are frequently criticized for, is a high degree of stability. Again, the health sector may be a bit different from the kinds of sectors in which one is more comfortable talking about markets. We have all heard that some substantial proportion of private firms fail in any given year; for a healthy market economy, a high degree of attrition among unsuccessful competitors is not only necessary but also desirable. Imagine, on the other hand, a world in which a quarter of the nursing homes, a quarter of the hospitals, or a quarter of the health insurers or HMOs went bankrupt in any given year.

ACCOUNTABILITY

Whatever the failures in the process, governmental regulators do retain a substantial degree of political accountability to the general public. That accountability may be imperfect and highly attenuated; yet it is often strong and direct. Indeed, many of the things for which regulators are most severely criticized (for example, the political nature of some CON decisions) suggest a high degree of accountability. Anyone who professes a faith in democratic self-government would be hard pressed to argue against a policy mechanism that legitimately claims the advantage of increased responsiveness to the expressed interest of voters.

One of the things that has been wrong with the discussion of regulation versus competition in the health sector has been the failure to address this very basic characteristic of regulation: that it is an essentially political process. Market strategies are, of course, essentially political processes as well. They just tend to promote the political interests of different groups from those whose interests are served by regulation.

It may be a bit unfair, but not historically inaccurate, to suggest that market advocates have identified with the interests of the haves while regulatory advocates have sympathized, at least rhetorically, with some of the have-nots. It is no accident that regulators tend to be Democrats, and deregulators, academics and Republicans.

Regulation, in its most basic terms, constitutes the imposition of influence and power by those with a political majority on those who have customarily exercised power in a given sector of economic activity. Of course, the critics of regulation are immediately going to respond that most regulatory processes have more effectively served the interests of those already in power, particularly the providers of service, than of consumers. That is probably accurate. But, when there is no consumer sovereignty to begin with, surely consumers stand a better chance of getting their interests served in a competitive political environment than in an historically uncompetitive and anticompetitive market for health services.

CONCLUSIONS

All these virtues notwithstanding, regulation is hardly the answer to all of the problems of health care policy. It deals poorly with qualitative issues, for example (although the record of markets is hardly encouraging either), and tends to penalize the very best or most efficient institutions while focusing on the worst. More to the point, regulation is a rubric that encompasses, even within the health care sector, a wide diversity of activities of widely varying degrees of success. Indeed, beyond a certain point, it probably makes little sense to talk generically about regulation at all.

For ideological reasons, the debate between competition and regulation has heretofore been rather lopsided. It has also, more fundamentally, been profoundly misplaced. Both regulation and competition are, or should be, tools — means to an end. Neither is really worth very much as an end in itself. The real questions are what kind of health care system should we have and what kind of health care system, in the short run, given the constraints, can we have. How one answers those questions largely determines how much regulation one thinks is necessary.

Advocates of greater reliance on market forces in health care tend to talk a great deal about efficiency, economy, and consumer choice. Regulators tend to focus on access, equity, and governmental budgets. Basic value choices are at issue, down beneath several layers of rhetoric. It is an old quarrel, and one with no immediate end in sight. It may be useful, though, to remember what the fight is all about.

If health care — or at least access to a defined minimum set of health services — is a right, or at least something we have agreed that everyone in society should have, then it might be suggested that the protection of rights is something we are generally loath to leave to the marketplace. Indeed, there are economists who define rights as those activities determined to require insulation from market forces. A poll tax is unconstitutional; so is slavery. Although we health care regulators sometimes tend to forget it, some things are too important to be defined solely in terms of cost.

Alain C. Enthoven

Health Care Costs: Why Regulation Fails, Why Competition Works, How to Get There from Here

Health care costs continue to soar and strain public finances. What is new and different now is the sheer size of the outlays in the face of growing taxpayer resistance and concern over deficits and inflation (30 states called for a constitutional convention to balance the budget). Government will be forced to bring the costs under control.

Many factors contribute to the cost increase: general inflation (though health spending has grown at about twice the general inflation rate), better insurance coverage, new technology, aging population, etc. But there has also been much overutilization of services, overinvestment and waste.

The main cause of unnecessary and unjustified increase in costs in the complex of perverse incentives inherent in our dominant financing system for health care: fee-for-service for the doctor, cost-reimbursement for the hospital, and third-party insurance to protect consumers, with premiums usually paid entirely or largely by employers or government. This system rewards providers of care with more revenue for giving more and more costly care, whether or not more is necessary or beneficial to the patient. It leaves insured consumers with little or no incentive to seek a less costly health care financing or delivery plan. There are many cost-increasing incentives and virtually no reward for economy.

This is not the only way health care can be financed. There are *alternative delivery systems* in successful operation which reward providers of health care services for finding ways to deliver better care at less cost. In these systems, participating physicians accept responsibility for providing comprehensive care to their enrolled members, usually for a per capita payment set in advance. The list of such systems includes prepaid group practices, individual practice associations, primary care networks and health care alliances. There are many variations on each of these concepts, but each includes some reward for

Alain C. Enthoven, Ph.D., is the Marriner S. Eccles Professor of Public and Private Management in the Graduate School of Business at Stanford University, Stanford, California.

economy in the use of resources. Many comparative studies provide convincing evidence that prepaid group practices reduce total per capita costs (premium and out-of-pocket) by 10 per cent to 40 percent compared to the costs for similar people cared for under traditional insurance programs. In competition, other alternative delivery systems have achieved similar savings.

The main direction of public policy in the 1970s has been to protect the dominant fee-for-service, cost-reimbursement and third-party insurance system from fair economic competition by alternative delivery systems, and to try to limit the cost-increasing effects by direct controls over prices and capacity.

HOSPITAL COST CONTAINMENT

Since 1977, the Carter Administration has tried to enact an annual percentage limit on the growth of total hospital spending or hospital cost-per-case. The main thing wrong with hospital cost containment is that it does *nothing* to correct the existing perverse cost-increasing incentives. It does not help reform the financing and delivery system, and does nothing to encourage competing alternative delivery systems. It is a pure spending restraint that ignores health care quality, efficiency and equity.

In fact, this approach reinforces and creates now cost-increasing incentives. A hospital that thought it needed less than the proposed annual increase limit would be foolish to take less. To do so would diminish its "entitlement" to future increases.

Finally, the general history of economic regulation does not support the presumption that regulation reduces costs. The present moves to deregulate transportation are based on the clear evidence that regulation had *raised* costs to consumers. (Admittedly, the feasibility of a competitive alternative is more readily apparent in transportation than in health services. We cannot just "deregulate health care"; we have to reform the basic incentives.) Public utility-type regulation motivates overinvestment. Regulators become "captured by the regulated."

CERTIFICATE-OF-NEED

The other main regulatory structure is certificate-of-need (CON) regulation by the states, executed through local authorities called health systems agencies (HSAs), as required by the National Health Planning and Resources Development Act. HSAs must issue a permit before increases in hospital capacity can take place, Several broadly-based comparison studies have shown that CON has failed to ameliorate the problem of hospital overinvestment. This is not surprising. The leading experts cannot agree even on standards for the appropriate number of beds, not to mention for more esoteric technologies.

PRINCIPLES OF A SYSTEM OF FAIR COMPETITION

If government controls on prices and capacity will not solve the problem, what will? It makes sense to go back to the underlying causes and see what can be done to correct the perverse incentives inherent in today's dominant financing system. In a system of fair economic competition among various types of health plans (including traditional insurance and fee-for-service as one option), consumers who joined health plans that did a good job of controlling costs would pay lower premiums or receive better benefits. Health plans that did a poor job of controlling costs would lose customers and risk being driven out of business. In the long run, the surviving health plans would be the ones that offer a good value to their members. The health care system would be transformed, gradually and voluntarily, from today's system with built-in cost increasing incentives, to a system with built-in incentives for consumer satisfaction and cost control.

The essential principles of such a system of competition are:

1. *Multiple Choice:* Once a year, each consumer (individual or family) would be offered the opportunity to enroll for the coming year in any of the qualified health plans operating in his area.
2. *Fixed-Dollar Subsidy:* The amount of financial help each consumer gets toward the purchase of his health plan membership—from Medicare, Medicaid, employer, or tax laws—would be the same whichever plan he chooses. The subsidy might be more for poor than nonpoor, for old than young, families than individuals, etc., *but no more for people who choose more costly health plans*. The family that chooses a more costly health plan would pay the extra cost itself. Thus, it would have an incentive to choose wisely.
3. *Same Rules for All Competitors:* A uniform set of rules would apply to all health plans. Rules would govern premium-setting practices, minimum benefit packages, catastrophic expense protection, etc. The point of such rules would be to assure that all health plans are competing to provide good quality comprehensive care at a reasonable cost, and not profiting by such practices as preferred risk selection or deceptive, inadequate coverage.
4. *Doctors in Competing Economic Units:* Physicians would be organized in competing economic units so that the premium each group charged would reflect its ability to control costs.

The main problems in our health care economy rise from the fact that, for the most part, these principles are not applied today.

- *Multiple Choice?* Most people, when they come to work, are presented with a single employer-provided health insurance plan. The aged are locked into Medicare, the eligible poor got Medicaid, both based on fee-for-service and cost reimbursement. (To be sure, the HMO Act requires employers to offer their employees the option of joining one group practice and one individual practice HMO if such federally qualified organizations exist in their area. But HMOs are too few, too small, and too tightly regulated to be able to bring the benefits of competition to most Americans in the foreseeable future. And there are other potentially desirable alternative delivery systems that do not meet the HMO Act definition. We need a broader concept of alternative systems.)

- *Fixed Dollar Subsidy?* Today, Medicare, Medicaid, employers and tax laws systematically pay more on behalf of beneficiaries who choose more costly health care plans or providers. For example, in 1970, Medicare paid $202 per capita on behalf of beneficiaries cared for by cost-effective Group Health Cooperative of Puget Sound, but paid $356, or 76 per cent more, on behalf of similar beneficiaries in the same area who chose to get their care from the fee-for-service sector. Among those employers who do give their employees a choice, many pay the whole premium either way, and thus eliminate the employee's financial incentive to choose the less costly plan.

- *Same Rules for All Competitors?* Equal rules are not applied now. HMOs must practice community-rating while insurers are free to experience-rate. HMOs must offer a comprehensive package of prepaid benefits while insurers are free to cover fewer benefits and use more deductibles. In effect, HMOs are required to provide necessary services without limit. Insurers can and do limit the amount they will pay on behalf of someone with catastrophic illness. Some HMOs have received public subsidies not available to insurers. We are far from applying equal rules to all.

- *Doctors in Competing Economic Units?* The market is dominated by "free choice of doctor" insurance plans. The medical profession has traditionally insisted on this principle. The effect is that the consumer's premium payment is the same whether he goes to the most extravagant or the most efficient doctor — again depriving him of a reward for seeking out doctors who use health resources economically. As well as "free choice of doctor," consumers should have the right to agree to get all their care from a limited set of providers in an alternative delivery system in exchange for better benefits or lower premiums.

COMPETITION IS WORKABLE AND EFFECTIVE

There are some groups and some market areas in which these principles have been applied, substantially if not completely.

The Federal Employees Health Benefits Program (FEHBP), in successful operation since 1960, offers employees a multiple choice of alternative plans and a fixed dollar contribution toward the plan of their choice. The State of California and Stanford University offer their employees a similar choice. (Each has minor exceptions to the equal dollar subsidy principle.) HMOs and similar alternative delivery systems have done very well in such fair competition. For example, about half the federal and state employees in Kaiser's northern California service area belong to Kaiser. More than half the Stanford families choose either Kaiser or the Palo Alto Clinic prepaid plan in preference to the Blue Cross "free-choice-of-doctor" plan.

A comparison of the FEHBP and Medicare illustrates another important point. Medicare is based on fee-for-service and cost reimbursement. The Medicare law is 102 pages long: the regulations fill 400 pages of fine print. The FEHBP law is eight pages long; the regulations are 16 pages long. A recent study showed that administrative cost per claim processed in the FEHBP was 22 per cent below that in Medicare. Thus we have some large-scale practical examples to show that competitive systems are simple and workable.

LOW-COST INCREMENTAL PROPOSALS

Competitive principles could form the basis for a comprehensive national health insurance plan. But at a time of rising concern over deficits and inflation, government leaders are understandably wary of new programs that cost money and raise taxes.

Alternatively, we could adopt the same principle in a few low-cost measures that would greatly enhance competition and the performance of our private health care financing system.

Employer contributions to health benefits are excluded from the taxable incomes of employees, and a part of individual premium payments is tax-deductible. This favorable treatment is costing the federal and state governments roughly $13 billion this year in foregone tax revenues. In these laws, the government has an ideal lever to make the market achieve public purposes more effectively. It can set requirements and minimum standards for employee health benefits programs as a condition for the favorable tax treatment.

- *Multiple Choice:* Each employer should be required to include, in any health benefits program he offers to employees, a choice of no fewer than three distinct health insurance or delivery plans that meet minimum standards. Different corporate entities would be required, not merely different options with the same carrier. Competition is the goal. (Small employers could meet the requirement through multi-employer trusts.)

    This requirement would give employers a powerful incentive to seek out and offer competing alternatives. (The HMO Act is much less effective because it gives employers no incentive to help HMOs get started, and it puts the burden on the HMOs to enforce dual choice. HMOs are understandably reluctant to antagonize potential customers.)

- *Fixed-Dollar Subsidy:* The employer's premium contribution should have to be the same amount, whichever plan the employee chooses. The employer might contribute more on behalf of employees in different categories (e.g. individuals vs. families, different locations, bargaining units, etc.), but not more on behalf of the employee who chooses a more costly health plan. Employers would not be required to contribute at any particular level.

The same principles should be embodied in a "freedom of choice" provision in Medicare. Today, Medicare beneficiaries are locked into a fee-for-service cost-reimbursement system. They are vulnerable to large uncovered expenses and the risks of catastrophic expense. Yet they are not allowed to realize for themselves most of the savings generated by joining an efficient alternative delivery system. The law should be changed to permit any beneficiary to direct that the "adjusted average per capita cost" to Medicare for people in his actuarial category be paid, as a fixed premium contribution on his behalf, to the alternative delivery system of his choice provided it meets reasonable federal performance standards.

Eventually, the present Medicare system, with its extremely complex and rigid regulatory apparatus, should be replaced by a payment system based on fixed prospective per capita premium subsidies (based on actuarial category), and fair economic competition in the private sector. In other words, as of a certain date, new beneficiaries ought to be covered by a new system modelled on the FEHBP. The savings in paperwork alone would be immense. Medicaid should be replaced by a similar system, with premium subsidies related to income on a graduated scale.

Standards for Qualified Health Plans

Basic Minimum Benefits: All health plans that qualify as non-taxable fringe benefits or for Medicare premium contributions should have to cover a minimum uniform set of benefits such as the basic benefits defined in the HMO Act. This would standardize a lot of fine print, make health plans much easier for consumers to understand and compare and protect consumers from tricky and misleading exclusions of important services. It would help locus competition on quality and accessibility of services, and total cost. (This provision need not increase premiums or costs to employers; premiums could be reduced to offset its costs by raising the deductibles and coinsurance rate.)

Catastrophic Expense Protection: All qualified health plans should be required to limit consumer cost-sharing (coinsurance, copayments, deductibles) for basic benefits to a maximum annual amount such as $1,500 per family. That is, every family should have catastrophic expense protection. The infrequency of catastrophic illness expense makes this kind of insurance much less costly than "first dollar coverage." But, as much as possible, this should be done in the *private sector* where people can *voluntarily* choose among alternative systems of cost control. (Catastrophic expense protection on a public entitlement basis would only add to the cost increasing incentives.)

Continuity of Coverage: Qualified health plans should be required to continue coverage for at least 60 days to those who have been members of an insured group. This would apply to people such as the unemployed after termination of employment, dependents after death of an employed family member and divorcees after divorce. There should be automatic coverage of newborn children. The unemployed, survivors, divorced spouses and dependent children and dependent children upon attainment of majority, should be able to convert to individual coverage without proof of insurability. Their premiums should be at group rates plus a reasonable allowance for handling costs. Health plans should not be allowed to cancel coverage because of illness or any reason other than failure to pay premiums.

When people lose their health insurance, there can be serious individual hardships, and for this the private health insurance industry can be justly criticized. This proposal would add little to the cost of insurance, but would greatly enhance people's continuity of coverage, and substantially reduce the number of people without protection.

Doctors in Competing Economic Units: Would competition occur under these rules? There is good reason for confidence. First, there are already active alternative delivery systems in many communities despite the existing disincentives. The HMO idea has achieved enhanced legitimacy in recent years.

Second, alternative delivery systems have been sponsored by many types of institutions. Potential sponsors are in abundant supply in most communities. The list includes physician groups, industrial companies, insurance companies, Blue Cross and Blue Shield, unions, universities and consumer cooperatives. The proposed requirement of multiple choice would give employers a powerful incentive to help competitors enter their markets.

Third, a market situation in which every consumer is insured by a "free-choice-of-doctor" third-party insurance plan would be unstable under the proposed rules. The potential gains to providers and consumers from joining an alternative delivery system would be too great. The situation would attract innovators.

Finally, health services are gradually being brought under the rules of competition applied to the rest of American business. The Federal Trade Commission has substantially upgraded its expertise and has been achieving significant gains in applying anti-monopoly principles to this field. For example, the FTC staff has recommended that physician organizations be required to divest themselves of control of Blue Shield plans. The Ohio State Medical Society has just been forced to give up ownership of Ohio Blue Shield. Medical society control of individual practice associations, with its obvious monopolistic potential, is coming under similar challenge. An effective anti-monopoly strategy is already evolving to complement these "low-cost, incremental proposals."

The competition of alternative delivery systems with built-in incentives to deliver better care at less cost is rapidly gaining momentum. The most productive thing the federal government could do now would be to eliminate the main barriers to this desirable development.

The American public has been warned that medical care may soon have to be rationed . . . . The truth is that medical care is already rationed and it always has been. One of the disgraces of national policy is that the poor and unemployed who cannot afford to pay for medical care or have no medical insurance must often accept inferior treatment, if they can get it at all.

JOHN P. BUNKER
Stanford University

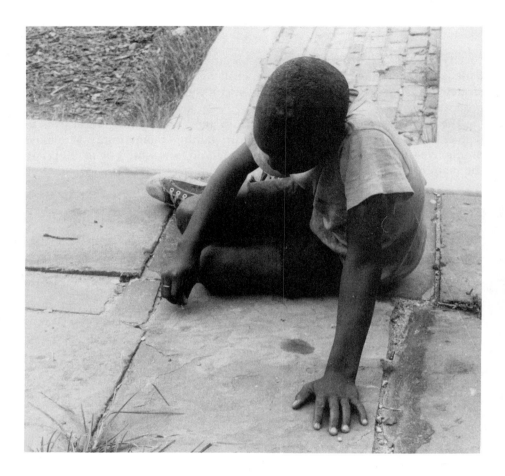

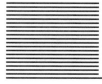

7

Inequities in Access
to Health Services

Aᴛᴛʜᴏᴜɢʜ national health expenditures have risen to 11.1 percent of the GNP, millions of people in this country still lack access to adequate health services. The common belief that health services are—and ought to be—available to every U.S. citizen is countered by the experience of individuals who receive infrequent health services of inadequate quality because of poverty, lack of insurance, unemployment, race, class, age, gender, geographic location, or health beliefs.

Many poor persons receive no benefits despite government-financed medical coverage through Medicare and Medicaid. More than 37 million Americans are without health insurance of any kind, and many of the insured fail to obtain services because they cannot afford required deductibles and copayments. Access is tangled in a complex knot of quality and cost, cost being the easiest aspect to measure and manipulate. Cost containment policy, which has had limited success in controlling costs, threatens to jeopardize access and quality. Improvements in the latter areas might in turn stimulate health cost inflation.

The concept of access includes process and outcome indices, but can be simply defined as a match of service, need, and affordable cost. Such a match depends on many elements—perception and identification of need; availability of the required service; knowledge of the service; a referral mechanism; common understanding of service usefulness; transportation; physically accessible location; information, motivation, and assistance to sustain treatment; and ability to cover costs. Although these are only some of the steps involved in gaining access to health services, they indicate the complexity of the issue.

Significant barriers to access are the lack of continuity among fragmented and complex health services and the inability of the present system to adapt services to varying ethnic, class, age, and gender requirements. Emergency and acute care continue to be more accessible than chronic and preventive services, which, if provided, might delay or prevent acute needs. Health-related non-medical services are particularly difficult to obtain. Availability of health services varies by geographic region, with prosperous states and urban areas providing a wider array of services than poor and rural areas offer. Differences in Medicaid coverage from state to state also create inequities.

This chapter examines the access question through the perspectives of demographic characteristics, individual reports, provider and financing influences, and alternative policy solutions.

Karen Davis and Diane Rowland illustrate the interaction of financial barriers, such as low income, unemployment, and lack of insurance, on access. In addition to insurance status, race and place of residence are significant determinants of ability to obtain health services. Individuals least able to bear the cost of poor health are most likely to be ill and uninsured. The uninsured are unlikely to have a regular source of care and must travel further and wait longer for services than insured persons do. Deaths have resulted from the transfer for financial reasons of uninsured patients from one hospital type to another. The authors make strong recommendations for resource development and access to primary and preventive care through comprehensive insurance or a cluster of interim financing mechanisms.

Signs of deterioration in access to medical services for the nation's poor, minorities, and uninsured are reported by Howard Freeman and colleagues. Even though the poor are experiencing more ill health than others, they receive fewer hospital and physician services. Equally serious, access to care for poor minorities has deteriorated in recent years. Despite problems faced by the poor, most people surveyed are satisfied with the care they receive. A surprising outcome of the research is that the aging population, the growing supply of physicians, and the number and quality of new technologies have not led to increases in visits (office, hospital) per person.

Uncompensated hospital care is a growing problem facing federal and state legislators, health providers, and society at large. Public hospitals bear an increasingly large share of the uncompensated care burden. In the past, cost shifting to other payer sources permitted community hospitals to care for nonpaying patients. As competition increased and third parties limited cost shifting within community hospitals, the burden was transferred to public hospitals. Gail Wilensky analyzes the advantages and disadvantages of solutions targeting providers, individuals, or localities. She suggests alternative revenue sources to cover costs and proposes policy directions that can be taken without restructuring the entire health service system.

In "Financing Charity Care in an Era of Competition" Lawrence Lewin and Marion Ein Lewin examine the impact of recent financing policies on the access to care of uninsured people. They report that "dumping" and "skimming" in the wake of market-driven price competition have left teaching and public hospitals with a disproportionate share of unpaid cases. The authors discuss the responsibility for financing health services for those who cannot pay, and propose a number of ideas for improved financing of indigent care.

Every society creates its own casualties.

J. N. MORRIS

Karen Davis/Diane Rowland

Uninsured and Underserved: Inequities in Health Care in the United States

The United States has one of the highest quality and most sophisticated systems of medical care in the world. Most Americans take for granted their access to this system of care. In times of emergency or illness, they can call upon a vast array of health resources from a family physician to a complex teaching hospital—assured that they will receive needed care and that their health insurance coverage will pick up the tab for the majority of bills incurred.

For a surprisingly large segment of the United States population, however, this ease of access to care does not exist. At any point in time, over 25 million Americans have no health insurance coverage from private health insurance plans or public programs. Without health insurance coverage or ready cash, such individuals can be and are turned away from hospitals even in emergency situations. Some neglect obtaining preventive or early care, often postponing care until conditions have become life-threatening. Others struggle with burdensome medical bills. Many come to rely upon crowded, understaffed public hospitals as the only source of reliable, available care.

The absence of universal health insurance coverage creates serious strains in our society. These strains are felt most acutely by the uninsured poor, who must worry about family members—a sick child, an adult afflicted with a deteriorating chronic health condition, a pregnant mother—going without needed medical assistance. It strains our image as a just and humane society when significant portions of the population endure avoidable pain, suffering, and even death because of an inability to pay for health care. Those physicians, other health professionals, and institutions that try to assist this uninsured group also incur serious strain. Demands typically far outstrip available time and resources. Strain is also felt by local governments whose communities include many uninsured persons, because locally funded public hospitals and

Karen Davis, Ph.D., is professor and chair of the Department of Health Policy and Management at Johns Hopkins University School of Hygiene and Public Health, Baltimore, Maryland.

Diane Rowland, Sc.D., is assistant professor, Department of Health Policy and Management at Johns Hopkins University School of Hygiene and Public Health, Baltimore, Maryland.

health centers inevitably incur major financial deficits. In recent years, many of the public facilities that have traditionally been the source of last-resort care have closed, thereby intensifying the stresses on other providers and the uninsured poor.

It is especially timely, therefore, to review what we know about the consequences of inadequate health insurance coverage for certain segments of our population. The first section of this paper presents information on the number and characteristics of the uninsured, while the second section describes patterns of health care utilization by the uninsured. The third section assesses the policy implications of these facts and offers recommendations for future public policy to ensure access to health care for all.

WHO ARE THE UNINSURED?

A snapshot view of the uninsured at a given point in time understates the number of people who spend some portion of the year uninsured. At any one time, there are over 25 million uninsured Americans, but as many as 34 million may be uninsured for some period of time during the year. Approximately 18 million are without insurance for the entire year, and 16 million are uninsured for some portion of the year.

The 34 million uninsured are persons of all incomes, racial and ethnic backgrounds, occupations, and geographic locations. In some cases whole families are uninsured, while in others coverage is mixed depending on employment status and eligibility for public programs. However, the poor, minorities, young adults, and rural residents are more likely than others to be uninsured. Over one-quarter of all blacks and minorities are uninsured during the year—a rate 1½ times that of whites. This disparity holds across the demographic and social characteristics of the uninsured.

Age

The uninsured population, whether covered for all or part of a year, is almost entirely under age 65. Nearly one-fifth of the non-aged population is uninsured for some or all of the year. Less than 1 percent of the aged, barely 200,000 persons, are uninsured during the year. This is attributable primarily to Medicare which provides basic coverage for hospital and physician services to most older Americans.

Examination of the uninsured by age group reveals that young adults are the group most likely to be uninsured. Almost one-third of all persons aged 19 to 24 are uninsured during the course of a year. Roughly 16 percent of this age group are without coverage all year, and an additional 14 percent lack coverage at least part of the year. This rate is nearly double that of other age groups. A variety of factors undoubtedly contribute to this situation. Young adults frequently lose coverage under their parents' policies at age 18. Many young adults may elect to forego coverage when it is available, since coverage is costly and they assume themselves to be relatively healthy. High youth unemployment, as well as employment in marginal jobs without health benefits, make insurance difficult to obtain or afford for this group.

Employment

Employment status and occupation are important factors in assessing the likelihood of being uninsured for all or part of a year. Most American workers receive their health care coverage through the workplace, but insurance coverage varies widely depending on the type of employer. Employees of small firms are less likely to be insured than employees of large firms. For example, 45 percent of employees in firms of 25 or fewer employees do not have employer-provided health insurance compared with only 1 percent in firms with more than 1,000 employees. Yet, small firms employ over 20 percent of all workers. Unionized firms are six times more likely to have employee health insurance than are nonunionized firms.

Insurance status varies by type of employment. Nearly one-quarter of all agricultural workers are uninsured during the year, with 16 percent uninsured for the entire year. As expected, white collar workers are the most likely to be insured, while blue collar and service workers fare only somewhat better than agricultural workers. Among blue collar and service workers, insurance coverage is low in the construction industry, wholesale and retail trades, and service industries, and high in manufacturing. Of manufacturing employees, 96 percent have health insurance through their place of employment.

Residence

These trends in coverage by employment are reflected in the regional picture of insurance status. In the heavily industrial and unionized Northeast and north central regions of the country, the percentage of uninsured during the year is half that of the South and the West. In these areas where agricultural interests are strong and unionization less extensive, over 20 percent of the population is uninsured during the course of a year. Of those living in the South and West, 11 percent are uninsured throughout the year compared with 5 percent in the Northeast and north central regions. Similarly, people in metropolitan areas are more likely to be insured than people living outside metropolitan areas.

Income and Race

However, while nature of employment and unionization may explain some of the regional variations, a critical underlying factor in the analysis is the distribution in the population of poverty and minorities. Residents of the

South comprise 32 percent of the total population under age 65. Yet 48 percent of the nation's minorities live in the South. The higher concentration of poor and minority persons in the South in comparison with other parts of the country helps explain the high level of uninsured individuals.

Poverty and lack of insurance are strongly correlated. Of poor families with incomes below 125 percent of the poverty line, 27 percent are uninsured. The near-poor, with incomes between 125 and 200 percent of poverty, fare only slightly better, with 21 percent uninsured during the year. The poor are always more likely to be uninsured than the middle and upper income groups.

The limited health insurance coverage for the poor and near-poor demonstrates the limits of coverage of the poor under Medicaid. Many assume that Medicaid finances health care services for all of the poor. However, many poor persons are ineligible for Medicaid due to categorical requirements for program eligibility and variations in state eligibility policies. Two-parent families are generally ineligible for Medicaid and single adults are covered only if they are aged or disabled. Moreover, many states have established income eligibility cutoffs well below the poverty level. Many states have not adjusted income levels to account for inflation, resulting in a reduction in the number of individuals covered over the last few years. As a result of the restrictions on Medicaid coverage, about 60 percent of the poor are not covered by Medicaid.

Thus, while the poor are obviously the least able to pay for care directly, they are the most likely to be without either Medicaid or private insurance. The poor are twice as likely to be uninsured as the middle class and three times as likely as those in upper income groups. Lack of insurance is inversely related to ability to bear the economic consequences of ill health.

Blacks, Hispanics, and other minorities are also more likely to be uninsured than whites regardless of their income; poor blacks are the most likely to be uninsured. Nearly one-third of poor blacks are uninsured during a year. If you are poor and a member of a minority group, your chances of being uninsured are four times as great as for a high income white.

Thus, health insurance coverage in the U.S. is to some extent a matter of luck. Those fortunate enough to be employed by large, unionized, manufacturing firms are also likely to be fortunate enough to have good health insurance coverage. Those who are poor, those who live in the South or in rural areas, and those who are black or minority group members are more likely to bear the personal and economic effects of lack of insurance and the consequent financial barriers to health care.

UTILIZATION OF HEALTH SERVICES BY THE UNINSURED

With the investment in primary care made by federal programs in the late 1960s and 1970s, significant progress in improving access to primary care for the poor and other disadvantaged groups was achieved. Virtually all of the numerous studies examining trends in access to health care conclude that differentials in utilization of physician services and preventive service by income have narrowed.

In the early 1960s the nonpoor visited physicians 23 percent more frequently than the poor even though the poor, then as now, were considerably sicker than the nonpoor. By the 1970s the poor visited physicians more frequently than the nonpoor, and more in accordance with their greater need for health care services. Blacks and other minorities also made substantial gains over this period. Utilization of services by rural residents also increased relative to urban residents.

However, use of preventive services by the poor, minorities, and rural residents continues to lag well behind use by those not facing similar barriers to health care. Some studies have also found that these differentials continue to exist for all disadvantaged groups even when adjusted for the greater health needs of the disadvantaged.

Ambulatory Care

Most striking is the extent to which insurance coverage affects use of ambulatory care. The insured receive 54 percent more ambulatory care from physicians than do the uninsured. However, the differential between the insured and uninsured for physician visits may understate the actual differential because variations in scope of coverage among the insured population are not accounted for. Some of the insured may only have insurance coverage for inpatient hospital care, not ambulatory care. Thus, although their utilization pattern is considered in the insured category, such individuals are actually uninsured for physician visits. Better data on ambulatory-care insurance coverage of the insured population therefore might indicate even greater differentials in use of ambulatory care.

Residence and race also affect utilization of ambulatory services. The lowest utilization of ambulatory care occurs for uninsured blacks and other minorities, including Hispanics. These persons use far less than more advantaged groups. For example, uninsured blacks and other minorities in the South make 1.5 physician visits per person annually, compared with 3.7 physician visits for insured whites in the South. That is, to be advantaged leads to a utilization rate almost 2.5 times that of individuals who are disadvantaged.

These data point to the importance of financial and physical barriers to access. It is not the case that the uninsured manage to obtain ambulatory care comparable in amount to that obtained by the insured by relying on public clinics, teaching hospital outpatient clinics, nonprofit health centers, or the charity of private physicians. Without insurance, many simply do without care.

Hospital Care

Despite the common perception that all disadvantaged persons can obtain hospital care from some charity facility, tremendous differentials in use of hospital care also exist by insurance status, residence, and race. The insured receive 90 percent more hospital care than do the uninsured. Differentials by insurance status are particularly marked in the South and in rural areas. In the South, insured persons receive three times as many days of hospital care annually as uninsured persons, regardless of race or ethnic background.

These hospital utilization differentials clearly demonstrate that the insured fare much better than the uninsured in obtaining health care services. Since those with insurance are likely to have basic coverage for hospitalization, the hospital utilization data provide a more accurate assessment of the role of insurance coverage in the use of health care services than do the ambulatory care differentials in the previous section.

These differentials remove any complacency about the accessibility of inpatient care. They reinforce similar findings by Wilensky and Berk who find that the insured poor use more hospital care than the uninsured poor. They find the biggest differences between those always uninsured and those on Medicaid all year. Those on Medicaid part of the year used fewer hospital services than those on Medicaid all year. The uninsured also used less hospital care than those privately insured. The analysis here extends these results to examine racial and regional differentials.

Health Status and Use of Services

Lower utilization of ambulatory and inpatient care by the uninsured is not a reflection of lower need for health care services. Instead, as measured by self-assessment of health status, the uninsured tend to be somewhat sicker than the insured. Fifteen percent of the uninsured under age 65 rate their health as fair or poor, compared with 11 percent of the insured. Blacks and other minorities in the South systematically rate their health the worst. Of insured blacks and other minorities in the South, 19 percent assess their health as fair or poor, compared with 9 percent of insured whites outside the South.

One possible explanation of the higher rate of poor or fair health among the uninsured is that the lack of insurance is itself related to health status. Those who rate their health as poor or fair are more likely to be unable to work because of illness than those who rate their health good or excellent. Since insurance coverage in the United States is related to employment, those who are unemployed due to poor health are also likely to be without insurance. Under an employment-based insurance system, the working population enjoys both good health and insurance coverage, while those too ill to work suffer both lack of employment and lack of insurance.

The sick who are uninsured use medical care services less than their insured counterparts. Utilization of ambulatory services, adjusted for health status, shows that the insured in poor health see a physician 70 percent more often than the uninsured in poor health. Physician visits per person under age 65 in fair or poor health average 6.9 among the insured, compared with 4.1 visits for the uninsured with similar health problems. Blacks and other minorities with fair or poor health who are insured receive twice as much care as their uninsured counterparts.

Among the uninsured in poor or fair health, the differentials in physician visits by race and residence are especially noteworthy. Uninsured whites have greater access to physician services than do uninsured minorities. A southern white in fair or poor health sees a physician twice as often as a southern minority person in fair or poor health. The same relationship exists for utilization of physician services in metropolitan areas. However, the utilization differential between whites and minorities narrows in areas outside the South and in nonmetropolitan areas.

The number of physician visits by the uninsured versus the insured in fair or poor health warrants further examination. It is expected that the individual in fair or poor health would require frequent physician visits for diagnosis and treatment of the condition. The average of five to seven visits annually by the insured would appear to provide a reasonable level of physician contact. But for uninsured minorities in the South in fair or poor health, the average number of visits is two per year. This rate would provide no more than an initial visit and one follow-up visit, which might be insufficient to treat serious or complex illnesses. Thus, lower rates of physician visits could impair adequate treatment and follow-up to promote a rapid recovery.

POLICY IMPLICATIONS

The utilization differentials between the insured and uninsured underscore the importance of financial barriers to health care. Lack of insurance coverage is the major barrier. It markedly affects the amount of both ambulatory and inpatient care received. Without insurance coverage, many individuals obviously do without care. Those able to obtain care incur substantial travel and waiting times.

Lack of insurance coverage has three major consequences: it contributes to unnecessary pain, suffering, disability, and even death among the uninsured; it places a financial burden on those uninsured who struggle to pay burdensome medical bills; and it places a financial strain on hospitals, physicians, and other health care providers who attempt to provide care to the uninsured.

Research is limited on both the health of the uninsured and the health consequences of having no insurance. Extensive data on utilization patterns by the uninsured desegregated by residence and race are presented for virtually the first time in this report. But a number of recent studies have shown that medical care utilization has a dramatic impact on health. A recent Urban Institute report by Hadley explores the relation between medical care utilization and mortality rates. It contains persuasive evidence that utilization of medical care services leads to a marked reduction in mortality rates. A recent study by Grossman and Goldman at the National Bureau of Economic Research has found that infant mortality rates have dropped significantly in communities served by federally funded community health centers. This growing body of evidence does provide considerable support to the importance of medical care utilization in assuring a healthy population — and at least indirectly provides a basis for concern that the lower medical care utilization of the uninsured contributes to unnecessary deaths and lowered health status.

Lack of insurance coverage also imposes serious financial burdens on those who try to make regular payments to retire enormous debts incurred in obtaining medical care. With the average cost of a hospital stay in the United States now in excess of $2,000, few individuals can afford to build payments for hospital care into their monthly living allowance. Yet, since the uninsured are more likely to be poor, the economic consequences of lack of insurance fall heaviest on those least able to bear the burden.

In addition to its consequences for the uninsured, lack of insurance also takes its toll on the health care system. One result is that the financial stability of hospitals and ambulatory care providers willing to provide charity care for those unable to pay is jeopardized. Health care providers serving the uninsured — particularly inner city community and teaching hospitals, county and municipal clinics, and community health centers — absorb much of the cost of this as charity care or a bad debt. Yet this burden is not evenly distributed among hospitals and other providers. A recent study by the Urban Institute found that one-seventh of a national sample of hospitals studied provided over 40 percent of the free care.

For many of the uninsured, community health centers and migrant health centers have helped to fill the gap in access created by the lack of insurance. This was especially important for those ineligible for Medicaid. However, simultaneously with the cutbacks in Medicaid, major reductions were made in these service delivery programs.

Financial strains on public hospitals and clinics supported by state and local governments are leading to further curtailment of services. Preadmission deposits, often sizeable in amount, impose serious barriers for many of the uninsured seeking hospital care. Teaching hospitals that have for years maintained an open-door policy are reevaluating the fiscal viability of continuing such a policy. In many areas, hospitals are beginning to transfer nonpaying

patients to public facilities, further expanding the charity load of those facilities and reducing their ability to remain solvent.

Public hospitals, traditionally the care provider of last resort, are under new
pressures to close or reduce services as local governments respond to shrinking
revenues. Yet, shifting the responsibility of public hospitals to community
hospitals will not solve the problem of caring for the uninsured. Recent hearings have documented the refusal of community hospitals to take uninsured
patients, even in emergency situations. This has led to documented cases of
deaths that could have been avoided with prompt medical attention.

Such disparities in access to care are unacceptable in a decent and humane
society. Several actions are required to assure progress toward adequate access
for all. Medicaid coverage should be expanded to provide basic insurance
coverage for all low-income individuals. The Medicaid programs in southern
states have tended to have very restrictive eligibility policies leaving many of
the poor uncovered. Expanded coverage of the poor through Medicaid would
improve the scope of coverage in the South and could help to alleviate some of
the extreme utilization differentials between the South and non-South. A
minimum income standard set at some percentage of the poverty level would
be an important first step. In 1979, 23 states, including most of the southern
states, had income eligibility levels for Medicaid below 55 percent of the
poverty level. Texas, Alabama, and Tennessee had the lowest standards in the
nation—less than $2,000 for a family of four. Coupled with implementation of
a minimum income standard, Medicaid coverage should be broadened to
include children and ultimately adults in two-parent families. Such steps
would help assure access to care for the nation's poorest families.

Yet, the near-poor and working poor without insurance cannot be forgotten.
Today, under Medicaid, only 29 states cover the medically needy to provide health
coverage for those with large medical expenses. In effect, this catastrophe coverage provides some measure of protection to working families and is undoubtedly
the source of care for many of the "sometimes insured." Coverage for the
medically needy is currently very limited in the South; implementation of coverage
for the medically needy would be another step toward reducing the disparities
between the South and the rest of the country. Expansion of this coverage option
is an important component of a positive health care agenda.

Finally, the extensiveness of unemployment in today's economy under-
scores the need to refine the link between employment and health insurance
coverage. "Out of work" ought not to translate to "without health care
services." Often, health needs are greatest during periods of stress related to
unemployment. Health insurance coverage should be extended through employer plans for a period following unemployment, and guaranteed through
public coverage until reemployment. Employers should also be encouraged to

provide comprehensive coverage, including prevention and primary care services, to all workers and their families.

These measures would help to provide protection and improved access to care for the 34 million or more Americans now without health care insurance. However, as the metropolitan and nonmetropolitan differentials among the insured demonstrate, financing alone is not enough to correct access differentials. Resources development must be coupled with improved financing in underserved areas to assure that needed providers are available. Continued funding and expansion of the community and migrant health center programs to assure physical access to services for residents of high poverty, medically underserved communities is an essential adjunct to broadened financing for low-income populations. Other important ways to provide expanded insurance coverage without perpetuating the cost inefficiencies of the existing system include: reform of Medicaid, Medicare, and private health insurance plans to encourage ambulatory care in cost-effective primary care programs; and experimentation with capitation payments to individual primary care centers, networks of centers, hospitals, or other major primary care providers for providing ambulatory and inpatient services to Medicaid beneficiaries.

This agenda of improved financing and resource development represents a positive strategy that can be employed to reduce major inequities in American health care. Today, some will argue that this agenda is too ambitious and costly and would instead opt for a more targeted and incremental approach. For example, instead of expanding Medicaid coverage, advocates of the incremental approach would favor renewed support to public hospitals and financial aid to hospitals serving large numbers of uninsured to mitigate the worst problems. These approaches are piecemeal, however, and do not address the fundamental problems identified in this paper. Such targeted approaches focus on protecting institutions serving the uninsured rather than protecting the uninsured themselves. Thus, they provide for the continued existence of a source of care for the uninsured seeking care, but do not provide comprehensive coverage to the uninsured to encourage early and preventive services. The poor and uninsured who do without care either because they do not live near an "aided facility" or do not know they could obtain free care from a hospital with a financial distress loan would still suffer inequitable health care differentials.

This paper demonstrates that lack of insurance makes a difference in health care utilization. Studies such as the recent work by Hadley point out the positive impact of medical care on mortality. Society ultimately bears the burden for care of the uninsured. The choice is between paying up front and directly covering the uninsured or indirectly paying for their care through subsidies to fiscally troubled health facilities, higher insurance premiums, and increased hospital costs to cover the cost of charity care and pay for the ill health caused by neglect and inadequate preventive and primary care. Thus, the best and most pragmatic approach is to provide health insurance coverage to the uninsured and to use targeted approaches to improve resource distribution and to remove remaining differentials. The inequities in health care in the United States described here will deepen unless a positive agenda is pursued.

In health there is freedom. Health is the first of all liberties.

HENRI FREDERIC AMIEL (1879)

Howard E. Freeman/Robert J. Blendon
Linda H. Aiken/Seymour Sudman
Connie F. Mullinix/Christopher R. Corey

Americans Report on Their Access to Health Care

In developing its initial grantmaking program in the early 1970s, The Robert Wood Johnson Foundation chose to emphasize improving access to health care in the United States. There were many press accounts at the time about the difficulties Americans experienced obtaining medical care, but there was little timely and systematic information about the overall magnitude of the problem, its distribution among various population groups, and changes over time. To acquire this information, the Johnson Foundation supported three independent national studies in 1976, 1982, and 1986 to measure the extent to which individuals were experiencing problems obtaining medical care. These surveys built on a research approach first implemented by the Committee on the Costs of Medical Care in the early 1930s, which was later extended and refined by Odin Anderson, Ronald Andersen, and their colleagues at the University of Chicago.

This paper highlights results from the recently completed 1986 survey of access to and use of health services. Six findings are of particular significance: (1) Between 1982 and 1986, Americans' overall use of medical care declined in terms of hospitalization and per capita physician visits. (2) Access to physician care for individuals who were poor, black, or uninsured decreased between 1982 and 1986, particularly for those in poor health. (3) Hospitalizations have

Howard E. Freeman, Ph.D., is professor of sociology, University of California, Los Angeles, California.

Robert J. Blendon, Sc.D., is professor and chair, Department of Health Policy and Management, Harvard University School of Public Health, Boston, Massachusetts.

Linda H. Aiken, R.N., Ph.D. is trustee professor of nursing and sociology, and associate director, Leonard Davis Institute of Health Economics, University of Pennsylvania, Philadelphia, Pennsylvania.

Seymour Sudman is professor of sociology at the University of Illinois, Urbana, Illinois.

Connie Flynt Mullinix, R.N., M.P.H., M.B.A., is clinical assistant professor, School of Nursing, University of North Carolina, Chapel Hill, North Carolina.

Christopher R. Corey is a doctoral student at the University of California, Los Angeles, California.

also declined for these disadvantaged groups, but the reduction is comparable to that experienced by the entire population. However, the uninsured and black and Hispanic Americans continue to receive less hospital care than might be appropriate given their higher rates of ill health. (4) Though much has been written about the overuse of medical care, this study found signs of underuse of important health services among key population groups. (5) The long-standing gap in receipt of medical care between rural and urban residents appears to have been eliminated. (6) Most Americans continue to be highly satisfied with their physician and inpatient hospital care. In addition, emergency care, which was a source of some dissatisfaction in 1982, received higher marks in 1986.

METHODS

Data reported in this article come from two telephone surveys conducted in 1982 and 1986, using similar research instruments and design. Each respondent was interviewed for approximately twenty-five minutes about various aspects of access to medical care: the availability of a personal physician or usual source of care; the actual use of doctors, other health professionals, and hospitals; self-reports of health status; the presence of serious health conditions; problems in paying for care; and the degree of satisfaction with the care received. Supplemental face-to-face interviews were conducted in 1986 with a small sample of people without telephones in three geographically dispersed communities. The findings of this survey confirm, as others have concluded, that if households without telephones were added to those surveyed by telephone, the findings would not be significantly different.

The 1986 study consisted of interviews with 10,130 people in the continental United States, 76 percent of those selected for interviews. People with chronic and serious illnesses were oversampled; the study group was weighted, however, so that the findings represent the U.S. population. Proxy interviews with a parent were conducted in order to obtain information on children under age seventeen. Also in cases where the respondent was too sick or otherwise unable to be interviewed, a proxy interview with another person in the household was completed. The 1982 data are from the previous foundation-supported survey undertaken by Louis Harris and Associates in conjunction with the University of Chicago. The study group consisted of approximately 6,700 adults and children. The 1982 sample was reweighted for the purposes of this analysis to be consistent with the procedures used for the 1986 sample; thus, there are small differences in the 1982 results reported here and in previous publications from the study.

The average number of physician visits reported in these two surveys differs somewhat from those reported by the National Center for Health Statistics because telephone consultations are not counted as visits in our two surveys. Also, the interviewers in our surveys probed to gain information on all visits to specialists, including mental health professionals, in 1986, which is not usually done in other national surveys.

DECLINE IN THE USE OF MEDICAL CARE

Between 1982 and 1986, the average use of medical care declined across all population groups. As illustrated in Exhibit 1, the percentage of Americans hospitalized one or more times in the year prior to the survey declined by 22 percent. One-third of Americans did not visit a physician even once in the year prior to the survey, a major change since 1982. Average per capita visits to physicians declined by 10 percent, a consequence of the reduced portion of the population with any ambulatory contacts in 1986. It should be noted, however, that mean physician visit rates reported in the 1982 survey were higher than other studies undertaken that year, including the Health Interview Survey. Hence, the difference in visits between our 1982 and 1986 data may overstate somewhat the actual decline in physician utilization.

Over the past two decades, a larger proportion of Americans have reported having access to a regular source of care, usually a particular private physician. Studies have suggested that patients may receive more appropriate and effective health care when they have a simple source for care—a place where there is some continuing knowledge of their health status and problems over time. However, as Exhibit 1 shows, a larger proportion of Americans in 1986 compared with 1982 report having no single usual source of care (18 percent compared to 11 percent). Even among people who report having a usual source of care, there appears to be more use of multiple physicians and settings. For example, of those who had a particular personal physician in 1982, 95 percent reported seeing that doctor on their last visit. In 1986, only 79 percent went to their regular doctor on their last visit.

The surveys do not provide data that permit a full explanation of the reduced use of physician and hospital care. The changes are consistent, however, with a number of trends in health care nationally including greater

EXHIBIT 1 The Use of Medical Care by Americans, 1982 and 1986

	1982	1986
Percent without a physician visit in the past year	19%	33%
Average number of per person physician visits within the past year	4.8	4.3
Percent hospitalized during the past year	9%	7%
Percent without a usual source of care	11%	18%

use of coinsurance and deductibles in private health insurance plans, increased out-of-pocket medical care costs, more widespread use of hospital preadmission screening, an increase in ambulatory surgery, and the rapid growth of urgent care centers.

DETERIORATING ACCESS FOR THE POOR, MINORITIES, AND UNINSURED

Data on the number of visits people make to doctors' offices and hospitals do not tell us all we wish to know about the accessibility of health care in the United States. For example, visit rates tell us little about the appropriateness of treatment received. Visit rates do provide one window, however, on the accessibility of personal health services to different groups in the country. Moreover, the usefulness of this measure of accessibility can be enhanced by taking into account individuals' relative need for health care. The President's Commission for the Study of Ethical Problems in Medicine and Biomedical and Behavioral Research in its 1983 report recommended that adjustments be made for health status in all comparisons of physician utilization rates between groups. Earlier studies have shown that a person's self-assessment of health status is a reasonably sensitive indicator of actual need for medical care, including the presence of chronic conditions and disabilities, the number of specific health problems and symptoms, sensory impairment and immobility, and limitations of normal activities due to illness.

The following exhibits, then, report utilization of physician and hospital care by health status for the poor, minorities, and the uninsured. Two types of comparisons are made: (1) the percent change between 1982 and 1986; and (2) the gap in receipt of care between different groups. The gap is the percent difference between two groups using the majority group as the standard against which the other is compared.

Low-income Americans.   The earliest access study, undertaken in 1931, found that people with low incomes saw physicians 50 percent less frequently than did those with higher incomes. This gap was of particular concern because of evidence that serious illness was more common among the poor. By the mid-1970s, after decades of gradual progress, this inequity in the frequency of use of physician services had been largely eliminated. Indeed, individuals from lower income groups were actually seeing physicians slightly more often than those of higher incomes, which reflected their higher burden of illness.

However, between 1982 and 1986, this improved situation changed, particularly for low-income groups who were in poorer health. The nation's low-income citizens received less physician care, on average, in 1986 than comparable groups did in 1982. Between 1982 and 1986 as shown in Exhibit 2, physician visit rates for low-income individuals in poorer health declined by

8 percent while visit rates for the nonpoor of similar health status increased by 42 percent. This widened a gap that had all but disappeared. By 1986, the poor had 27 percent fewer physician visits than did the nonpoor of the same health status. This suggests a significant reversal in the longstanding trend toward greater equity in the accessibility of physician care.

Low-income adults, particularly those under age sixty-five, have experienced marked declines in physician visits since 1982 (Exhibit 3). The average number of physician visits declined by 30 percent for poor adults under age sixty-five while no change was found for the nonpoor. By 1986, poor and nonpoor adults under age sixty-five were seeing physicians at roughly the

EXHIBIT 2 Mean Number of Physician Visits by Income and Health Status, 1982 and 1986

Income	Fair and poor health		Percent change
	1982	1986	1982 to 1986
Poor and near poor[a]	9.1	8.4	−8%
Nonpoor	8.1	11.5	+42%
Gap (percent)[b]	+12%	−27%	
	Excellent and good health		
Poor and near poor	4.1	3.3	−20%
Nonpoor	4.2	3.8	−10%
Gap (percent)	−2%	−13%	

[a]Less than 150 percent of poverty level.
[b]Percent difference in visits by poor compared to nonpoor.

EXHIBIT 3 Mean Number of Physician Visits and Perceived Health Status by Age and Income, 1982 and 1986

	Physician visits		Percent change	Percent in fair/poor health
	1982	1986	1982–1986	1986
Children below 17:				
Poor/near poor	3.8	3.9	+3%	13%
Nonpoor	4.5	3.8	−16	4
Gap (percent)	−16%	+3%		
Adults 17–64:				
Poor/near poor	6.7	4.7	−30	21
Nonpoor	4.5	4.5	0	8
Gap (percent)	+49%	+4%		
Elderly 65+:				
Poor/near poor	6.0	4.8	−20	42
Nonpoor	5.7	4.9	−14	25
Gap (percent)	+5%	−2%		

EXHIBIT 4 Percent Hospitalized One or More Times in Year and Perceived Health Status by Income, 1982 and 1986

Income	Percent hospitalized		Percent in fair/poor health
	1982	1986	1989
Poor and near poor	10.4	7.9	22%
Nonpoor	8.8	6.2	8
Gap (percent)	+18%	+27%	

same rates even though almost three times more of the poor reported themselves in only fair or poor health. If poor and nonpoor adults had comparable access to physicians, we would expect the poor to see physicians more often because a larger proportion are in ill health. The same trends in access are noted for the elderly. Poor and nonpoor elderly saw physicians at the same rates in 1986 despite a higher proportion of poor elderly reporting themselves in ill health. Access to physician care for poor children remained about the same over the period, but physician use rates for poor children do not reflect that more poor children than nonpoor children are in ill health.

A number of changes in the organization and financing of hospital care occurred between 1982 and 1986. There has been much speculation about how these changes affected low income Americans. The national decline in hospital use mentioned earlier is reflected in a reduction of hospitalization among both poor and nonpoor Americans, as indicated in Exhibit 4. The poor were more likely than the nonpoor in both 1982 and 1986 to have been hospitalized at least once in a year, which appears to be justified in view of the larger proportion of low-income individuals in ill health. Our data do not permit an assessment, however, of whether the levels of hospital use by the poor in either 1982 or 1986 were appropriate to their actual levels of need.

Access for minorities.   An important measure of equity of access is the frequency of the use of health services by minorities. Hispanics, on average, see physicians at about the same rate as whites. For black Americans, however, the

EXHIBIT 5 Mean Number of Physician Visits by Ethnicity and Health Status, 1982 and 1986

Race	Fair and poor health		Excellent and good health	
	1982	1986	1982	1986
Black	7.6	6.8	4.5	2.8
White	8.6	10.1	4.2	3.8
Gap (percent)	−12%	−33%	+7%	−26%
Hispanic	9.7	9.8	3.9	3.9
White	8.6	10.1	4.2	3.8
Gap (percent)	+13%	−3%	−7%	+3%

EXHIBIT 6 Percent Hospitalized One or More Times in Year by Ethnicity, 1982 and 1986

Ethnicity	Percent hospitalized		Percent in fair/poor health
	1982	1986	1986
Black	7.6	6.2	15.3%
White	10.2	6.8	10.6
Gap (percent)	−25%	−9%	
Hispanic	6.3	4.5	19.4
White	10.2	6.8	10.6
Gap (percent)	−38%	−34%	

1986 survey portrays a picture of diminishing access to medical care. As indicated in Exhibit 5, physician visit rates for blacks declined between 1982 and 1986. Thus, by 1986, there was a difference of 33 percent between physician visit rates of blacks and whites in ill health, and about the same for those in good health. The growing gap in physician visits between blacks and whites is of particular concern in view of the evidence recently assembled by the National Institutes of Health showing that black Americans have a considerably higher mortality rate than whites have.

All ethnic groups were affected by the overall national decline in hospital use (Exhibit 6). However, the study shows that in both 1982 and 1986 there were significant gaps in receipt of hospital care for Hispanics compared to whites despite a greater proportion of Hispanics in ill health. Blacks were also less likely than whites to be hospitalized given their poorer health status.

Access for the uninsured.   Health insurance continues to be an important factor influencing access to medical care. The nation's uninsured population contains a somewhat larger share of people in fair or poor health than is found among those with health insurance. Thus, if there were no economic barriers to care, the receipt of physician services and hospital care by the uninsured

EXHIBIT 7 Mean Number of Physician Visits, Percent Hospitalized, and Perceived Health Status by Insurance Coverage for Persons under 65, 1982 and 1986

Insurance coverage	Physician visits		Percent in fair/poor health
	1982	1986	1986
Uninsured	3.8	3.2	12%
Insured	4.7	4.4	9
Gap (percent)	−19%	−27%	
	Percent hospitalized		
Uninsured	5.2	4.6	12
Insured	8.5	5.7	9
Gap (percent)	−39%	−19%	

would be expected to exceed that received by the insured. As can be seen in Exhibit 7, the uninsured had fewer physician visits and were less likely than the insured to be hospitalized in both 1982 and 1986. The gap between the uninsured and the insured in average number of physician visits widened substantially in 1986, suggesting that the uninsured are experiencing greater difficulty obtaining physician care. While the gap in receipt of hospital care narrowed over the period, a 19 percent difference still remains between the uninsured and the insured. In both 1982 and 1986, a smaller proportion of the uninsured was hospitalized than the higher burden of illness suggests might be appropriate.

Those surveyed were also asked if they had ever failed to obtain needed medical care for economic reasons. The results, presented in Exhibit 8, closely parallel the other findings. Of those interviewed, 6 percent, representing approximately 13.5 million Americans, reported not receiving medical care for financial reasons. An estimated 1 million individuals actually tried to obtain needed care but did not receive it. The majority of Americans experiencing these difficulties were poor, uninsured, or minorities.

UNDERUSE OF MEDICAL CARE

Growing concerns about the nation's rising health care bill have led to an almost exclusive focus by public and private sector policymakers on how to reduce the unnecessary overuse of costly health care. Less attention has been directed to the possibility of serious underuse of medical care by some people. The results from this study point to particular problems of underuse across the country.

Exhibit 9 presents data providing measures of potential underuse of medical care by different groups in the country. One in six Americans who had an identifiable chronic and serious illness (such as cancer, heart disease, diabetes,

EXHIBIT 8 Percent of Americans Not Receiving Care for Economic Reasons, 1986

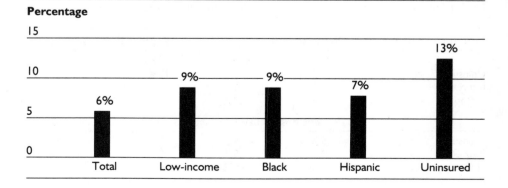

EXHIBIT 9 Indicators of Potential Underuse of Medical Care, 1986

Problem	U.S.	Low-Income	Black	Hispanic	Uninsured
Percent with chronic illness without physician visit in a year	17%	18%	25%	22%	20%
Among persons with one or more physician visits in year, percent with serious symptoms who did not see or contact a physician	41	42	39	53	67
Percent pregnant women without first trimester prenatal care	15	30	17	27	20
Percent of persons with hypertension without blood pressure check in a year	20	15	30	30	22
Percent without a dentist visit in a year	38	57	50	47	—

and stroke) did not see a physician even once during the year. Many physicians would agree that patients with such illnesses should be seen by a doctor at least annually.

The survey also asked respondents whether, over the past thirty days, they had experienced one or more symptoms judged by a panel of physicians to warrant care in most instances, and if so, whether they sought medical attention. These serious symptoms were adapted from an instrument developed by the University of Chicago, and subsequently modified for use in the Rand Health Insurance Experiment. Of those respondents who had at least one physician visit in the year, 41 percent reported the occurrence of one or more of five serious symptoms and did not see or tell a physician about the problem. These symptoms included bleeding, other than nosebleeds or menstrual periods, not caused by accidents; shortness of breath after light exercise; loss of consciousness, fainting, or passing out; chest pain when exercising; and weight loss of more than ten pounds (except for dieting). The large proportion of people who failed to visit or telephone a physician in the face of having these symptoms is of concern.

Likewise, the large proportion of pregnant women who did not seek prenatal care in the first three months of their pregnancy is troubling. Infant mortality has been reduced by half since 1960, but the rates of infant death in the United States still exceed those of many other comparable industrialized countries. A recent Institute of Medicine study concluded that early prenatal care leads to improved maternal and infant outcomes. It is therefore of concern to find that one in seven pregnant women surveyed in 1986 did not seek medical care early in pregnancy.

The study also found signs of underuse of medical care for persons diagnosed as having hypertension. This disease is associated with two of the nation's major killers—heart disease and stroke. Thus, it is of concern that 20

EXHIBIT 10 Mean Physician Visits, Percent Hospitalized, and Perceived Health Status for Urban and Rural Residents, 1982 and 1986

Residence	Physician visits		Percent in fair/poor health
	1982	1986	1986
Rural	4.4	4.4	14%
Urban	5.0	4.3	11
Gap (percent)	−12%	+2%	
	Percent hospitalized		
Rural	9.7	8.0	14
Urban	9.1	6.0	11
Gap (percent)	+7%	+33%	

percent of people with diagnosed hypertension surveyed in 1986 — and almost one-third of blacks and Hispanics with this condition — did not have their blood pressure checked at least once during the year.

Americans have traditionally underused dental services, and this trend appears to have continued. Thirty-eight percent of all respondents had not visited a dentist in a year; only half of low-income individuals reported a dental visit.

These data taken together suggest that a substantial number of Americans may not be getting as much health care as they need. The reasons may include social and cultural factors as well as financial barriers. However, the presence of signs of underuse among all segments of the population also suggests a lack of understanding of appropriate use of medical care and a need for improved public education.

OTHER FINDINGS

Improved access for rural Americans.   A positive finding in the 1986 survey is that rural Americans, on average, appear to be receiving as much medical care as their urban counterparts, as indicated in Exhibit 10. Closing the rural/urban gap in access to health services has been a national goal for many years. That goal now appears to have been achieved. This is not to say, of course, that residents of some isolated rural communities do not still experience problems obtaining timely medical care. The same is true for some inner-city residents. However, it is clear that major strides have been made in improving the geographic accessibility of physician and hospital services.

Satisfaction with medical care.   Despite substantial disparities among various groups in their access to medical care, most Americans remain highly satisfied with the care they receive from physicians and hospitals. Even the modest levels of dissatisfaction with emergency care found in 1982 had declined by 1986 (Exhibit 11).

EXHIBIT 11 Percent Dissatisfied with Their Use of Medical Care, 1982 and 1986

Type of visit	Percent dissatisfied	
	1982	1986
Most recent emergency visit	11%	5%
Most recent physician visit	3	2
Most recent hospitalization	4	4

CONCLUSION

The results of the 1986 University of California, Los Angeles survey, the largest supported by The Robert Wood Johnson Foundation to date, are both surprising and disturbing. Many of the nation's forecasters in health have clearly not been on the mark. An aging population, a growing supply of physicians, and more and better medical technologies have not, as predicted, led to significant increases in use of health care per person. Rather, this study suggests that there has been a decline in visits to physicians and in the proportion of people hospitalized. This trend cuts across all groups within our country and is difficult to fully explain. Some will obviously associate this with the many changes now occurring in health care arrangements that emphasize lower utilization of health care resources, including health maintenance organizations, preferred provider organizations, utilization review, and diagnosis-related groups.

This study cannot answer the critical questions of whether Americans are sicker or remain in ill health longer because they receive less medical care today than they did in 1982. There are, however, significant numbers of individuals who have serious and potentially life-threatening illnesses who do not appear to use health care appropriately. This may prove to be a problem requiring more public education or it may reflect unrecognized financial or professional barriers to care.

On the positive side, after many years of national attention to achieving a more equitable geographic distribution of health resources, rural Americans, on average, appear to be receiving as much medical care as urban residents. While some isolated rural communities clearly have continuing problems that should not be overlooked, we can take some pride in knowing that medical care is reasonably accessible nationwide. Also on a positive note, Americans continue to express a high level of satisfaction with the medical care they receive.

Clearly, the most disturbing findings relate to the signs of deterioration in access to medical care for the nation's poor, minorities, and the uninsured. In particular, the poor and black Americans have experienced a reversal of the gains in access to physician care made over the previous two decades, moving us further from securing more equitable access to care for all.

Gail R. Wilensky

Solving Uncompensated Hospital Care: Targeting the Indigent and the Uninsured

Uncompensated hospital care is not a new policy issue, but it has received an increasing amount of attention. Factors responsible for this include the recent recession which brought a sharp rise in unemployment, the increased emphasis placed by policymakers on prudent-buyer concepts, the heightened awareness of medical care costs by employers in their role as major purchasers of health care, and the anticipated decline in hospital revenues resulting from Medicare's prospective payment system. While some may argue that uncompensated hospital care naturally results from increased reliance on market principles—a hallmark of the Reagan administration—there is widespread agreement that these market-oriented reforms cannot succeed without more explicit treatment of the uncompensated care issue. However, designing appropriate public policies requires not only an understanding of why uncompensated care represents a threat to the use of market-oriented reforms, but also of why uncompensated care is generated, how much there is, and who receives it.

Much of the public policy discussion of uncompensated care assumes that it is synonymous with indigent care. This is an unwarranted assumption. Many of the people who generate uncompensated care are not poor. This implies that at least two policy strategies are necessary: one for the poor with little or no insurance coverage, and a second for those who are not poor but who either have little or no insurance coverage, or do not pay their bills.

HOW BIG IS THE PROBLEM?

The amount of dollars spent on uncompensated hospital care is surprisingly small. According to the American Hospital Association's "Annual Survey of Hospitals," community hospitals provided $6.2 billion of uncompensated care in 1982. This amount was made up of $4.5 billion of bad debt (costs for

Gail R. Wilensky, Ph.D., is administrator of the Health Care Financing Administration, Department of Health and Human Services, Washington, D.C., and a former vice president of the Center for Health Affairs, Project HOPE, Millwood, New Jersey.

[320]

patients who were expected to pay but who for some reason did not pay) and $1.7 billion of charity care (cost for patients who were not expected to pay). While there is little question that the amount of uncompensated care provided by community hospitals increased from 1978 to 1982, the size of the increase is less clear. The problem is that the amount of increase is very sensitive to the deflator used in constructing the time series estimate. Using the consumer price index as the deflator, uncompensated care increased from 4.5 billion in 1978 to 6.2 billion in 1982. If the GNP deflator is used, the increase is larger—from 4.2 billion to 6.2 billion—and if hospital prices are used as the deflator, the increase is smaller—from 5.2 billion to 6.2 billion.

While the total amount of uncompensated care is not large—6 percent of total community hospital payments and 5 percent of community hospital charges—it is not evenly distributed among hospitals, as shown in Exhibit 1. Both teaching hospitals and government hospitals (teaching and nonteaching) provided a substantially greater proportion of uncompensated hospital care.

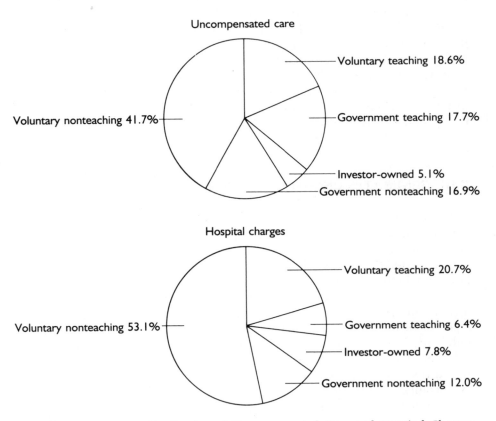

EXHIBIT 1 Percentage Distribution of Uncompensated Care and Hospital Charges by Hospital Type, 1982

Teaching hospitals, for example, accounted for 27 percent of total hospital charges but 35 percent of the uncompensated care. The disparity between hospital charges and uncompensated care is even more striking for government teaching hospitals, which account for 6 percent of the hospital charges and almost 18 percent of the uncompensated care, just as the public hospitals and teaching hospitals bear a disproportionately larger share of the uncompensated care, the nonteaching voluntary hospitals and investor-owned hospitals bear a disproportionately small share of the uncompensated care expenses. The discrepancy is substantial for the voluntary nonteaching hospitals, which are responsible for 53 percent of the charges and 42 percent of the uncompensated care.

WHO PAYS FOR UNCOMPENSATED CARE?

For the most part, hospitals have financed uncompensated care by shifting costs among private third-party payers. Public hospitals often use appropriated monies to cover the cost of this care. The ultimate payer under cost-shifting is difficult to determine and will vary from hospital to hospital according to both the amount of uncompensated care provided as well as the revenue sources. However, hospitals which attempt to cover their uncompensated care costs by increasing their revenues from their privately insured patients can expect to lose those patients as employers increasingly exercise their roles as prudent buyers and search out the lowest costs of care. Thus, the growing emphasis on price competition will render this option impractical in the future.

WHO GENERATES UNCOMPENSATED CARE?

Little is known directly about the characteristics of individuals who receive care for which the provider is not compensated. To obtain this information, one would need to sample the hospital discharge records of individuals who had generated bad debt or charity care and then interview these individuals to find out whether they had insurance, whether insurance had been available to those without insurance, the extent of their insurance coverage, and their income and work status. We do, however, have information available about the types of hospitals that experience uncompensated care, such as the urban public teaching hospitals, other teaching hospitals, and, to a lesser extent, the voluntary hospitals and proprietary hospitals. Both the Sloan study and The Urban Institute study have indicated that hospitals with high concentrations of uncompensated care have disproportionate numbers of patients who are uninsured and low income.

As suggested by the patient populations of the hospitals that provide uncompensated care, the individuals most likely to generate uncompensated care are the uninsured and, to a lesser extent, the underinsured. Unlike the data on uncompensated care, much is known about the uninsured population. A limited amount of information is available about the underinsured.

There are several characteristics of those who are always uninsured which are worth noting: (1) the age group most likely to be uninsured are the young adults age eighteen to twenty-four; (2) one-third of the uninsured are under age eighteen; (3) one-half of the uninsured are from families with (1977) incomes above $15,000; and (4) over half were employed all or part of the year.

An examination shows that the popular image of the uninsured as predominately poor and unemployed or out of the labor force is not accurate. The uninsured are disproportionately poor — nearly one-third are poor or near poor; nonetheless, two-thirds of the uninsured are not poor, and one-half are in families with incomes that are at least twice the poverty level. Similarly, while the uninsured are disproportionately out of the labor force, over three-quarters of the uninsured are employed or are the dependents of employed workers. These workers tend to be lower wage earners with lower levels of education than the labor force as a whole and in almost all cases were not offered insurance by their employers. While young adults are disproportionately represented in the employed uninsured, almost half of this group are over thirty years old. Similarly, compared to the rest of the working population the employed uninsured are more likely to be employed part-time or self-employed, but in absolute terms two-thirds are full-time workers.

To summarize, neither the care nor the people generating the uncompensated hospital care are homogeneous. The care itself is a combination of inpatient catastrophic care, outpatient care, and normal uncomplicated stays. As best we can tell, the people generating uncompensated care are a mix of the poor and the nonpoor uninsured, individuals with inadequate insurance, and individuals who do not pay their deductibles and coinsurance. In view of the diversity of the population at risk for generating uncompensated care, it is unlikely that a single solution will be appropriate.

WHAT CAN AND SHOULD BE DONE ABOUT UNCOMPENSATED HOSPITAL CARE?

There are four basic strategies we can consider in dealing with uncompensated care: targeting providers, targeting individuals, providing grants to states, and doing nothing.

Targeting providers. The most commonly discussed strategy for attacking uncompensated care is by targeting providers, either by reimbursing them directly through an all-payer system, or indirectly by granting additional revenues to hospitals from a fund of pooled resources. The most direct way to reimburse providers is through an all-payer rate-setting system which includes an allowance for charity and bad debt in each payment made to hospitals. Maryland and New Jersey reimburse providers of uncompensated care through this mechanism.

The all-payer rate-setting system is highly regarded by some policymakers for several reasons: it limits reimbursement to those who would otherwise generate uncompensated care rather than to all those without insurance, it is administratively feasible, all payers of health care contribute a share of the cost, and it does not appear as an additional line item in a governmental budget. Offsetting these advantages are several major disadvantages. The all-payer system pays for care at whatever hospital the individuals use as opposed to directing them to providers who may be the most efficient. More important, many believe that all-payer systems provide little incentive for competitive innovation and that they reinforce existing relationships between payers and hospitals. All-payer systems are also highly regulatory and are therefore not attractive to states with political climates which favor a less imposing government role. Nonetheless, all-payer systems address the problem directly and thus will remain an attractive option in political arenas which make government the primary allocator of resources.

Another way of targeting providers is to grant funds to providers from a common pool of revenues. New York, an all-payer state, has had such a mechanism in place for the last year. Florida, not an all-payer state, has recently introduced legislation that would provide funds for uncompensated care from a common pool of revenue. Targeting providers through the use of revenue pools could have most of the advantages of the all-payer system with fewer of the disadvantages. Since they need not be tied to all-payer systems, they need not be as highly regulated a system as the all-payer system. In addition, revenue pools could be used to encourage competitive innovation by reimbursing cost-effective providers at a higher rate than less efficient providers. Unfortunately, most systems that target providers have compensated hospitals according to their existing patterns of utilization whether those patterns reinforce efficient delivery of care or not.

Targeting individuals. A second strategy for financing uncompensated hospital care is to target individuals—that is, to make sure that individuals without adequate insurance acquire coverage so that they can pay their bills. There are a variety of options for implementing this strategy: catastrophic illness insurance, state-sponsored insurance for high-risk individuals, insurance for the unemployed or other special populations, and insurance for the indigent.

Grants to local governments. Rather than specifying a national program either to target providers or individuals as a way of covering some or all uncompensated care, another possibility is to let each respective state or local government decide the type of program it wants. Assuming that whatever federal responsibility exists is primarily related to the indigent population, a matching or block grant could be provided states with the amount of the grant based primarily on the number of individuals in that state who are below the poverty line. An adjustment might also be made for unusually high levels of unemployment as well. The state, or preferably the local government after receiving a pass-through grant from the state, could then decide whether to reimburse hospitals directly through all-payer rate setting or by lump sums from a pool of revenues, or whether to attempt to provide the uninsured with insurance through a variety of means such as catastrophic illness programs, expanded medically needy programs, or a voucher system. The primary reason to direct grants through the state rather than to local governments is that the levels of responsibility of local governments for the provision of services for the needy varies across the United States. However, as long as states give local jurisdictions the choice as to how the funds are to be distributed, the primary advantages of local decision making would remain.

The major disadvantage of the intergovernmental grant approach is that there would be higher direct costs and higher administrative costs than in a program limited to providers and which therefore only reflected current users. However, the grants approach has several major advantages: it can be used to channel funds to those individuals who are in need, it does not establish a new entitlement program for individuals, it reflects both the needs and desires of local community, and it gives local communities the autonomy to determine their own levels of competition and innovation.

Doing nothing.   A final short-run option is to do nothing. This, however, is not a solution in the long run. The competitive pressures resulting from Medicare, Medicaid, and employers adopting prudent-buyer techniques, will focus increased attention on individuals who are without insurance coverage and who generate uncompensated care. Since we as a nation will not allow these individuals to go without the most necessary medical care, some method will be adopted to compensate hospitals providing care for these individuals.

RAISING REVENUE

Most of the programs discussed will require some increased level of public expenditures on health care. This raises the question of the type of taxes which would be used to support additional expenditures. The most likely options available include general fund financing, a tax on insurance premiums, an excise tax on hospital bills of insured patients, a tax cap on employment-related health insurance, and an excise tax on alcohol and tobacco.

A general tax such as a consumption tax or an income tax is an attractive revenue source, but in an era of high federal deficit they are politically unrealistic. Excise taxes on alcohol and tobacco are less desirable than general fund taxes and are also being discussed as deficit reduction measures. Should this not be the case, they would be regarded as an attractive mechanism for providing some of the needed revenue. The tax cap, also if not earmarked for other purposes, is a desirable revenue source for funding a risk pool and perhaps a portion of indigent care. An excise tax on premiums is an acceptable approach for financing some or all uncompensated care. A tax on hospital revenue financed by private payers is a less preferred variation on the excise tax on insurance premiums. However, any of the above explicit taxes are preferable to the current method of financing uncompensated care through cost shifting, which will become untenable in the long run.

PROPOSED POLICY DIRECTIONS

While there is not detailed information on who generates uncompensated care, there is suggestive evidence that they are individuals with no insurance or limited insurance. More data are available on the uninsured and these make it clear that many of the individuals without health insurance are not poor. This suggests that direct financing of uncompensated care is more than a problem of financing care for the indigent. Financing care for the indigent, however, is an important component of uncompensated care.

Recognition that uncompensated care reflects a heterogenous population suggests a two-pronged approach: a program for the indigent and a program for the nonindigent uninsured. Although indigent care can be financed through a variety of policy options, the most promising is the use of grants to state governments with funds passing through to local governments. This would allow communities the ability to assess their own particular circumstances and to decide whether vouchers, direct reimbursement to providers, an expansion of Medicaid or medically needy programs, or some other program would be best for them.

Those individuals who are not poor but are uninsured need to have insurance made available to them at reasonable rates. Risk pools seem to be an attractive way to do this. However, the risk pool should be subsidized by the state or federal government on the grounds that these individuals, unlike the vast majority of nonaged individuals who have employment-related insurance, are not currently receiving any subsidy from the tax exclusion accorded employment-related insurance. Additionally, unless limited subsidization is provided, it is likely that such insurance would be prohibitively expensive. There is a danger, however, that if the subsidy were substantial, employers might encourage their employees to get insurance from the risk pool. Given the substantial advantages associated with the current tax exclusion, this is unlikely to be an issue unless the level for the tax cap was set very low and the subsidy was set very high. These two programs might be financed by a combination of tax capping to support the risk pools and excise taxes on insurance premiums, hospital revenues, or tobacco and alcohol to support additional financing of indigent care.

The two-pronged approach suggested here is not without potential problems. Grants to state governments might not always result in the proper distribution to local government levels, and grants to local governments may be difficult to implement given differing local government structure. Given flexibility, some state and local governments will adopt more equitable or efficient programs than others, thus leaving some of the indigent better off than others. Furthermore, not all eligibles may take advantage of a risk pool. Some individuals, particularly the young adults, may be willing to engage in "free-rider" behavior, especially if they know that grants are being made to finance uncompensated care. Finally, some of the care currently being provided is uncompensated care which might not be covered by this type of insurance. Nonetheless, the two-pronged program suggested here is a way of addressing what is currently a major policy issue and it does so in ways that may be politically acceptable because it does not require major restructuring of the entire health care delivery system.

Our retrograde health care system reserves its greatest hardships for the following groups: the poor and near-poor, workers (including those in agriculture), the unemployed, the disabled, displaced, homemakers, the elderly, and children.

HEALTH CARE USA: 1984

Lawrence S. Lewin/Marion Ein Lewin

Financing Charity Care in an Era of Competition

For most of the 1980s, the health care industry has been in the throes of a major effort to see whether the market discipline of price competition can lead to a more cost-effective and responsive health care system. Few predicted that the road would be a smooth one, and, in recent years, the problem of financing charity care has emerged as a major threat to support for competition in the minds of employers as well as elected political officials.

As more and more Americans confront difficulty in gaining access to and paying for care, a backlash against further development of market forces is emerging. There is growing talk of mandating insurance benefits and of renewed interest in proposals for some type of national health insurance. In addition, attempts to further deregulate the health care industry are being challenged as inappropriate until charity care financing and access problems are ameliorated. While earlier efforts in state legislatures to adopt an all-payer rate setting as a solution appear to have abated, the indigent care issue has obstructed efforts in several states to curtail Certificate of Need.

In an effort to reduce hospital costs, payers are moving from paying charges as billed to paying negotiated rates. The cost of charity patients, and those with large uncompensated charges, thus is spread among fewer payers. In such an environment, hospitals committed to serving the uninsured poor are forced to increase their charges, while those with low or declining charity care burdens can gain a significant price-competitive advantage solely by avoiding charity care. The result has been an erosion of the genteel arrangement of cross-subsidies (cost shifting) that historically allowed hospitals to provide charity care without serious financial penalty or competitive handicap. As the pressures of competition among hospitals and prudent purchasing by payers squeeze those providing charity care, some have begun to reduce or limit their commitments. Indeed, Feder and Hadley documented such actions as early as 1980. An even more serious shortfall exists in primary and preventive care.

Lawrence S. Lewin is president of Lewin/ICF, Washington, D.C.
Marion Ein Lewin is director of the Pew Health Policy Fellowship Programs, Institute of Medicine, National Academy of Sciences, Washington, D.C.

Efforts to avoid charity care cases did not, of course, begin with the advent of price competition. Patient dumping and skimming are by no means new phenomena, nor are the disproportionate charity care roles played by teaching and public hospitals. What is new is that the tendency to shift uninsured patients to public hospitals or to severely limit charity care has accelerated where competitive forces have escalated. The pressure to reduce unsponsored care has also intensified as hospitals in general have developed an increased preoccupation with producing "bottom lines" or total margins. In the past, most nonprofits were content to set charges to break even. Now, hospital executives and their trustees worry about producing large enough margins (profits) to retain favorable bond ratings and thus low-cost access to capital, and to ensure that they will have sufficiently deep pockets to ride out the storm of declining demand and tough competition. The result is a tension between margin and mission that is manifesting itself in hospitals' attitudes toward charity care.

PUBLIC OR PRIVATE RESPONSIBILITY?

Although some support shared public-private responsibility for financing charity care, the popular view seems to be that it is first and foremost the responsibility of government. This view, which is particularly popular among the most ardent advocates of competition, poses some ironic and painful twists for its proponents and has some serious flaws.

First, the call for expanded public responsibilities runs counter to prevailing conservative thinking that government's role in the domestic economy, and especially the health care sector, is already too large, and that big government leads inevitably to increased regulation. This view also runs counter to the Reagan administration's efforts to strengthen voluntarism as a viable alternative to government. Ironically, the position that the government should be responsible for the indigent care problem provides strong support for national health insurance and similar approaches that rely on mandates and regulations.

Second, as a practical matter, increased government spending on a scale that would "solve" the charity care financing problem is highly improbable given the present federal deficit and the requirements of the Gramm-Rudman Act. In this climate, the proponents of a substantially larger federal financial role appear either naive or disingenuous.

Third, the call for increased government financing of charity care provided by hospitals suggests that the highest priority for new tax revenues should be to increase hospital income, when the more serious health care problem may not be uncompensated hospital care, but unrendered or deferred primary and preventive care. The problem is not that there are too few dollars in the health care system for hospitals to provide charity care, but rather that the unequal distribution of the charity care burden is creating competitive handicaps for those serving the uninsured poor, forcing providers to either curtail their commitments or risk pricing themselves out of the market.

Fourth, arguments in favor of expanding government responsibility also ignore the long-standing and predominantly charitable character of the hospital industry. A recent public opinion poll conducted by Cambridge Reports, Inc., for *Health Management Quarterly*, reported that the vast majority of the American public (85 percent of those sampled) believes that hospitals "should provide care to everyone regardless of patients' ability to pay." One of the underlying historical purposes of tax-exempt status is to attract and preserve capital for those nonprofit institutions providing vital social services that government otherwise would have to provide or finance. Those who currently enjoy the benefits of tax exemption should carefully consider the financial and political consequences if the government should take over the provision or financing of hospital-based charity care.

Finally, arguments to rely primarily on government financing imply that there are no other ways to bring about fair competition, to retain medical care resources already in place, and to improve access to primary and preventive care. As this article seeks to prove, this is assuredly not the case. There are already in practice a number of approaches that are not only feasible, but, given the larger goals of the health care system, more appropriate and realistic than a major shift to government financing would be. In general, the financing of charity care can be improved in three ways: (1) expanded private and public insurance; (2) increased support for public hospitals and clinics and other programs aimed at underserved priority groups; and (3) an equitable sharing of the financial burden of providing charity care.

EXPANDING THE REACH OF INSURANCE

Altered federal policies, changes in the labor force, and a more competitive, price-oriented health care environment are rapidly rending the fabric of public and private health insurance coverage. Both Medicaid and Medicare are the targets of increased cost-control efforts by federal and state governments, leaving vulnerable groups — low-income mothers, children, and the elderly — without needed coverage. In the private sector, businesses are shifting insurance costs, especially for dependents, increasingly to their employees. The mounting out-of-pocket costs that result may be encouraging workers to drop their dependents from the insurance rolls. In 1982, 36.3 percent of uninsured children lived with parents who had insurance. Changing trends in the labor force will place the insurance problem into sharper view, as high-paying, value-added manufacturing jobs give way to a service economy with fewer fringe benefits, lower wages, and more part-time workers.

Broadening the reach of insurance is viewed by many as one way to improve access to care. At least twenty states have expanded their Medicaid programs, with federal support.

States, providers, and private employers have found it in their interest to support Medicaid expansion. For states, the program funds are matched by at least a 50 percent federal contribution. For providers, Medicaid covers services that in most cases would end up as charity or bad debt. And for employers, financing care of the indigent through Medicaid also spreads the burden across the business community through state taxes; the tax rate businesses pay is far below the amount they pay through cost shifting. In spite of these efforts, however, Medicaid coverage for the poor remains inadequate.

Another target group in the expansion of insurance are those without insurance who are employed. Urban Institute data show that three-fourths of the 37 million in this country who lack insurance are either employed or dependents of employed persons. Many of these work for small businesses, which are not required to provide insurance benefits. Such benefits for small employers often are more costly and less comprehensive than are products marketed to larger groups. To address these problems, efforts are under way nationwide to develop insurance products for this segment of the population.

INCREASING INSTITUTIONAL SUPPORT FOR DEDICATED PROVIDERS

Public hospitals and clinics bear a disproportionate share of the burden of care for low-income uninsured persons. In many cities, they represent the principal source of inpatient care for the indigent and the only source of primary and preventive services.

Why not, then, simply increase the funding for these public programs as a means of assuring access to care for the medically indigent? In many cases, doing so would be a productive response, and may be the only sensible solution. But overreliance on this option also has its shortcomings. Public hospitals are not always easily accessible, especially to persons in rural areas; such hospitals tend to serve primarily the poor and thus result in a two-class system of care.

Sadly, our public institutions have fallen behind in the adequacy of both physical and human resources. As a result, forcing the medically indigent to rely increasingly on public hospitals and clinics without making a major commitment to upgrading these facilities is tantamount to institutionalizing a two-class system of care. Additionally, a greatly expanded commitment not only seems improbable given today's budget crisis, it also appears wasteful given the excess capacity that exists in the private system. Improved access to, and efficient use of, the resources already in place seems a more sensible approach.

Direct grants to dedicated caregivers, rather than the traditional fee-for-service market, succeed more often in providing the appropriate type of care (often both medical and social services) to seriously underserved populations. This seemingly contradicts the conventional wisdom that improved access via expanded insurance is always the preferred approach. But given the very low physician payment rates in most state Medicaid programs, increasing access for specific target groups would almost certainly require increasing payment levels for all physicians to make treating already underserved patients more appealing. While this may be justified in theory, it is most unlikely to occur in practice.

SHARING THE BURDEN EQUITABLY: INDIGENT CARE FUNDS

In the absence of universal coverage or a secure, stable public-sector safety net, some segment of the population will continue to be uninsured. While most local governments operate or support public hospitals, clinics, health centers, and related programs that serve the uninsured, usually based on income, one-third of the nation's largest cities lack a publicly mandated, tax-supported provider of care for the poor. As a result, some level of uncompensated hospital care and unrendered primary care will remain for the foreseeable future.

In efforts to preserve and increase resources for indigent care, and to promote fair competition, a number of states have looked at indigent care funds or pools as a way of ameliorating the problem of unsponsored charity care, at least for the present, until more systematic financing reforms can be implemented. Indigent care funds as an approach have generated a great deal of attention and debate.

What is an indigent care pool? An indigent care pool collects funds from a variety of possible sources and redistributes them primarily to those who bear a disproportionate share of the uncompensated charity care burden. Its basic objectives are: (1) to forestall the erosion of the system of cross-subsidies that has traditionally financed a significant portion of hospital-based charity care; (2) to prevent those who avoid charity care from thereby gaining an advantage in price-competitive markets; and (3) to permit a targeting of resources on indigent care, especially for primary and preventive care. Indigent care funds can take a variety of forms, differing in who pays into the pool; the nature and extent of federal, state, and local financial participation; how the funds are to be used (for example, to expand Medicaid, to reduce hospital uncompensated care, to fund primary care programs, to support high-risk insurance pools, and so on); and how and by whom the pool is administered.

Isn't this really a sick tax by another name? While the pool assessment is in reality a form of taxation, it is not a new tax. The so-called sick tax has always been with us in the form of the cost-shift mechanism, which is a kind of implicit cross-subsidy. The effect of the pooling mechanism is to preserve these funds in the system, but to distribute them more fairly in the form of a rational, explicit cross-subsidy. In fact, in an efficient market where price competition is really effective, this "tax" can prove to be budget-neutral. That is, the higher net levies on low charity providers that are passed on to the insurer should be offset by the reduction in charges by high charity providers who benefit from the pool. Unless the intent is to generate new dollars, the pool will not necessarily result in a net increase in total premiums.

Moreover, the term "sick tax" suggests that this tax is levied only on those who go to the hospital. In reality, the tax is primarily through, more than on, hospitals and is effectively a tax on health benefits, since hospitals that pay more into the pool than they receive from it will have to raise their charges, which in turn will require the insurer or third party administrator to increase premiums unless there are offsetting reductions from other hospitals. Thus, as is the case in any insurance plan, the increased premium costs, if any, are spread among all members, not just those who go into the hospital.

Why not just tax benefits directly?   It would be highly desirable to tax insurance benefits directly as many health economists have urged. Doing so, however, would mitigate the positive incentive the pooling mechanism offers hospitals to provide charity care in order to avoid a net tax. Unfortunately, the federal Employee Retirement and Income Security Act (ERISA) of 1973, as currently written, expressly prohibits states from exercising tax or regulatory jurisdiction over self-insured plans.

Since the ERISA exemption prohibits a direct tax on benefits, the indirect tax via the pool is the next best choice. Not only does it extend to health maintenance organizations (HMOs) and preferred provider organizations (PPOs), which are major factors in eroding the implicit cross-subsidies, but it offsets the preference these plans might otherwise have for hospitals that avoid charity care. Finally, there is an equity rationale for even indirectly taxing health benefits given the more than $40 billion in federal income tax deductions that recipients of these benefits and their employers enjoy.

Why should funds taken from hospitals be used to pay for physicians' services? Little is known about the amount and distribution of charity care by physicians in the 1980s. The few studies that have been done suggest that most physicians do provide at least some charity care, and that it is unevenly distributed. Nevertheless, a large portion of the uninsured poor rely heavily on hospital emergency rooms and public clinics rather than physicians' offices for much of their care.

There is, however, good reason to use the pool's proceeds for other than hospital services whether or not physicians contribute directly. The most important reason is that access to primary and preventive care services appears to be especially problematic. In addition, our studies have shown that uncompensated outpatient services make up a large proportion of total uncompensated care in many states, especially for the high-burden hospitals. In one city, for example, uncompensated costs for Medicaid and other outpatient services were found to be more than twice as high as for inpatient care.

How does pooling avoid propping up inefficient providers?   By itself, the pooling mechanism cannot accomplish this important objective. Strategies that include Medicaid managed care systems, such as California's selective contracting and Pennsylvania's experimental "Buy Right" program, among others, are more direct means for improving the efficient purchase of health care for the medically indigent. However, the flexibility available to those administering the fund makes it possible for them to take advantage of these tools. In addition, pooling makes it more difficult for providers to mask their inefficiency through lower prices by avoiding charity care, compared to efficient providers who would have to charge higher prices if they have high charity care burdens.

Won't state and local governments use the tax on providers to replace public appropriations?   It is true that an improperly constructed statute permits all levels of government to view the pooling arrangement as a replacement for public funds.

A more complicated issue is whether to require maintenance of effort at the county or municipal level, where there is a potential for significant displacement of local government contributions to public hospitals and clinics. The issue arises because public general hospitals usually receive a large share of the fund's disbursements. Because the financing of these facilities accounts for a large share of local government budgets, it may be appropriate to allow for a limited amount of displacement of these funds. If limits on such displacement are deemed desirable, there are two approaches that might be useful. The first would be to cap the amount of disbursements specific public hospitals or clinics could receive from the fund, as New Jersey does, leaving the amount above the cap as a county or municipal responsibility. The other would require any local government in a position to reduce its level of financial support to allocate a designated percentage of this amount to primary and preventive care projects in its jurisdiction or adjacent areas.

Isn't this procompetitive approach regulation in disguise?   No disguise is intended; the pooling arrangement is a form of regulation as is any form of taxation designed to redistribute income or create incentives for economic or social purposes. Where the pooling approach differs from other forms of taxation is that it keeps the proceeds within the health care system and that it explicitly seeks to promote fair competition, not just competition per se. In this regard, the pooling approach is in the tradition of many regulatory activities in our society that are designed to preserve the integrity and viability of the market system while protecting valued social goals.

ADVANTAGES OF POOLING

In summary, the pooling approach, although not without its risks, does have three major advantages. First, if the problem in a state or a regional market is less one of access to hospital services by the medically indigent, and more one of unfair competition because of unequal distribution of charity care, the fund permits a leveling of the playing field without raising general revenue tax funds to do so. That is, it can accomplish this goal not by reducing the total amount of uncompensated hospital care, but simply by redistributing dollars among hospitals to neutralize the competitive advantages and handicaps that result from these differences. By avoiding the need for new general tax revenues for this purpose, it frees those dollars to meet more serious needs such as primary and preventive care. Second, pooling offers flexibility in how funds are raised: who contributes to the fund and the conditions of participation. For example, to avoid the timing and cash flow problems that have plagued Florida's program, a fund could operate on reconciliation, using cash transactions only periodically to reconcile accounts, and retaining only enough cash in the fund to operate the program. Funds can be used to support Medicaid expansion, offset uncompensated care differences, subsidize high-risk pools or small employer insurance programs, support primary care grants, and pay for special studies, among others. Finally, pooling offers flexibility on the delivery side, permitting choice among many options as to the kinds of services to fund, whether to operate statewide or in a regional market, whether to use direct purchase of services, grants, contracts, and so forth.

In a world of universal health insurance and assured financial access, halfway technologies such as the pooling mechanism should be unnecessary. But, as this article has suggested, we are, and for some time are likely to remain, some distance from these worthy goals. Until we reach them, we must find ways of allowing competition and improved access for our nation's medically indigent to coexist. The indigent care fund may not be an appropriate solution for all communities, but it deserves careful consideration by many.

The rise and growth of competition is surely one of the most significant developments in the health care sector in the last decade.

LAWRENCE D. BROWN
University of Michigan

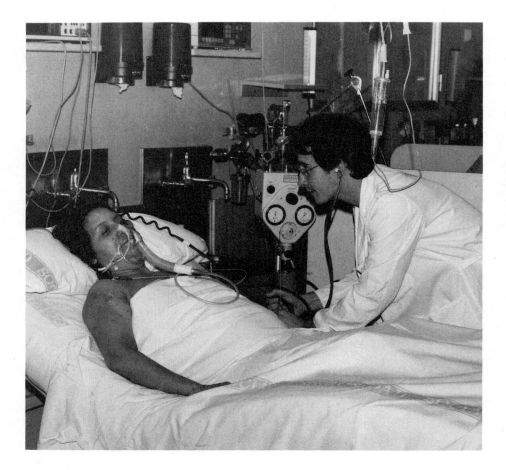

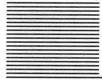

8

Quality, Effectiveness, and Appropriateness of Care

ONCERNS ABOUT ACCESS TO HEALTH CARE SERVICES and the costs of care of necessity raise questions about quality. Initial studies of quality focused on the process of care and the structure of services. In recent years, however, investigators are emphasizing effectiveness, appropriateness, and outcomes of care. Because of the complexity of emerging treatment modes, physicians face uncertainty about whether the benefits of a particular treatment outweigh the risks. Because our knowledge is incomplete, we see an increased emphasis on outcomes rather than process in order to produce the capacity to better inform physicians and assist them and their patients in decision making and thus ultimately improve the quality of care.

This initiative in health services places new burdens on the federal government to support studies related to outcomes and to inform physicians of the findings. All of our authors stress the importance of federal agencies' role in funding studies and disseminating findings in health services research. Thus far, the level of funding has been sadly inadequate to address the need.

In "Health Services Research: Is It Good for You and Me?" veteran investigator Robert Brook takes a historical view of this applied research field. His conclusions verify the increased usefulness and effectiveness of these studies both at the policy and the patient care levels. He welcomes the contributions of health services research in providing better information to patients and physicians to assist them in engineering the best possible treatment results.

In "Variations in Physician Practice: The Role of Uncertainty" physician/ mathematician David M. Eddy discusses his interest in reducing uncertainty in medical care and determining the most efficacious treatments. He describes the factors at play in his research applying probability theory to the uncertain decision making process in medical therapeutics.

Peter E. Dans calls the reticence of the government and others to fund health services research "a national disgrace." He points to the potential value of such studies in providing a solid foundation for regulation and suggests that payers, institutions, and professionals join together in an effort to measure the effects of their treatment.

The whole earth is our hospital.

T. S. ELIOT

Robert H. Brook

Health Services Research: Is It Good for You and Me?

Health services research is an applied science that operates at a patient or population level and asks questions such as: Does this technology work? Is it cost-effective? What is the impact of DRGs on quality?

It is important to mention two principles that shape an applied research field such as health services research. First, studies can be classified as methods (how should quality be measured?), descriptive (what is the level of quality in this academic institution?), analytical (do teaching hospitals provide better quality than nonteaching hospitals?), or experimental (after randomizing patients to an HMO or the fee-for-service system, in which system is the quality of care better?). Second, health services research is conducted at two levels. Research studies can answer questions at the doctor-patient level, such as, "Will changes in interviewing style improve patient compliance?" and at the policy level, for example, "How will factors such as providing reimbursement for medications affect patient compliance?" To understand the impact of health services research, it is important to keep in mind whether the focus is on descriptive research at the patient level or experimental research at the policy level.

When I became an intern at Baltimore City Hospitals, one of my first rotations was in the emergency room. We worked 24 hours — off 8, on 12, off 8, on 16, off 8, and so on. The State of Maryland was not in the business of regulating interns' on-call hours. For me, the rotation through the emergency room was a second motivational force to ask some hard questions. Was all this work necessary? What did we accomplish? I vowed to find out.

AN EARLY STUDY

When my first elective came, I drew a systematic sample of patients and followed them up six months after they had completed their initial emergency room visits. All sorts of findings emerged: First, we did not do as much as we

Robert H. Brook, M.D., is chief, Division of Geriatrics, and professor of medicine and public health, Center for the Health Sciences, University of California, Los Angeles, and senior staff researcher, The Rand Corporation, Santa Monica, California.

thought. Professionals, myself included, believe in ourselves, and this belief can result in overestimations of our efficiency, efficacy, and effect. In my emergency room follow-up study, I learned that we were not terribly productive. We generally saw only a few patients but spent a lot of (probably too much) time with them. Second, by six months we lost to follow-up many if not most of our patients, even those who had chronic disease. For instance, of 141 patients who were sick enough at their initial emergency room visits to require a follow-up barium enema, upper-gastrointestinal x-ray, or gallbladder study, 67% completed their x-rays. Of those completing their x-rays, 38% knew whether they were normal or not; and of those who had abnormalities, 37% received adequate therapy. In summary, about a fourth of the entire group received effective care.

Our academic mega-workups that were performed during the initial emergency room visits had been largely for naught. Some of these disappointing outcomes were the result of lack of compliance on the part of patients, but most of the time the system in which I practiced had failed. Follow-up appointments were not given because an appointment desk was closed, laboratory slips containing important abnormal results mysteriously disappeared, and providing continuous, coordinated care over time was difficult. Some gastric and duodenal ulcers went untreated, and a few cancers were not removed. My awareness of and participation in health services research had moved to the descriptive phase. It still had a long way to go, however, as I realized that the results of the study could not be generalized beyond the one institution in which it was conducted.

INADEQUACIES IN HEALTH CARE

Since that time, many health services researchers, myself included, have spent considerable effort learning how to define and measure better quality of care. The dimensions of quality have been defined. We have applied these definitions and proven that a substantial fraction of care we deliver is inadequate, and that there are variations in the amounts of care and in the appropriateness and outcomes of care that we provide that are too large to be ignored. For example:

1. The probability that a man has had a prostatectomy by the time he reaches the age of 80 varies from 20 percent to 60 percent, depending on the New England town in which he lives. For a woman, the corresponding figures for loss of her uterus by the age of 70 are 20 percent and 75 percent. These variations are not just local phenomena but also occur statewide. For example, depending on the state in which they reside, some people over the

age of 65 have a threefold increased probability of undergoing coronary artery bypass surgery. Respective figures for carotid endarterectomy, pacemaker insertion, and coronary angiography are four-, three- and two-fold.

2. Among all continuing patients being treated in 16 academic internal medicine primary care practices, 30% of those who should have received a flu vaccination actually received one. The range among practices was 4 to 83%. Corresponding figures for giving pneumococcal vaccinations, teaching breast self-examination, and discussing birth control were 19% (range 2–54), 50% (range 35–63), and 56% (range 0–82).

3. Based on a random sample of Medicare patient records, a fourth of upper-gastrointestinal endoscopies and coronary angiographies and two-thirds of carotid endarterectomies were performed for clinically equivocal or inappropriate reasons. Almost half of carotid endarterectomies performed in five academic VA hospitals were also considered to have been performed for medically equivocal or inappropriate reasons, as were two-fifths of the coronary artery bypass surgeries performed in a random sample of three hospitals in one western state. In addition, appropriateness varied by hospital, with one hospital's staff operating for appropriate indications 78% of the time, and another's, 37% of the time.

4. An analysis of clinical data from a large hospital chain demonstrated that over a fourth of deaths from cerebrovascular accidents, pneumonia, or myocardial infarction might have been preventable. Sophisticated clinical adjustment for case severity disclosed that mortality from coronary artery bypass surgery varied 20-fold among 16 academic institutions.

OUTCOMES AND APPROPRIATENESS OF CARE

Although much more methods research is needed, advances in health services research, in general, and the science of measuring the appropriateness and outcomes of care, in specific, have made it possible for studies of quality to move from the descriptive to the analytical and experimental level. This, in turn, has resulted in a fundamental change in the nature of discussions concerning the future of the medical system. Whereas previously attention was focused almost exclusively on determining levels of health care expenditures and on ascertaining whether use of services was equitably distributed among segments of the U.S. population, today it is possible to introduce the concept of outcomes and appropriateness of care. Models have been tested that relate quality to policy, taking into account clinical and organizational variables. These models can permit us to monitor the impacts of policy changes and governmental regulation on quality of care. For example, we are now in a position to understand at a clinical level whether and how the prospective payment system and diagnosis-related groups (DRGs) — the development of the DRG system itself is a testimony to the effect of health services research —

have affected the quality of care delivered to hospitalized patients; whether paying physicians on a salary versus fee-for-service basis affects quality; and the degree to which changes in a patient's insurance status can have an impact on care.

For instance, a typical example of modern health services research was prompted by actions in California in 1982, when 270,000 medically indigent adults who had previously been covered by MediCal (Medicaid in California) were suddenly disenfranchised. Because of the previous investment in developing and validating measures of quality of care and the availability of a strong, clinically aware group of health services researchers at an academic center, Lurie and colleagues were able quickly to organize a study to determine the impact of this policy action. They showed unequivocally that it increased the blood pressures and impaired the health of these poor, chronically ill people and probably caused the deaths of some. Specifically, before termination of medical benefits, 3% of the 186 adults studied had diastolic blood pressures greater than 100 mm Hg, one year later, the corresponding figure was 19%. General health status fell nine points on a 100-point scale; seven of the 186 people died, many after they depleted their supplies of medications. Satisfaction with care declined from 97% satisfied to 40% satisfied, and about half of the population (versus 92% before termination of benefits) had a regular doctor to whom they could go for care.

EVALUATING CURRENT AND PROPOSED POLICIES

We are now in a position, if we so choose, to monitor with clinical precision a wide variety of current or proposed policy actions and to assess their beneficial or harmful effects in terms of quality and health status. In fact, we can evaluate whether the world is moving closer to the goal of the World Health Organization of achieving good health for all by the year 2000.

The motivation for mounting such evaluations and making them a routine part of academic health centers is substantiated by the work described above. In addition, we know from other health services research studies that changing economic incentives can have a profound effect on use of services. Unfortunately, such changes appear to affect the use of both medically appropriate and inappropriate services. For instance, patients' deductible charges and coinsurance charges can reduce use of services substantially, as shown in the RAND Health Insurance Experiment. This reduction had no impact on the health of the average person enrolled in the experiment, but it did worsen the health of people who were both poor and sick. People taking advantage of the free care plan had had 40% more episodes of ambulatory care for conditions for which care is highly effective, but they also had had 50% more episodes of care for conditions for which care is rarely effective. Free care had increased the per person, per year use of penicillin by 70%, narcotics by 90%, and minor tranquilizers by 50%. (The use of antibiotics is related more to a person's insurance status than to the presence of a bacterium. This fact is not routinely taught in medical school.) In another study of insurance benefits, payment for drugs was restricted to three drugs per month. This policy reduced the use of medications of limited efficacy by 58%, but it also reduced use of essential medications by 28%; for example, use of insulin fell 28%, and use of digoxin fell 45%.

In order to perform high-quality health services research studies, academic health centers and other governmental and policy organizations must welcome multidisciplinary teams of well-trained researchers and help provide them with adequate funding. The agency that has the major mission in the federal government for funding health services research, the National Center for Health Services Research, has not done well in the latter regard. In constant dollars, from 1975 to 1985 this agency lost 75% of its extramural budget (for comparison purposes, the National Institutes of Health's budget grew by 27%). In 1985, the National Center awarded 39 investigator-initiated grants (compared with 2,500 from the NIH). The National Center's budget in 1975 was 0.9% of the NIH's budget; in 1985, it was 0.2%. The Health Care Financing Administration also supports research at the federal level. Its research is targeted to answer questions that pertain to Medicare and Medicaid patients, but its research budget was less than 0.03% of its service budget.

IMPACTS OF HEALTH SERVICES RESEARCH

Turning from the policy level and issues of funding to health services research at the patient level, advances in how to measure quality have also resulted in, and will in the future continue to result in, changes in how we educate medical students and residents. Health services research studies have documented that patient compliance can be affected by what physicians do. In particular, it is important that physicians routinely assess compliance with medications or other treatment modalities, allow patients to express concerns about what bothers them, and encourage patients to participate actively in their care. For example, scales for measuring physician instruction and effort in increasing compliance have been developed. In low-income populations, if physicians exert high effort (for instance, asking about noncompliance, responding to patient problems), compliance with medications is over 80%, while with low effort it is 15%. If physicians write out medication instructions and hand them to their patients, compliance is over 50%; if not, compliance is less than 30%. In addition, techniques that help to involve diabetic patients actively in their own care have been shown in a randomized controlled clinical trial both to improve the patients' functional status and to reduce concentrations of glycosylated hemoglobin.

Health services researchers have proven that tailoring a patient's daily medication regimen results in increased compliance, and we have demonstrated that the complexity of a medication regimen has a direct relationship to compliance. Much remains to be done. Better methods for measuring quality are required. Better and more conceptually sound interventions are needed. More experiments must be done. Nonetheless, courses that use findings from these research activities have been developed and have become a standard part of the curricula of some medical schools and residency programs. However, such courses represent only a beginning. For instance, doctors of the future will need more than just a brief acquaintance with the principles and methods of quality assurance.

Work in measuring quality at both the patient level and the policy level is beginning to change, fundamentally, relationships between the public and the profession. We are on the verge of becoming comfortable with disclosing to the public information about our performance. Measurement tools that can be used to assess appropriateness of care, disease severity, and outcomes of care and statistical tools that allow adjustment for differences in disease severity across populations have made this possible.

DISCLOSING OUTCOME OF CARE

To date, the agency responsible for administrating the Medicare program has released two reports on hospital mortality and is committed to releasing an updated mortality report annually. Last year's report lists for each hospital in the United States the hospital's overall mortality experience and its mortality experiences for 16 disease-specific categories. Sophisticated statistical tests are used to indicate when a hospital's performance is below or above average. As the field of health services research matures and as experience with adjusting for differences in case mix and severity among patients and hospitals grows, the validity of these comparisons will increase, and they will become more useful.

People (patients) can already obtain copies of last year's report, for it is available for a nominal charge from the Government Printing Office. After reading such a report, patients may ask their physicians questions such as: "Why do you admit to this hospital, as opposed to the one down the block that has a lower mortality rate?" "What do you know about your hospital's mortality rate, and why is it so high?" "Has your hospital's mortality rate changed recently?" How will the medical students that we educate answer such questions?

In the future, mortality information could be used by third-party payers when they decide which hospitals should be part of a preferred provider group or should be part of their health insurance plan. Mortality data could be made available when people decide in which health plan to enroll. They could be used to examine cost-quality trade-offs. If cost of care is twice as high in one hospital as in another, but the outcomes are the same, why should public or pre-tax money be used to pay for care in the more expensive hospital?

DEVELOPING INFORMATION ABOUT PRACTICE STANDARDS

In addition to information about the outcome of care, data such as those described above on the appropriateness of care and the availability of decision analysis and meta-analysis tools will almost certainly lead to the development, use, and public release of information about practice standards. These standards will represent clinical guidelines by which decisions regarding whether a service should be either performed or paid for may be judged. The development of these standards or guidelines will change the way medicine is taught and practiced, and I hope academic centers will play a major role in this activity.

ADVANCES IN RESEARCH

Before leaving this discussion of the impact of health services research, its effects on other aspects of medicine must be considered. For instance, two major changes have occurred in conducting clinical research. First, the efforts of health services researchers have resulted in the development of better experimental and quasi-experimental designs by which clinical interventions such as prostatectomy can be evaluated. Nonintrusive methods for data collections have been introduced. Better ways of combining information from independently conducted small trials have been developed. In addition, advances in clinimetrics have made us better at categorizing patients into clinically homogeneous groups.

Critically important to clinical research, however, has been the work performed in advancing the measurement of health status and patient function. After a decade of research in the health status area we are fortunate to have witnessed the development of a number of good measures. Not only can these measures be used to assess whether changes in health policy can affect quality of life, but they can be used to determine whether clinical interventions work. Thus, for patients undergoing treatment for mild hypertension, we can measure the effect of therapy, not only in lowering blood pressure, and thus extending life expectancy, but also on the quality of life. We can ask whether a therapy that may not extend life improves its quality, and we can even determine whether therapies produce trade-offs — decreases in length of survival but increases in quality of life, or vice versa. Clinical trials in the future will most assuredly include health status measures as outcome measures, and thus clinicians will have available to them more relevant information in helping their patients decide whether to undergo a particular intervention or receive a particular service. In order to use such information wisely, medical students and physicians will need to acquire new skills, including how to assess a patient's preferences or utilities for one health status state or another. Performing work of this nature will require the active participation of many academic health centers.

CONCLUSION

Doing good health services research, which is still a new and rare activity, is complicated, depends upon teams of physicians and social scientists working together, and produces complex, not simple, results. It requires the involvement of the entire university and the development of strong medical school divisions in which physician-health services researchers live and work. Thanks largely to the Clinical Scholars Program of the Robert Wood Johnson Foundation, physicians to staff such divisions exist. However, if we are to use them optimally, the national funding for health services research must be increased, and the local intellectual climate and working conditions must be improved. It is worth the effort. It will make a difference. The health of the American people has already benefited and will continue to benefit from such an effort.

The fact that physicians and medical organizations are more interested in disease than in health might be regarded as an expression of professional bias, but this attitude corresponds in reality to a widespread human trait.

RENE DUBOS

David M. Eddy

Variations in Physician Practice: The Role of Uncertainty

Why do physicians vary so much in the way they practice medicine? At first view, there should be no problem. There are diseases — neatly named and categorized by textbooks, journal articles, and medical specialty societies. There are various procedures physicians can use to diagnose and treat these diseases. It should be possible to determine the value of any particular procedure by applying it to patients who have a disease and observing the outcome. And the rest should be easy — if the outcome is good, the procedure should be used for patients with that disease; if the outcome is bad, it should not. Some variation in practice patterns can be expected due to differences in the incidence of various diseases, patients' preferences, and the available resources, but these variations should be small and explainable.

The problem of course is that nothing is this simple. Uncertainty, biases, errors, and differences of opinions, motives, and values weaken every link in the chain that connects a patient's actual condition to the selection of a diagnostic test or treatment. This paper describes some of the factors that cause decisions about the use of medical procedures to be so difficult, and that contribute to the alarming variations we observe in actual practice. It examines the components of the decision problem a physician faces, and the psychology of medical reasoning, focusing in particular on the role of uncertainty. Finally, it suggests some actions to reduce uncertainty and encourage consistency of good medical practice.

Uncertainty creeps into medical practice through every pore. Whether a physician is defining a disease, making a diagnosis, selecting a procedure, observing outcomes, assessing probabilities, assigning preferences, or putting it all together, he is walking on very slippery terrain. It is difficult for nonphysicians, and for many physicians, to appreciate how complex these tasks are, how poorly we understand them, and how easy it is for honest people to come to different conclusions.

David M. Eddy, M.D., Ph.D., is Alexander McMahon Professor of Health Policy and Management, Duke University, Durham, North Carolina.

DEFINING A DISEASE

If one looks at patients who are obviously ill, it is fairly easy to identify the physical and chemical disorders that characterize that illness. On the other hand, a large part of medicine is practiced on people who do not have obvious illnesses, but rather have signs, symptoms, or findings that may or may not represent an illness that should be treated. Three closely related problems make it difficult to determine whether or not a patient actually has a disease that needs to be diagnosed or treated.

One problem is that the dividing line between "normal" and "abnormal" is not nearly as sharp as a cursory reading of a textbook would suggest. First, the clues on which we base the diagnosis of many diseases can be very difficult to see, with frequent errors in both directions (missing an existing disease and "finding" a nondisease). Second, even if the diagnosis were correct and a disease were acknowledged to be present, the "disease" might not actually cause the patient any harm.

A second problem is that many "diseases," at least at the time they are diagnosed, do not by themselves cause pain, suffering, disability, or threat to life. They are considered diseases only because they increase the probability that something else that is truly bad will happen in the future. This raises two more sources of uncertainty. (1) If a condition presages a bad outcome, one must judge the probabilities. Most conditions of this type do not always cause a "real" disease, and the "real" disease can usually occur without the condition. In situ lobular carcinoma of the breast presages a future invasive breast cancer less than 50 percent of the time, and the great majority of invasive breast cancers occur without a history of in situ lobular carcinoma. (2) Just because a condition can precede a "real" disease and can indicate a higher probability that the disease will develop, does not necessarily mean that it causes the disease, or that treating the condition will prevent it from occurring. Ocular hypertension and glaucoma are good examples; loss of visual field and blindness appear to occur whether or not the ocular pressure is lowered.

The difficulty of defining a disease is compounded by the fact that many of the signs, symptoms, findings, and conditions that might suggest a disease are extremely common. If a breast biopsy were performed on a random sample of senior citizens, fully 90 percent of them could have fibrocystic disease. If obesity is a disease, the average American is diseased. By the time they reach seventy, about two-thirds of women have had their uteruses removed. Because the average blood pressure increases with age, some physicians feel a need to relabel "hypertension" to keep the majority of older people from having this disease.

And the ambiguities grow worse as medical technology expands. More and more diseases are being defined by an abnormal result on some test, leaving uncertainty about its real meaning to a patient and the appropriate treatment. Silent gallstones were silent until the oral cholecystogram was introduced, dysplasia of the cervix did not exist before the Pap smear, and many people's coronary artery disease showed up only on a treadmill test. Finding "diseases" early may be worthwhile, but it is difficult to know what else is being scooped up in the net.

Given these uncertainties about what constitutes a disease, it should not be surprising that there are debates about the definitions of many diseases, and when there is agreement about a definition, it is often blatantly and admittedly arbitrary. A quick review of the literature reveals multiple definitions of glaucoma, diabetes, fibrocystic disease of the breast, coronary artery disease, myocardial infarction, stroke, and dozens of other conditions. Morbid obesity is defined as 100 percent above the ideal weight. But what is "ideal," and why 100 percent? The lesson is that for many conditions a clinician faces, there is no clear definition of disease that provides an unequivocal guide to action, and there is wide room for differences of opinion and variations in practice.

MAKING A DIAGNOSIS

Suppose everyone agreed that a particular collection of signs, symptoms, and test results constituted an unequivocal definition of a disease. Would this eliminate the uncertainty? Unfortunately, even when sharp criteria are created, physicians vary widely in their application of these criteria—in their ability to ask about symptoms, observe signs, interpret test results, and record the answers.

SELECTING A PROCEDURE

The task of selecting a procedure is no less difficult. There are two main issues.

First, for any patient condition there are dozens of procedures that can be ordered, in any combination, at any time. The list of procedures that might be included in a workup of chest pain or hypertension would take more than a page, spanning the spectrum from simply asking questions, to blood studies, to x-rays. Even for highly specific diagnostic problems, there can be a large choice of procedures.

Second, adding to the uncertainties of defining and choosing a procedure is the fact that the value of any particular procedure depends on who performs it, on whom it is performed, and the circumstances of performance. The potential for variability in the people who perform procedures can be appreciated by considering one of the procedures, the Pap smear. A gynecologist reviewed the technique used by sixty of his colleagues to take a Pap smear, and found that only fifteen of them performed the test properly. With this amount of slippage in such a simple test, one can only imagine the variation in quality that occurs with a more complicated procedure like coronary artery bypass surgery. Each procedure has many faces, and many factors influence the quality and consequences of its use.

OBSERVING OUTCOMES

In theory, much of the uncertainty just described could be managed if it were possible to conduct enough experiments under enough conditions, and observe the outcomes. Unfortunately, measuring the outcomes of medical procedures is one of the most difficult problems we face. The goal is to predict how the use of a procedure in a particular case will affect that patient's health and welfare. Standing in the way are at least a half dozen major obstacles. The central problem is that there is a natural variation in the way people respond to a medical procedure.

One consequence of this natural variation is that to study the outcomes of any procedure it is necessary to conduct the procedure on many different people who are thought to represent the particular patients we want to know about, and then average the results. This in turn raises additional problems. First, many of the diseases are fairly rare, and it is necessary to average over many people to get a sample large enough to yield reliable results. This usually requires using many physicians, drawing patients from many settings, and performing the experiments at different times. Each of these elements introduces additional variation.

An additional problem is that most procedures have multiple outcomes and it is not sufficient to examine just one of them. For example, a coronary artery bypass may change the life expectancy of a sixty-year-old man with triple vessel disease, but it will also change his joy of life for several weeks after the operation, the degree and severity of his chest pain, his ability to work and make love, his relationship with his son, the physical appearance of his chest, and his pocketbook. Pain, disability, anxiety, family relations, and any number of other outcomes are all important consequences of a procedure that deserve consideration. But the list is too long for practical experiments and many of the items on it are invisible or not measurable at all. We either lack suitable units (for example, for anxiety or pain), or the units exist but no experiments are fine enough to detect a change (for example, the increased incidence in breast cancer due to radiation from mammography).

Beyond this, many of the outcomes needed to evaluate a medical procedure take years to observe. Finally, even when the best trials are conducted, we still might not get an answer.

Unable to turn to a definitive body of clinical and epidemiological research, a clinician or research scientist who wants to know the value of a procedure is left with a mixture of randomized controlled trials, nonrandomized trials, uncontrolled trials, and clinical observations. The evidence from different sources can easily go in different directions, and it is virtually impossible for anyone to sort things out in his or her head. Unfortunately, the individual physician may be most impressed by observations made in his or individual practice. This source of evidence is notoriously vulnerable to bias and error. What a physician sees and remembers is biased by the types of patients who come in; by the decisions of the patients to accept a treatment and return for follow-up; by a natural desire to see good things; and by a whole series of emotions that charge one's memory. On top of these biases, the observations are vulnerable to large statistical errors because of the small number of patients a physician sees in a personal practice.

The difficulty of measuring outcomes has three important implications: We are uncertain about the precise consequences of using a particular procedure for a particular patient. We cannot, over the short term at least, resolve this uncertainty. And whatever a physician chooses to do cannot be proved right or wrong.

ASSESSING PREFERENCES

Now assume that a physician can know the outcomes of recommending a particular procedure for a particular patient. Is it possible to declare whether these outcomes are good or bad? Unfortunately, no. The basic problem is that any procedure has multiple outcomes, some good and some bad. The expected reduction in chest pain that some people will get from coronary artery bypass surgery is accompanied by a splitting of the chest, a chance of an operative mortality, days in the hospital, pain, anxiety, and financial expense. Because the outcomes are multiple and move in different directions, tradeoffs have to be made. And making tradeoffs involves values.

Just as there is a natural variation in how each of us responds to a medical procedure, there is a variation in how we value different outcomes. The fact that General Motors alone produces more than fifty distinct models of automobiles, not to mention dozens of options for each model, demonstrates how tastes about even a single item can vary. Imagine the variation in how different people value pain, disability, operative mortality, life expectancy, a day in a hospital, and who is going to feed the dogs.

To the inherent variation in values individual patients place on different outcomes must be added two additional sources of uncertainty and variation in assessing values. First because decisions about procedures are typically made by physicians on behalf of their patients, the physicians must infer their patients' values, and keep them distinct from their own personal preferences. This raises the second problem, communication. It is difficult enough to assess one's own values about the outcomes of a complicated decision (think about switching jobs); consider having someone else try to learn your thoughts and do it for you. The room for error in communication can be appreciated by returning to the experiment in which four physicians asked 993 coal miners about cough, shortness of breath, pain, and sputum. The variation in the reports of responses to a simple question like, "Do you have a cough?" was large; imagine a question like, "How do you feel about operative mortality?"

PUTTING IT ALL TOGETHER

The final decision about how to manage a patient requires synthesizing all the information about a disease, the patient, signs and symptoms, the effectiveness of dozens of tests and treatments, outcomes, and values. All of this must be done without knowing precisely what the patient has, with uncertainty about signs and symptoms, with imperfect knowledge of the sensitivity and specificity of tests, with no training in manipulating probabilities, with incomplete and biased information about outcomes, and with no language for communicating or assessing values. If each piece of this puzzle is difficult, it is even more difficult for anyone to synthesize all the information and be certain of the answer. It would be an extremely hard task for a research team; there is no hope that it could occur with any precision in the head of a busy clinician. Hence the wide variability in the estimates physicians place on the values of procedures.

CONSEQUENCES

The view of anyone who wants a close look at the consequences of different medical procedures is, at best, smoky. Some procedures may present a clear picture, and their value, or lack of it, may be obvious; putting a finger on a bleeding carotid artery is an extreme example. But for many, if not most medical procedures, we can only see shadows and gross movements. We usually know the direction in which various outcome measures can move when a medical activity is undertaken, but we typically do not know the probabilities they will move in those directions, or how far they will move. We certainly do not know how a particular individual will respond. Words like "rare," "common," and "a lot" must be used instead of "one out of 1,000," or "seven on a scale of one to ten."

There is also a strong tendency to oversimplify. One of the easiest ways to fit a large problem in our minds is to lop off huge parts of it. In medical decisions, one option is to focus on length of life and discount inconvenience, pain, disability, short-term risks and financial costs. A physician can also draw on a number of simplifying heuristics. Anyone uncomfortable dealing with probabilities can use the heuristic, "If there is any chance of (the disease), the (procedure) should be performed." If one cannot estimate the number of people to be saved, one can use the heuristic, "If but one patient is saved, the effort is worthwhile." If one cannot contemplate alternative uses of resources that might deliver a greater benefit to a population, there is the heuristic, "Costs should not be considered in decisions about individual patients." There is a general purpose heuristic, "When in doubt, do it." Or as one investigator wrote, "An error of commission is to be preferred to an error of omission." Unfortunately, a large number of incentives encourage simplifications that lead to overutilization. It is time-consuming, mentally taxing, and often threatening to colleagues for a physician to undertake a deep analysis of a confusing clinical problem. A physician is less likely to be sued for doing too much than too little. Most physicians' incomes go up if they do more, and go down if they do less. Hospitals get to fill more beds and bill for more procedures, laboratories collect more money for services, and companies sell more drugs, devices, and instruments. The more that is done, the more the providers win. The losers are patients, consumers, and taxpayers—anyone who has to undergo a valueless procedure or pay the bill.

In the end, given all the uncertainties, incentives, and heuristics, a physician will have to do what is comfortable. If it is admitted that the uncertainty surrounding the use of a procedure is great, and that there is no way to identify for certain what is best, or to prove that any particular action is right or wrong, the safest and most comfortable position is to do what others are doing. The applicable maxim is "safety in numbers." A physician who follows the practices of his or her colleagues is safe from criticism, free from having to explain his or her actions, and defended by the concurrence of colleagues.

This tendency to follow the pack is the most important single explanation of regional variations in medical practice. If uncertainty caused individual physicians to practice at random, or to follow their personal interpretations and values, without any attempts to match the actions of their neighbors, the variations in practice patterns would average out, and no significant differences would be observed at the regional level. Differences between regions are observed because individual physicians tend to follow what is considered standard and accepted in the community. A community standard evolves from statements published in national journals and textbooks, from the opinions of established physicians, and from new ideas brought to the community by new physicians. The community standards themselves exist because enough is known to enable the leaders of a community to develop opinions which, when followed by their colleagues, become community standards. The differences between community standards exist because not enough is known to establish which opinion is correct. We call the community standards for a particular practice clinical policies, and anyone who makes an unambiguous recommendation about a medical practice is a policymaker.

WHAT HARM IS DONE?

First, it should be clear that some variation in practice is appropriate. The differences in patients' risks, signs and symptoms, responses to treatment, and values are real. Differences in physicians' talents and the available facilities are also real. If physicians were able to tailor their practices to take these individual differences into account, variations would be both inevitable and desirable. The problem is that uncertainty so clouds every aspect of this problem that many of the appropriate variations cannot occur, and many of the variations we see are not motivated by logic or a deep understanding of the issues.

There is no doubt that uncertainty about the consequences of different medical activities can harm both the quality and cost of medical practice. It is also true, however, that most of the simplifications and heuristics point in one direction, toward overutilization. When this happens the price is paid in terms of inconvenience, pain, distress, days in the hospital, unnecessary risks, and money.

CONCLUSIONS

Many of the problems described in this paper are insurmountable. There is no way to shorten the time needed to observe ten-year survival rates, and there is no way to increase the frequency of rare diseases, reduce the number of outcomes that are important to a patient, or decrease natural variations in response to treatment. Nor do we want to suppress the differences that exist in patients' preferences.

However, while we can not eliminate uncertainty, we can decrease the amount of it and develop strategies to minimize its damage. In fact, the profession and society have not begun to exploit the available techniques for reducing uncertainty and maximizing expected outcomes. The evaluation of medical practices and the development of clinical policies deserve much more attention and a higher priority than they currently get.

First, physicians can do more to admit the existence of uncertainty, both to themselves and to their patients. While this will undoubtedly be unsettling, it is honest, and it opens the way for a more intensive search for ways to reduce uncertainty.

Second, people who want to promote policies regarding the use of medical procedures can learn the necessary languages.

Third, physicians who follow existing policies can examine more carefully the supporting evidence and logic. The mere fact that a policy is established and accepted does not make it correct.

Fourth, to encourage and assist the two previous actions, any policy statement, whether it be made by an individual physician at a hospital conference, or a third-party payer considering reimbursement, should be accompanied by (1) a list of medical and economic outcomes that were considered in making the policy, (2) the policymaker's estimates of what can be expected to happen with respect to each of the listed outcomes if the policy is followed, and (3) the supporting evidence for those estimates. Any policy-maker unable to supply that information should not be making policies.

Fifth, editors and reviewers of journals can encourage publication of good papers that synthesize existing information, estimate the outcomes of different policies, and present the rationales for different actions. Such work, while not traditional, is both difficult and important.

Sixth, editors and reviewers can require that any author who recommends a policy supply the information listed in action 4. No good journal today will report the results of an experiment without a description of the design and methods; it is no less important to describe the reasoning behind a policy statement.

Seventh, the government can support far more evaluation research to analyze medical practices.

Finally, patients can push the process by asking questions.

I believe these actions should be taken. Some of the uncertainty and the resulting variations in practice patterns that exist are unavoidable, but much of the uncertainty can be managed far better than is done now. The problems that exist today are not the fault of any individuals; the fault lies with the profession and society as a whole for not developing the traditions and methods needed to assess medical practices. Today the problem is bad; five years from now, if not improved, it will be a tragedy.

The body reflects the attitude of the mind. Improve the function of the body and you must improve the state of the mind.

MOSHE FELDENKRAIS

Peter E. Dans

The Health Care Revolution: A Preliminary Report from the Front

A financial officer at The Johns Hopkins Hospital recently said to me, "Medicine is a simplistic name for an evolving creature that no more resembles what it was 20 years ago than the U.S. resembles the original 13 colonies." Paul Starr may have put it more eloquently, but my friend is right. There is and has been a quiet revolution going on in American medicine. In 1957, when I entered medical school, many hospitals were segregated by race and class as well as sex. At one teaching hospital at which I trained, ambulance drivers were asked to wait until patients were preliminarily assessed to be ready to transport them to a municipal hospital, if they were not considered instructive admissions. At another, patients clearly needing hospitalization balked at being admitted because they lacked financial coverage. The length of stay for myocardial infarction had been halved in that decade but was still three weeks, *if the patient survived*. The hospital charges and the corresponding wages of the many fewer health care workers and administrators were much lower.

Medicare, Medicaid, and expanding employer health insurance coverage changed all that. For better and worse, medical care became synonymous with health care. Hospitals increased in size and scope as they competed to provide the "best" and the latest in technology. Even without correcting for inflation, The Johns Hopkins Hospital budgets of 1936 ($1.8 million), 1961 ($15 million), and 1988 ($265 million) reflect the enormity of these changes. Access was broadened; wages of health care workers increased; services once donated were reimbursed; technology and our ability to treat many conditions were enhanced. The average length of stay for myocardial infarction was halved again, and survival rose. While all patients appear to have gained, this was especially true for the poor and the elderly. In the process, hospitals became more than just sites for health care, education, and research; they became major employers and community resources for coping with problems society relegates to the shadows—traditionally the province of municipal and eleemosynary hospitals.

Peter E. Dans, M.D., is associate professor of medicine and director of Medical Practice Evaluation, Johns Hopkins Hospital, Baltimore, Maryland.

In the mid-1970s, increasing budgetary constraints and the health care system's own successes shifted attention to its perceived failures. Huge expenditures for acute-care services became harder to justify as the course of diseases was altered and people who would have died experienced prolonged periods of chronic illness. Geographic variations in health care services, although not new, seemed to provide opportunities for cost savings. As a result, payers have issued a confusing array of regulations regarding admission, length of stay, and intensity of service. Rarely have these been accompanied by any assessment of their effect on quality of care or on the health care institutions and professions. In many cases, "dollars saved" appears to be the only measure of outcome.

Consequently, it is refreshing to see the study by Imperiale et al of the effect of one such regulation, that of preadmission screening, on the quality of care to Medicare patients in Connecticut during the winter of 1986. They quite correctly call their results preliminary. In fact, their most striking finding is that so few requests for elective admissions (105 of 28,450) were disapproved, and even then 22 patients were admitted anyway. As they note, the regulation could have been cost-effective only if physicians were deterred from requesting admissions that would have been routine before. In the absence of evidence of such a "sentinel effect," the wholesale intrusion on professional autonomy hardly seems justified.

Despite the small sample size, their failure to detect major adverse outcomes is encouraging. However, some patients did experience problems whose significance may be perceived differently by payers and those on or near the front lines (patients, families, care givers, and lawyers). Like the generals, payers and policymakers focus on aggregate statistics at a distance from the front, whereas to those in the trenches, what happens to individuals matters most. The anterior-chamber hemorrhage in the patient mobilized after cataract extraction is similar to the endophthalmitis in a Maryland patient whose physician wondered if the denied overnight admission would have prevented it. How many excess admissions can be justified to prevent such complications is a question worthy of much greater study, as is how physicians set such cut-off points. This is referred to by Nightingale as "risk preference" and by Feinstein as the "chagrin factor." Clearly, admission to hospital is not risk free, but chagrin is especially keen when catastrophes happen after patients are sent home against better judgment. For payers and policymakers, distance and large numbers tend to insulate them (or make them more objective, if you prefer).

Physicians are also more likely to remember those patients who were admitted after an abortive attempt at outpatient treatment. The fact that the patients ultimately did well is reassuring in retrospect, but the outcome was not so clear in the anxious moments surrounding the delayed admission. That the mentally retarded patient whose admission for a breast biopsy was denied and who then refused the same-day surgery had an apparently benign mass 15 months later is comforting. However, what if it had not been benign? Payers usually respond by saying that they only issue guidelines and that physicians must use their best judgments to pick out exceptions. However, physicians operate under considerable uncertainty and cannot be absolutely sure which patient will or will not do well. Third-party reviewers have the benefit of hindsight.

A more tangible problem is the shifting of financial and social costs to the family and the patient, as happened in some of the cases. Where social support systems are adequate, acute-care hospital admissions to solve social problems are inappropriate. However, in the absence of community facilities or home health care services, the disposition of elderly debilitated patients brought to emergency departments on nights, weekends, or holidays is often very difficult. The patient, the family, the physician, and the hospital are caught in a no-win situation. Such problems are becoming even more acute for non-Medicare homeless patients as well as for those with the acquired immuno-deficiency syndrome or the consequences of intravenous drug abuse. The downsizing and reduced funding of the municipal and state hospital systems have weakened the society's safety net.

Because of the variability in the mix of patients, providers, and institutions, as well as the expectations of the communities in which they reside, most health services research studies should not be extrapolated beyond their time and place. This study is no exception. Its major importance lies in illustrating what ought to be routinely carried out in all medical service areas. In fact, given the extent of the current health care revolution in America, the amount of money and time spent in research and development relating health care process to outcome is a national disgrace. As little as 0.5% of health care expenditures, if put into research and development, would give a much more solid foundation for the numerous regulations ostensibly aimed at more effective and efficient care.

In the new business climate, it is fashionable to invoke the perversion of the golden rule, "He who has the gold makes the rules." Whether one likes it or not, third-party payers are now in the catbird seat. They can retrospectively deny payment even for what they agree is necessary care. Ironically though, "quality of care" has become a hot topic among payers—partly because of its marketing potential. However, defining and measuring quality of care are not easy. If this is to be more than just "lip service," payers should join together and work with health care institutions and professional societies in each medical service area to measure the effect of their interventions. This is beginning to happen in a few areas. One would hope that a large-scale commitment to such an enterprise is not antithetical to the new competition ethic (Federal Trade Commission—please take note).

Blendon and Rogers put it best when they echoed the physicians' primary operating principle, "First, do no harm," in warning against harming the health care system. Unfortunately, there is mounting anecdotal evidence that access problems are again rearing their ugly heads, especially for the poor, the elderly, and those patients whose characteristics, medical conditions, or both render them "undesirable." To illustrate this, one need only look at the long overdue attention being given to the problem of alcohol and drug abuse. While competition is keen for the drug-impaired affluent, the resources available to help the underclass with the same problems are relatively minuscule. The rising problems of the acquired immunodeficiency syndrome in this population add to its basic inequity in making this poor social policy.

In commenting on the reemergence of problems in obtaining rural emergency care, one Colorado legislator cited the politics of scarcity as favoring those whose voices can be heard. In the old days of federal largesse and cost-shifting, adjustments could be made to provide care to the uninsured. Now, each payer wants to pay only what it deems necessary or what it says its bottom line permits. This self-interest ethic leaves little room for altruism.

Enlightened self-interest, however, should lead payers to be concerned that the whole may ultimately be less than the sum of the parts. Attention narrowly focused on their quarterly statements and their own patients may lead to disastrous long-term effects. They should be concerned about the viability of health care institutions and the attractiveness of the health care professions. Increasing shortages of nurses and other hands-on personnel in some acute-care settings do not bode well for the future of a balanced health care system in some rural and inner-city areas. Recent attention to long house-staff hours, if carried to its inevitable conclusion, will mean more, not less, money will be needed, at least in the short term. That more physicians are expressing disgruntlement about the practice of medicine may please some, but the increasing "deprofessionalization of medicine" is being too widely recognized to be ignored. Unless these issues are carefully and systematically studied, the health care system, as imperfect as it may be, will surely erode, quietly but inexorably. Even the affluent and the well-connected may find it will not be there when they need it. In this regard, the Colorado legislator went on to say: "There are places in this state where you better pray you don't have an accident." If true, this is indeed a sad commentary on health care in 1980s America.

The rank and file of doctors are no more scientific than their tailors. Doctoring is an art, not a science: Any layman who is interested in science sufficiently to take in one of the scientific journals and follow the literature of the scientific movement knows more about it than these doctors (probably a large majority) who are not interested in it and practice it only to earn their bread.

GEORGE BERNARD SHAW

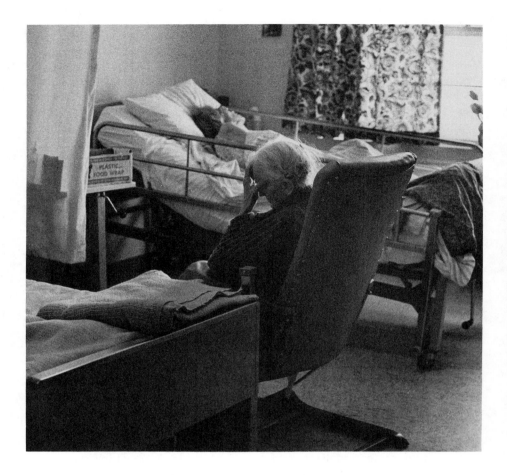

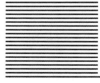

9

Chronic Illness, Aging, and Long-Term Care

R EPRESENTING 11.3 PERCENT of the population or 26 million people in 1980 and projected to reach 21.1 percent or 64 million by 2030, older Americans bear a disproportionate burden of chronic illness and disability. People in the U.S. are living longer than ever before, and as they get older they develop more and more chronic illnesses and disabilities. The burden of chronic illness and disability increases progressively in old age. The problems are increasing as this group grows faster than the rest of the population, and the oldest old subgroup, aged 85 and over, expands the fastest. Despite the improvement in the economic status of the majority of the elderly in the past 20 years, the situation of many elders in society is precarious.

Advancing age requires difficult life transitions at best. For most people it means an abrupt, sometimes involuntary retirement, a substantial drop in income, and other social adjustments. The hardships of this major life transition are exacerbated by the lack of support provided old people just when they are required to give up their employment income. Individuals are living longer but face many uncertainties, particularly because of the probability that illness and disability will become a serious problem.

In recent years, social science research has uncovered major evidence about health and disease in old age and has driven home the central character of social, economic, and family circumstances as major factors influencing the health of people over 65 years of age. More than one-fourth of the old people in this country survive at or near the poverty level. Their health is depleted by their living conditions.

[361]

The tragedy of old age described by Robert Butler is not the fact of aging and death, nor necessarily even the experience of chronic illness, but the combined effects of poverty, illness, social isolation, and ageism. Countering the negative myths perpetuated by this society about growing old, Butler illustrates the results of systematic stereotyping and discrimination on people in late life. He recommends broad public educational efforts and concentrated study of all that produces and supports healthy mental and physical development throughout the life cycle.

Carroll Estes and Juanita Wood paint an alarming picture of the threatened disappearance of nonprofit community-based health and social service providers for the elderly in the U.S. Policy shifts and medical care cost containment are challenging the private, nonprofit agencies that have traditionally provided noninstitutional health and social services to the elderly. At issue is the ability of communities to maintain a viable service sector predicated on full access for all individuals with chronic and long-term health and social service needs. Unlike the existing highly discrete, medicalized, fragmented service delivery system available only to those who can pay, an improved nonprofit community-based system will require innovative policymaking, professional leaders, and public sponsorship.

In "Medical Care at the End of Life" Ann Scitovsky and A. M. Capron focus on the high medical expenses of the elderly, especially those incurred in the last year of life. In response to economic and ethical questions about the appropriateness of expenditure and the possibility of overtreatment, the authors review current knowledge about health services and costs in the final years of life. The conclusions fail to support common assumptions and raise new issues for consideration.

In an upbeat closing to the chapter, Anne Sommers and Victoria Weisfeld set new goals for improving the health of the elderly and postponing old age. A comprehensive set of recommendations to federal, state, and local governments, health professions, the insurance industry, the labor market, and the media outline policies to support health goals. Objectives include reducing the number of elders in nursing homes, the number of bed disability days experienced, and the proportion of elders unable to function independently. Increases in health status, labor force participation, and other productive activities complete this optimistic set of objectives.

An everchanging, rhythmic biotic adventure of varying individuals, health is a part of the weave of life, coloring it brightly here, subtly shading it there, obvious in one place, obscure — almost lost — in another.

BENJAMIN A. KOGAN

Robert N. Butler

The Tragedy of Old Age in America

What is it like to be old in the United States? What will our own lives be like when we are old? Americans find it difficult to think about old age until they are propelled into the midst of it by their own aging and that of relatives and friends. Aging is the neglected stepchild of the human life cycle. Though we have begun to examine the socially taboo subjects of dying and death, we have leaped over that long period of time preceding death known as old age. In truth, it is easier to manage the problem of death than the problem of living as an old person. Death is a dramatic, one-time crisis while old age is a day-by-day and year-by-year confrontation with powerful external and internal forces, a bittersweet coming to terms with one's own personality and one's life.

Those of us who are not old barricade ourselves from discussions of old age by declaring the subject morbid, boring or in poor taste. Optimism and euphemism are other common devices. People will speak of looking forward to their "retirement years." The elderly are described respectfully as "senior citizens," "golden agers," "our elders," and one hears of old people who are considered inspirations and examples of how to "age well" or "gracefully." There is the popularly accepted opinion that Social Security and pensions provide a comfortable and reliable flow of funds so the elderly have few financial worries. Medicare has lulled the population into reassuring itself that the once terrible financial burdens of late-life illnesses are now eradicated. Advertisements and travel folders show relaxed, happy, well-dressed older people enjoying recreation, travel and their grandchildren. If they are no longer living in the old family home, they are pictured as delighted residents of retirement communities with names like Leisure World and Sun City, with lots of grass, clean air and fun. This is the American ideal of the "golden years" toward which millions of citizens are expectantly toiling through their workdays.

But this is not the full story. A second theme runs through the popular view of old age. Our colloquialisms reveal a great deal: once you are old you are "fading fast," "over the hill," "out to pasture," "down the drain," "finished,"

Robert N. Butler, M.D., is Brookdale Professor and chair of the Gerald and May Ellen Ritter Department of Geriatrics and Adult Development, Mount Sinai Medical Center, New York, New York. He served as director of the National Institute on Aging, National Institutes of Health, and is author of *Sex After Sixty* and *Why Survive? Being Old in America*.

[363]

"out of date," an "old crock," "fogy," "geezer" or "biddy." One hears children saying they are afraid to get old, middle-aged people declaring they want to die after they have passed their prime, and numbers of old people wishing they were dead.

What can we possibly conclude from these discrepant points of view? Our popular attitudes could be summed up as a combination of wishful thinking and stark terror. We base our feelings on primitive fears, prejudice and stereotypes rather than on knowledge and insight. In reality, the way one experiences old age is contingent upon physical health, personality, earlier life experiences, the actual circumstances of late-life events (in what order they occur, how they occur, when they occur) and the social supports one receives: adequate finances, shelter, medical care, social roles, religious support, recreation. All of these are crucial and interconnected elements which together determine the quality of life.

Old age is neither inherently miserable nor inherently sublime—like every stage of life it has problems, joys, fears and potentials. The process of aging and eventual death must ultimately be accepted as the natural progression of the life cycle, the old completing their prescribed life spans and making way for the young. Much that is unique in old age in fact derives from the reality of aging and the imminence of death. The old must clarify and find use for what they have attained in a lifetime of learning and adapting; they must conserve strength and resources where necessary and adjust creatively to those changes and losses that occur as part of the aging experience. The elderly have the potential for qualities of human reflection and observation which can only come from having lived an entire life span. There is a lifetime accumulation of personality and experience which is available to be used and enjoyed.

But what are an individual's chances for a "good" old age in America, with satisfying final years and a dignified death? Unfortunately, none too good. For many elderly Americans old age is a tragedy, a period of quiet despair, deprivation, desolation and muted rage. This can be a consequence of the kind of life a person has led in younger years and the problems in his or her relationships with others. There are also inevitable personal and physical losses to be sustained, some of which can become overwhelming and unbearable. All of this is the individual factor, the existential element. But old age is frequently a tragedy even when the early years have been fulfilling and people seemingly have everything going for them. Herein lies what I consider to be the genuine tragedy of old age in America—we have shaped a society which is extremely harsh to live in when one is old. The tragedy of old age is not the fact that each of us must grow old and die but that the process of doing so has been made unnecessarily and at times excruciatingly painful, humiliating, debilitating and isolating through insensitivity, ignorance and poverty. The potentials for satisfactions and even triumphs in late life are real and vastly underexplored. For the most part the elderly struggle to exist in an inhospitable world.

Are things *really* that bad? Let's begin by looking at the basic daily requirements for survival. Poverty or drastically lowered income and old age go hand in hand. People who are poor all their lives remain poor as they grow old. Most of us realize this. What we do not realize is that these poor are joined by multitudes of people who become poor only after growing older. When Social Security becomes the sole or primary income, it means subsistence-level life styles for many, and recent increases do not keep up with soaring costs of living. Private pension plans often do not pay off, and pension payments that do come in are not tied to inflationary decreases in buying power. Savings can be wiped out by a single unexpected catastrophe.

It has been estimated that at least 30 percent of the elderly live in substandard housing. Many more must deprive themselves of essentials to keep their homes in repair.

The American dream promised older people that if they worked hard enough all their lives, things would turn out well for them. Today's elderly were brought up to believe in pride, self-reliance and independence. Many are tough, determined individuals who manage to survive against adversity. But even the tough ones reach a point where help should be available to them.

Age discrimination in employment is unrestrained, with arbitrary retirement practices and bias against hiring older people for available jobs. Social Security penalizes the old by reducing their income checks as soon as they earn more than $2,400 a year. Job-training programs don't want the elderly (or the middle-aged, for that matter), so there is no opportunity to learn new skills. Employers rarely make concessions for the possible physical limitations of otherwise valuable older employees, and instead they are fired, retired or forced to resign.

It is obvious that the old get sick more frequently and more severely than the young, and 86 percent have chronic health problems of varying degree. These health problems, while significant, are largely treatable and for the most part do not impair the capacity to work. Medicare pays for only 45 percent of older people's health expenses; the balance must come from their own incomes and savings, or from Medicaid, which requires a humiliating means test. A serious illness can mean instant poverty. Drugs prescribed outside of hospitals, hearing aids, glasses, dental care and podiatry are not covered at all under Medicare. There is prejudice against the old by doctors and other medical personnel who don't like to bother with them. Psychiatrists and mental-health personnel typically assume that the mental problems of the old are untreatable. Psychoanalysts, the elite of the psychiatric profession, rarely accept them as patients. Medical schools and other teaching institutions find them "uninteresting." Voluntary hospitals are well known for dumping the "Medicare patient" into municipal hospitals; municipal hospitals in turn funnel them into nursing homes, mental hospitals and chronic disease institutions without the adequate diagnostic and treatment effort which might enable them to return home. Persons who do remain at home while in ill health have serious difficulties in getting social, medical and psychiatric services brought directly to them.

Problems large and small confront the elderly. They are easy targets for crime in the streets and in their homes. Because of loneliness, confusion, hearing and visual difficulties they are prime victims of dishonest door-to-door salesmen and fraudulent advertising, and buy defective hearing aids, dance lessons, useless "Medicare insurance supplements," and quack health remedies. Persons crippled by arthritis or strokes are yelled at by impatient bus drivers for their slowness in climbing on and off buses. Traffic lights turn red before they can get across the street. Revolving doors move too quickly. Subways usually have no elevators or escalators.

Old women fare worse than old men. Women have an average life expectancy of seven years longer than men and tend to marry men older than themselves; so two-thirds (six million) of all older women are widows.* When widowed they do not have the same social prerogatives as older men to date and marry those who are younger. As a result, they are likely to end up alone—an ironic turn of events when one remembers that most of them were raised from childhood to consider marriage the only acceptable state. The income levels of older working women are generally lower than those of men; many never worked outside the home until their children were grown and then only at unskilled, low-paying jobs. Others who worked all their lives typically received low wages, with lower Social Security and private retirement benefits as a result. Until 1973, housewives who were widowed received only 82.5 percent of their husbands' Social Security benefits even though they were full-time homemakers.

Black, Mexican-American and American Indian elderly all have a lower life expectancy than whites, due to their socioeconomic disadvantages. Although the life expectancy of 67.5 years for white men remained the same from 1960 to 1968, the life expectancy for black men *declined* a full year during that time (from 61.1 to 60.0). Blacks of all ages make up 11 percent of the total United States population, but they constitute only 7.8 percent of the elderly. The life expectancy for Mexican-Americans is estimated at 57 years, and for American Indians at 44 years. Most do not live long enough to be eligible for the benefits of Social Security and Medicare. Poverty is the norm. Scant attention is paid to their particular cultural interests and heritage.

Asian-American elderly (Chinese, Japanese, Korean, Filipino and Samoan) are victims of a public impression that they are independently cared for by their families and therefore do not need help. However, patterns of immigration by Asian-Americans to this country, the cultural barriers, language problems and discrimination they have faced have all taken a toll of their elderly and their

---

*Twenty percent of American women are widows by 60, 50 percent by 65, 66⅔ by 75.

families. This is particularly true of older Chinese men, who were not allowed to bring their wives and families with them to the United States or to intermarry.

MYTHS AND STEREOTYPES ABOUT THE OLD

In addition to dealing with the difficulties of physical and economic survival, older people are affected by the multitude of myths and stereotypes surrounding old age.

The Myth of Aging.   The idea of chronological aging (measuring one's age by the number of years one has lived) is a kind of myth. It is clear that there are great differences in the rates of physiological, chronological, psychological and social aging within the person and from person to person. In fact, physiological indicators show a greater range from the mean in old age than in any other age group, and this is true of personality as well. Older people actually become more diverse rather than more similar with advancing years. There are extraordinarily "young" 80-year-olds as well as "old" 80-year-olds. Chronological age, therefore, is a convenient but imprecise indicator of physical, mental and emotional status. For the purposes of this article old age may be considered to commence at the conventionally accepted point of 65.

We do know that organic brain damage can create such extensive intellectual impairment that people of all types and personalities may become dull-eyed, blank-faced and unresponsive. Massive destruction of the brain and body has a "leveling" effect which can produce increasing homogeneity among the elderly. But most older people do not suffer impairment of this magnitude during the greater part of their later life.

The Myth of Unproductivity.   Many believe the old to be unproductive. But in the absence of diseases and social adversities, old people tend to remain productive and actively involved in life. There are dazzling examples like octogenarians Georgia O'Keeffe continuing to paint and Pope John XXIII revitalizing his church, and septuagenarians Duke Ellington composing and working his hectic concert schedule and Golda Meir acting as her country's vigorous Prime Minister. Substantial numbers of people become unusually creative for the first time in old age, when exceptional and inborn talents may be discovered and expressed. What is most pertinent to our discussion here, however, is the fact that many old people continue to contribute usefully to their families and community in a variety of ways, including active employment. The 1971 Bureau of Labor Statistics figures show 1,780,000 people over 65 working full time and 1,257,000 part time. Since society and business practice do not encourage the continued employment of the elderly, it is obvious that many more would work if jobs were available.

When productive incapacity develops, it can be traced more directly to a variety of losses, diseases or circumstances than to that mysterious process called aging. Even then, in spite of the presence of severe handicaps, activity and involvement are often maintained.

The Myth of Disengagement.   This is related to the previous myth and holds that older people prefer to disengage from life, to withdraw into themselves, choosing to live alone or perhaps only with their peers, Ironically, some gerontologists themselves hold these views. One study, *Growing Old: The Process of Disengagement*, presents the theory that mutual separation of the aged person from his society is a natural part of the aging experience. There is no evidence to support this generalization. Disengagement is only one of many patterns of reaction to old age.

The Myth of Inflexibility.   The ability to change and adapt has little to do with one's age and more to do with one's lifelong character. But even this statement has to be qualified. One is not necessarily destined to maintain one's character in earlier life permanently. True, the endurance, the strength and the stability in human character structure are remarkable and protective. But most, if not all, people change and remain open to change throughout the course of life, right up to its termination. The old notion, whether ascribed to Pope Alexander VI or Sigmund Freud, that character is laid down in final form by the fifth year of life can be confidently refuted. Change is the hallmark of living. The notion that older people become less responsive to innovation and change because of age is not supported by scientific studies of healthy older people living in the community or by everyday observations and clinical psychiatric experience.

A related cliché is that political conservatism increases with age. If one's options are constricted by job discrimination, reduced or fixed income and runaway inflation, as older people's are, one may become conservative out of economic necessity rather than out of qualities innate in the psyche. Thus an older person may vote against the creation of better schools or an expansion of social services for tax reasons. His property—his home—may be his only equity, and his income is likely to be too low to weather increased taxes. A perfectly sensible self-interest rather than "conservatism" is at work here. Naturally, conservatives do exist among the elderly, but so do liberals, radicals and moderates. Once again diversity rather than homogeneity is the norm.

The Myth of "Senility."   The notion that old people are senile, showing forgetfulness, confusional episodes and reduced attention, is widely accepted. "Senility" is a popularized layman's term used by doctors and the public alike to categorize the behavior of the old. Some of what is called senile is the result of brain damage, but anxiety and depression are also frequently lumped within the same category of senility, even though they are treatable and often revers- ible. Old people, like young people, experience a full range of emotions, including anxiety, grief, depression and paranoid states. It is all too easy to blame age and brain damage when accounting for the mental problems and emotional concerns of later life.

Drug tranquilization is another frequent, misdiagnosed and potentially reversible cause of so-called senility. Malnutrition and unrecognized physical illnesses, such as congestive heart failure, may produce "senile behavior" by reducing the supply of blood, oxygen and food to the brain. Alcoholism, often associated with bereavement, is another cause. Because it has been so con- venient to dismiss all these manifestations by lumping them together under an improper and inaccurate diagnostic label, the elderly often do not receive the benefits of decent diagnosis and treatment.

Actual irreversible brain damage, of course, is not a myth, and two major conditions create mental disorders. One is cerebral arteriosclerosis (hardening of the arteries of the brain); the other, unfortunately referred to as senile brain disease, is due to a mysterious dissolution of brain cells. Such conditions account for some 50 percent of the cases of major mental disorders in old age, and the symptoms connected with these conditions are the ones that form the basis for what has come to be known as senility. But, as I wish to emphasize again, similar symptoms can be found in a number of other conditions which are reversible through proper treatment.

The Myth of Serenity.   In contrast to the previous myths, which view the elderly in a negative light, the myth of serenity portrays old age as a kind of adult fairyland. Now at last comes a time of relative peace and serenity when people can relax and enjoy the fruits of their labors after the storms of active life are over. Advertising slogans, television and romantic fiction foster the myth. Visions of carefree, cookie-baking grandmothers and rocking-chair grandfathers are cherished by younger generations. But, in fact, older persons experience more stresses than any other age group, and these stresses are often devastating. The strength of the aged to endure crisis is remarkable, and tran- quility is an unlikely as well as inappropriate response under these circumstances. Depression, anxiety, psychosomatic illnesses, paranoia, garrulousness and irrita- bility are some of the internal reactions to external stresses.

AGEISM—THE PREJUDICE AGAINST THE ELDERLY

The stereotyping and myths surrounding old age can be explained in part by lack of knowledge and by insufficient contact with a wide variety of older people. But there is another powerful factor operating—a deep and profound prejudice against the elderly which is found to some degree in all of us. In thinking about how to describe this, I coined the word "ageism" in 1968:

> Ageism can be seen as a process of systematic stereotyping of and discrimination against people because they are old, just as racism and sexism accomplish this with skin color and gender. Old people are categorized as senile, rigid in thought and manner, old-fashioned in morality and skills. . . . Ageism allows the younger generations to see older people as different from themselves; thus they subtly cease to identify with their elders as human beings.

Ageism makes it easier to ignore the frequently poor social and economic plight of older people. We can avoid dealing with the reality that our productivity-minded society has little use for non-producers—in this case those who have reached an arbitrarily defined retirement age. We can also avoid, for a time at least, reminders of the personal reality of our own aging and death.

Ageism is manifested in a wide range of phenomena, both on individual and institutional levels—stereotypes and myths, outright disdain and dislike, or simply subtle avoidance of contact; discriminatory practices in housing, employment and services of all kinds; epithets, cartoons and jokes. At times ageism becomes an expedient method by which society promotes viewpoints about the aged in order to relieve itself of responsibility toward them. At other times ageism serves highly personal objectives, protecting younger (usually middle-aged) individuals—often at high emotional cost—from thinking about things they fear (aging, illness, death).

The elderly's part in eliciting the kind of response which they receive from the young and from society at large is often a subtle but powerful factor in the public's generally disparaging views of them. They collaborate with their ostracizers. Some individuals act "senile"; others may deny their true feelings in an attempt to "age graciously" and obtain the approval which is otherwise denied them. Psychologist Margaret Thaler Singer observed similarities between the Rorschach test findings in members of a National Institute of Mental Health sample of aged volunteers who were resigned in the face of aging and those in American GI prisoners of war who collaborated with their captors in Korea.

Other self-sabotaging behavior can be a refusal to identify oneself as elderly at all. One sees older persons who affect the dress and behavior patterns of the young, pretending like Peter Pan that they have never grown up. Older women can be seen engaging in sad, frantic attempts to appear young, as if this would ensure appreciation and acceptance in the eyes of others.

A significant minority of older people conceal their age from themselves as well as from others. In a study of 1,700 elderly persons, Taves and Hansen found that one-sixth thought of themselves as old between the ages of 54 and 69, one-third between the ages of 70 and 79, and only 40 percent by age 80 and over. About one person in seven said they never thought of themselves as old.

In a study by Tuckman and Lorge that queried over 1,000 persons from 20 to 80, those under 30 classified themselves as young, and of those between 30 and 60, most classified themselves as middle-aged. At age 60 only a small proportion classified themselves as old, and at age 80 slightly over half called themselves old. A small percentage of the 80-year-olds persisted in describing themselves as young.

Of course, considering oneself "young" is not simply a prejudice or a delusion. Healthy older people do feel strong and vigorous, much as they did in their earlier days. The problem comes when this good feeling is called "youth" rather than "health," thus tying it to chronological age instead of to physical and mental well-being.

Lack of empathy is a further reaction by the elderly to their experiences in the larger culture. Out of emotional self-protection many healthy, prosperous, well-educated old people feel no identification with or protectiveness toward the poor elderly. A lack of compassion is of course not unique to the aged, but it has a special irony here with the advent of catastrophic illnesses or the exhaustion of resources that goes with a long life, they too run a high risk of finding themselves among the poor, facing similar indifference from their wealthier peers.

Older people are not always victims, passive and fated by their environment. They, too, initiate direct actions and stimulate responses. They may exploit their age and its accompanying challenges to gain something they want or need, perhaps to their own detriment (e.g., by demanding services from others and thus allowing their own skills to atrophy). Exploitation can backfire; excessive requests to others by an older person may be met at first, but as requests increase they are felt as demands—and may indeed be demands. Younger people who attempt to deal with a demanding older person may find themselves going through successive cycles of rage, guilt and over-protectiveness without realizing they are being manipulated. In addition to his "age" the older person may exploit his diseases and his impairments, capitalizing upon his alleged helplessness. Invalids of all ages do this, but older people can more easily take on the appearance of frailty when others would not be allowed this behavior. Manipulation by older people is best recognized for what it is—a valuable clue that there is energy available which should be redirected toward greater benefit for themselves and others.

It must also be remembered that the old can have many prejudices against the young. These may be a result of their attractiveness, vigor and sexual prowess. Older people may be troubled by the extraordinary changes that they see in the world around them and blame the younger generation. They may be angry at the brevity of life and begrudge someone the fresh chance of living out a life span which they have already completed.

Angry and ambivalent feelings flow, too, between the old and the middle-aged, who are caught up in the problems unique to their age and position within the life cycle. The middle-aged bear the heaviest personal and social responsibilities since they are called upon to help support—individually and collectively—both ends of the life cycle: the nurture and education of their young and the financial, emotional and physical care of the old. Many have not been prepared for their heavy responsibilities and are surprised and over-whelmed by them. Frequently these responsibilities trap them in their careers or life styles until the children grow up or their parents die. A common reaction is anger at both the young and the old. The effects of financial pressures are seen primarily in the middle and lower economic classes. But the middle-aged of all classes are inclined to be ambivalent toward the young and old since both age groups remind them of their own waning youth. In addition—with reason—they fear technological or professional obsolescence as they see what has happened to their elders and feel the pressure of youth pushing its way toward their position in society. Furthermore, their responsibilities are likely to increase in the future as more and more of their parents and grandparents live longer life spans.

STUDYING THE OLD

We have put precious little work and research into examining the last phase of life. What research has been done has concentrated primarily on studies of the 5 percent of elderly who are in institutions. The few research studies on the healthy aged living in the community have produced exciting new looks at the possibilities and problems of this age group. But on the whole medicine and the behavioral sciences seem to have shared society's negative views of old age and have quite consistently presented *decline* as the key concept of late life, with *neglect* forming the major treatment technique and research response.

Ultimately interest must focus on clarifying the complex, interwoven ele-ments necessary to produce and support physical and mental health up to the very end of life rather than our present preoccupation with "curing" ills after they develop. Understanding what interferes with healthy development throughout the life cycle gives us a chance to prevent problems, instead of rushing frantically and often futilely to solve them after they occur. Life is a continuing process from birth until death and it seems strange that it so seldom occurs to us to study life as a whole.

Finally, from a philosophic view, a greater understanding and control over the diseases and difficulties of later life would hopefully make old age less frightening and more acceptable as a truly valuable last phase of life. The relief of human suffering has merit in itself, but it also releases human beings from the fears and defenses they build up around it.

WHOSE RESPONSIBILITY ARE THEY?

Are older Americans entitled to decent income, health, housing, transportation and opportunities for employment as well as to social status and participation in society? Who should see to it that they get them? Why can't they manage their lives themselves? The struggle to decide on the place of the old in a culture has been familiar throughout history. Cultural attitudes have ranged from veneration, protectiveness, and sentimentality to derogation, rejection, pity and abandonment.

Older Americans of today—indeed the old people in any society—contributed to the growth of the society in which younger people live. One might assume that they would have a justifiable expectation of sharing in what is referred to as America's affluence. All of us, whatever our age, are now contributing taxes and services to our nation and are collectively preparing for our own old age. What will the future bring for us? Will anyone help us if we cannot adequately help ourselves?

The Depression of the 1930s convinced many rugged individualists that forces beyond the control of the individual could bring widespread devastation and poverty. A legislative landmark of Roosevelt's New Deal was the inauguration of Social Security in 1935, a consequence of many pressures. . . . Perhaps the final impetus came from the need to have the old retire in order to provide employment for the young. Thus, years after most Western European industrial nations had introduced it, the United States made its decision for the collective insurance-policy form of income maintenance for the disabled and retired. Eighty-five cents ($0.85) of every federal dollar now expended annually for programs for the elderly derive from Social Security trust funds to which we all contribute—as did the majority of the present elderly themselves in their working days.

Social Security, Medicare and federal housing programs have helped to gain for the elderly *some* income security, *some* health care and *some* housing. But the task has not been finished and the efforts do not match the needs.

Health is a continuing property in the sense that it is present from the ovum until death; it does not disappear during an illness to return on recovery, but the level of health changes throughout life.

J. R. AUDY and F. L. DUNN

Carroll L. Estes/Juanita B. Wood

The Non-profit Sector and Community-based Care for the Elderly in the U.S.: A Disappearing Resource?

INTRODUCTION

This article addresses social justice and equity issues in the allocation of resources for the development of a health and social service system—a system that aims to provide appropriate services to meet the needs of the elderly residing in communities throughout the United States. For more than a decade, national attention has been focused on developing equitable and effective ways of providing and paying for health care and supportive social services to meet the needs of a growing aging population. Many federally funded studies and service demonstrations, along with considerable political rhetoric, have argued for a move away from institutional care supported by Medicare (in hospitals) and Medicaid (in nursing homes) toward the provision of community-based care. The goal of such a shift is to enable older Americans to remain in their homes and communities as long as possible.

Historically, the non-profit service delivery sector has been important in understanding conditions faced by older Americans. Also referred to as the independent sector, the third sector, and the voluntary sector, it is important to the elderly because one of its major functions is the delivery of comprehensive, coordinated delivery systems of community care.

Three major points need to be made at the outset:

First, the importance of the non-profit sector in the delivery of community-based health and human services must be acknowledged. Consider the following: in 1980, approximately half (46%) of all publicly financed health dollars went to non-profit sector institutions including hospitals, and almost 90% of all publicly financed social service dollars went to non-profit organizations. In other words, non-profit sector institutions and agencies have filled a key role in the delivery of federally supported health and human services.

Carroll L. Estes, Ph.D., is professor of sociology, chair of the Department of Social and Behavioral Sciences, and director of the Institute for Health and Aging, School of Nursing, University of California, San Francisco.

Juanita B. Wood, Ph.D., is associate specialist in social and behavioral science at the Institute for Health and Aging, School of Nursing, University of California, San Francisco.

Second, viewed as a proportion of total revenues for the non-profit sector itself, the governmental role in supporting this sector has been quite significant. For example, in 1980, 43% of all revenues in non-profit sector health and human service agencies originated from government sources. Further, government funding exceeds private giving for health and human services by two to three times. Largely as a result of federal support, the non-profit service sector grew faster than the economy as a whole from 1975 to 1980. This period was characterized by an increasing dependence on governmental funding by all charitable service organizations in the non-profit sector.

Third, as a proportion of non-profit sector activity, health and social services play a very large role. For example, approximately 40% (40,983) of the 106,791, charitable non-profit organizations listed by the Census of Service Industries in 1977 were delivering social services, and 12% (12,307 organizations) were delivering health services. Thus, half of all organizations in the non-profit sector deliver health and social services. Social service agencies comprise the single largest proportion (38%) of all organization types operating in the non-profit sector. As early as 1977, fully 70% of the expenditures of charitable non-profit sector organizations were for health and social services ($8.3 billion for Social Services and $44 billion for health). Sixty-nine percent of the employees of the non-profit sector were working in health and human services.

The value of the non-profit sector

Recent literature indicates a growing consensus that the traditional role of the non-profit sector is currently being challenged, or threatened as never before. This concern is reflected in the creation of yet another voluntary organization, Independent Sector (IS), founded in 1980 "to preserve and enhance" the "national tradition" of giving, volunteering and not-for-profit initiative.

Traditionally and historically, the value of the for-profit sector has been embedded in the notions that business is to be operated in terms of self-interest and economic profitability. In contrast, the non-profit sector has been embedded in the notion that there are non-economic motivations in the society; that altruism and values of "community" stand as an important part of the society. Another justification for the non-profit sector has been that it represents an important vehicle of pluralistic expression of particularistic interests and citizen participation in American life via voluntary association. Alexis de Tocqueville wrote exquisitely about this in the 1840s. In U.S. society, the significance of voluntary action is demonstrated by the fact that at least 47% of Americans volunteer regularly in some kind of organized fashion, contributing an estimated $65 billion to the gross national product.

The conventional theoretical rationale for this sector has been squarely lodged in the pluralistic tradition, with the central arguments in favor of the non-profit sector focused on the dual limitations of the state and the hazards of the market. As early as Edmund Burke's reflections on the French Revolution in 1790, family, church and gild were venerated as exerting "a civilizing influence beyond anything the state could ever provide . . . a source of order, a fabric for social life, and a basis for resisting the tyranny of majority" in what appears to be an "anti-statist" hostility to government. Sociologists Robert Nesbit and Peter Berger have echoed similar themes of concern with the decline of community, those "intermediate associations" and "mediating institutions" that operate in between the individual and the larger institutions of society. As a valued "buffer" between the for-profit sector and a growing welfare state, it has been argued that the private non-profit sector has grown vigorous because it has functioned precisely to constrain the growth of the public sector.

Changes in federal support

In spite of their ideological value in reinforcing self-reliance and charity in the individual and collective conscience, non-profit social service and health agencies have, in the aggregate, experienced public funding erosions since 1981. Overall, federal support to non-profit organizations (excluding Medicare and Medicaid) during 1982–1985 dropped $17 billion below what it would have been, had FY 1980 spending levels been maintained. Projections for the next four years (1986–1988) are for another $18 billion loss in federal funds — or a total cumulative loss below FY 1980 levels (in constant dollars) of −30% (again, excluding Medicare and Medicaid).

Among the deepest cuts for the 1982–1988 period are in social services (−42%) and community development (−39%). The seriousness of a 42% cut in federal funding is apparent in view of the fact that, not only are private non-profit social services involved in running public programs and publicly funded services, these organizations currently draw more revenues from the Federal government than from all of private giving combined.

Statistical projections show that private giving would have had to increase 147% between 1981 and 1985 to offset projected federal budget cuts in non-profit fields of activity—a growth rate exceeding ten times the historic peak of giving. As Salamon and Abramson report, "During the first three years of the Reagan administration, private giving . . . offset only about 17% of estimated revenue losses of non-profits." Since there is no indication that private giving is increasing significantly, the conclusion must be that the private sector is not making up for lost federal resources to community health and social service agencies that provide care to the elderly.

TRENDS AFFECTING THE PRIVATE NON-PROFIT SECTOR

Three major trends in U.S. society and public policy are relevant to the currently challenged role of the private non-profit sector. First, and of growing importance, are the economic problems of corporate America. While some businesses are making spectacular profits, many U.S. corporations are recording low profit-margins relative to prior years. Historically, what tends to occur in periods of serious economic downturns such as the recent one, is that corporate restructuring occurs, which is characterized by the weeding-out of "inefficient" businesses as well as corporate consolidation and centralization.

A second phenomenon affecting the non-profit sector is the emphasis on deregulation initiated by the Reagan Administration beginning in 1981. Deregulation has facilitated the entry of for-profits in health and human services, on the theory that it would reduce costs and increase cost effectiveness.

A third factor is the increasingly important policy objective of medical care cost containment. Non-profit health and social service organizations are affected by the external factors of price competition and cost control in the health industry, factors that traditionally have not played a major part in the non-profit service sector organizations in the U.S. It is not difficult to imagine that the incentives and the traditional functions served by non-profit organizations in providing non-institutional home-based and community care will change accordingly, as these organizations themselves are required to become both competitive and "profitable."

RESEARCH FINDINGS ON THE NON-PROFIT SECTOR, 1983–84

Based on the authors' research in 1983 and 1984 of 335 agencies in 32 large U.S. urban communities that were purposively drawn from the largest states within each of eight geographically dispersed federal regions, the following changes appear to be occurring among the home health, homemaker/chore, and adult day health agencies; senior centers, nutrition, and information and referral programs; community health and community mental health centers; and local health departments:

First, in all but the home health agencies, losses of public financing have been reported, and funding cuts generally appear to be greater for the social, as opposed to medical services.

Second, the community delivery system of non-profit agencies is being restructured. Evidence of this restructuring is in (a) the weeding out of the weaker, less competitive, inefficient, non-profit agencies, (b) the consolidation of agencies, (c) the concentration of services, and (d) the diversification of organizational structures, with the entry of for-profit entities, attached to non-profit organization entities.

Both vertical and horizontal integration are occurring, as single service agencies are becoming part of multi-institutional chains, and hospitals are extending their own service array to incorporate home health services, extended care and skilled nursing services, enabling them to channel and track patients throughout the health care system.

Another process also appears to be occurring. It is the "absorption" or non-profit service agencies by the proprietary organizations, with the dramatic growth of for-profit sector agencies in the provision of certain types of community services (especially in home health and nutrition). Proprietary home health agencies, for example, have grown 539% in the past 5 years, and now comprise more than one-quarter of all such agencies.

Access to community-based health and social services is increasingly limited to those who are eligible under a very stringent Medicare policy, or to those who can afford to pay directly or through private insurance. The ability of non-profit agencies to continue serving the low income is threatened since these clients either have no reimbursement source or a low Medicaid reimbursement.

The process of informalization in which there is a transfer of functions from the formal to the informal economy is applicable to the recent changes in the health care sector. Care taking for the frail elderly by non-profit institutions, for example, is now being transferred to family care-givers in the home largely as a result of early hospital discharge policy. In the context of cost control and the family role in providing service, the social costs of such a shift will be experienced primarily by women, who are the major caregivers of the elderly. Although the family has played an important traditional role in caring for elders, the family's ability to meet the needs of the chronically ill will be constrained by the following major social trends: a decreasing parent-child ratio, the changing nature of the household economy with the movement of older women into the workforce, and the growing number of older women who themselves are single, living alone, and without the financial resources to meet the needs of their very old and chronically ill dependent spouses, siblings or parents.

The state's overriding objective of cost containment and the DRG Medicare policy designed to implement that goal is also having the effect of creating a new commercial market — the home. The medicalization of health care over the last two decades referred to the highly specialized, medical solutions to social problems and was limited largely to institutional settings. The authors' research data suggest that this medical care market is now expanding to include the community care service system which hithertofore had been deemed social in nature. The home is one aspect of the community-based system that is now regarded as potentially profitable. Hence, because of the medicalization of community care, the newest institution is becoming "the home." Many community-based service agencies that were oriented toward the delivery of comprehensive services are being altered and reshaped as providers of primarily medical or medically-related services due to medically biased reimbursement policies under Medicare (including the more "liberalized" Medicare home health policy).

The application and reimbursement of highly technical, specialized services under "home health" exemplifies this change of shift away from coordinated community-based services. The "unbundling" of services is an economic term to characterize a process where multi-services are no longer financially viable as a comprehensive package. Under this incentive scheme, home health agencies survive and thrive by offering highly distinct, specialized services to those who can afford to pay for them. To compete with a for-profit national corporation, a local non-profit home health agency cannot afford to continue to offer an array of services for which there is no reimbursement (e.g. transportation, outreach or telephone reassurance); they will not be competitive on the price of the home-health services offered. Agencies have responded by unbundling their services, offering the more easily reimbursable services.

The authors' survey data show that reimbursement is much more assured for medical compared to social services, at least partly as a result of a growing problem of claims that are being denied by Medicare fiscal intermediaries, particularly for those services that may be classified as socially-supportive. Fiscal intermediaries have tightened considerably on Medicare reimbursement for these home-health services to stem the cost rise; Medicare home health expenditure increased about 200% between 1978 and 1982. The result is a clear move away from the policy goals of the prior decade that were aimed at building comprehensive and coordinated community-based service delivery systems.

Another trend revealed by the authors' data is the polarization between the frail (very old) sick clients who are home-bound and those younger elderly in the community who need supportive services to avoid institutionalization. This trend is partially the result of prioritizing services for the frail elderly at the federal and state levels and the emphasis of Medicare reimbursement policies.

DISCUSSION

A major implication of cost containment and the increasingly competitive health and human services market is likely to be that non-profit agencies will serve fewer low-income elderly. Since 1981 there have been federal cuts in social services, as well as in Medicaid, and states have been unable (or unwilling) to make up or fill in the Medicaid cuts. Because Medicaid reimbursement tends to be extremely low for medical services to the poor, it is more profitable and cost-effective for non-profit service agencies to attract the higher reimbursement recipients (e.g. Medicare and private pay patients) while avoiding the Medicaid recipient. One potential result of the non-profits' adoption or the same business incentives as proprietary agencies is the emergence of a "no-care zone" for certain types of individuals who are unable to pay for their care.

Another result is that non-profit agencies are themselves being encouraged to create separate for-profit organizations to attract private-pay patients. These incentives are accelerating the "blurring" of the boundaries between the profit and non-profit sectors — a phenomenon that has been encouraged by the competitive ideology and dual pressures on non-profits to compete effectively in the contracting for clientele and their growing need generate additional revenues, as their public-service funding is cut. One unfortunate result is likely to be the further delegitimation of non-profit sector activity in itself. That is, insofar as non-profits look and behave just like for-profits (also avoiding low-income clients and generating income), what, then, would be the rationale for continuing non-profit organizations' special tax status?

In conclusion, the following issues of distributive justice and community care are raised:

1. How will client access be affected in the long run, particularly as the ability to pay for services is diminished for the low-income elderly? As services are unbundled? As the delivery system becomes more fragmented?
2. What will or can be the commitment of professionals who provide services and their ability to make independent decisions based on client need in the face of market pressures of the proprietary organization? In the face of national and regional proprietary market considerations, how will local needs fare?
3. What are the implications of the shift in non-profit sector policy from one which was to serve the general welfare or "public good" to one which is charged with purely economic values of competition and cost-containment?
4. What will be the human consequences for the frail and needy elderly who are likely to confront an increasingly medicalized and costly service delivery system?

Medicare cost-containment policies are being formulated and implemented apart from the broader understanding of the consequences of these policies to the larger system of community care. One of the most significant contributions of gerontology to the knowledge of social sciences and health policy research has been the understanding that highly specialized, fragmented, medical acute-care services alone are not sufficient to meet long-term care needs of the elderly. In fact, such a single-minded, biomedical approach will not only be extremely costly, but also will not achieve the goals of improved health or quality of life for older persons.

These concerns become more salient when viewed in the context of an increased demand on community agencies to meet the needs of an older and sicker population. Virtually all types of agencies interviewed in the authors' study in 1983 and 1984 reported dramatic increases in number of clients seeking their services and in the number of "old-old" clients (75 years of age and over). While some of this change may be attributable to overall growth in the elderly population, the most likely reason for the increased demand would appear to be medical cost containment pressures (and Medicare prospective payment) which is encouraging early hospital discharge or elderly patients.

The research reported here has identified a change in national focus in the name of decentralization—away from a primary concern for "community" and access to care, in the name of containment and cost effectiveness. At issue is the ability of communities to maintain a viable service sector predicated on service needs and service accessibility, as opposed to a highly discrete, medicalized, and disaggregated service delivery system that is available only to those who can pay (or for whom some reimbursement policy pays adequately). The challenge is considerable for policymakers, leaders in the non-profit sector, professionals, and the public.

States of health or disease are the expressions of the success or failure experienced by the organism in its efforts to respond adaptively to environmental challenge.

RENE DUBOS

Anne A. Scitovsky/Alexander M. Capron

Medical Care at the End of Life: The Interaction of Economics and Ethics

INTRODUCTION

The rising cost of medical care in the United States over the past quarter century has become a matter of growing concern for both private citizens and government at all levels. National health expenditures increased almost 12-fold between 1960 and 1982, from $26.9 billion to $322.4 billion, or from 5.3% of the gross national product (GNP) to 10.5%. Only a small part of this increase is attributable to the increase in the population, which grew by only, about 30% during this period. The major factors accounting for the increase in spending for medical care are the steady rise in medical care prices, which increased at a faster pace than did the prices of all other goods and services; greater use of health services because of higher real incomes and more comprehensive health insurance coverage: changes in medical technologies, such as the introduction of new and more expensive forms of treatment; and last but not least, the increase in the number and proportion of persons aged 65 years and older, who have higher medical care expenses per capita than younger persons.

It is this last problem, the high medical expenses of the elderly, which has been receiving special attention in recent years. One reason for this concern is the drain these expenses are putting on the Medicare Hospital Insurance Trust Fund, which is in danger of a deficit by the end of the century, unless changes are made in its benefit structure or financing or both. Various studies have shown another equally if not more important reason: A very large share of the elderly's medical care expenditures are incurred in the last year or even months of their lives; this has led to the question of whether scarce resources are being "wasted" on the dying, resources that could be spent more productively on other patients. Finally, doubts about the appropriateness of treatment are also voiced by people, like Eli Ginzberg, who are concerned "less with financial risk and more with the dangers threatening the aged from overtreatment in acute care hospitals."

Anne A. Scitovsky is chief of Health Economics at the Palo Alto Medical Foundation/ Research Institute, Palo Alto, California, and lecturer at the Institute for Health Policy Studies, School of Medicine, University of California, San Francisco, California.

Alexander M. Capron, L.L.B., is professor of law and medicine, University of Southern California Law Center, Los Angeles, California.

In this article we review the economic, ethical, and legal problems of the use and costs of medical care at the end of life. We begin with an overview of the general problem of health care and the elderly, their increasing numbers, their health status, their health care needs, and their health care expenditures. In the second section we examine what we know and do not know about medical expenditures of the elderly in their last years of life.

HEALTH CARE AND THE ELDERLY

The Aging of the Population

More Americans are living to age 65 and over than ever before. In 1950, there were 12.4 million elderly people in the United States, or 8.2% of the total population. By 1981 their number had grown to 26.1 million, or 11.4% of the population. By the year 2000 their number is expected to reach 35.1 million, or 13.1% of the population. Moreover, the proportion of the very old—those aged 75 years and over—has grown even more rapidly than that of the "young" elderly, those aged 65 to 74 years. In 1950, the "old old" accounted for only 2.6% of the total population and 31.7% of the total number of elderly, but by 1981 had increased to 4.5% of the total population and 40.2% of the elderly population.

During the first half of this century the major cause of the aging of the population was the decline in fertility, which reduced the proportion of young persons to older persons. In the second half of the century, the leading factor has been the decline in mortality across all age groups, resulting from improved living standards and medical advances in the prevention and treatment of infectious diseases that formerly were often fatal. The age-adjusted mortality rate for all ages declined from 8.4 deaths per 1000 population in 1950 to 5.4 deaths in 1982. During the same period, the rate for persons aged 65 years and over dropped from 62.7 per 1000 to 50.5. Similar declines occurred for each of the over-65 year age groups.

As a result of the decline in mortality rates, life expectancy—both at birth and at age 65—has increased substantially in the course of the past three decades. A child born in 1982 could expect to live almost six years longer than one born in 1950 and reach age 74.5 years compared to 68.2 years for a child born in 1950. Similarly, a person aged 65 years in 1982 could expect to live another 16.8 years—almost three years longer than the 13.9 years expected for a person aged 65 years in 1950. Female life expectancy has especially increased—a woman aged 65 years in 1982 can expect to live an additional 18.8 years on average compared to 14.4 years for a 65-year-old male. Thus, an increasing proportion of the elderly, and especially of the very old, is female.

Health Status and Health Needs of the Elderly

Although life expectancy at age 65 is now almost 17 years, what has been termed "active life expectancy" is considerably less. "Active life expectancy," is the projected number of years of functional well-being: the end point of "active life expectancy" is not death but "the loss of independence in the activities of daily living (ADL)." According to a study by the originators of the concept, a group of 65 to 69 year-old persons living in the community whose total life expectancy was 16.5 years had an "active life expectancy," of only 10.0 years. Moreover, they found that the proportion of dependent years increased with age, so that persons living independently at age 85 would need assistance for 60% of their remaining 7.3 years of life.

The reason for the increasing dependence of elderly people is the deterioration of their health due to the onset of chronic conditions that tend to become more disabling as they grow older. By every measure of health status, elderly people are worse off than younger people. National data show that almost half of all elderly people have some activity limitation, almost 40% are limited in their major activity, and almost 18% are unable to carry out their major activity. Elderly people average about 40 days of restricted activity per year, 14 of them bed disability days. Almost one third rate their health as fair or poor compared to that of others their age. The data also show the elderly's increasing dependence on others as they grow older. For example, while 53 of every 1000 persons aged 65 to 74 need some help in one or more basic activities of daily living, this number nearly triples (to 157) for those aged 75 and over.

Because the elderly suffer primarily from chronic conditions, they use more health care services than younger persons. In contrast to acute conditions, there is generally no cure for chronic conditions, but medical care can at least make symptoms more tolerable. As a result, the elderly's use of medical care tends to be high and to continue over many years. For example, persons aged 65 years and over average 6.3 physician visits per person per year compared to between four and five visits for those under 65 years. The differences in their use of hospital services are even more striking. The elderly average 396.5 hospital admissions and 4155.3 hospital days per 1000 population per year, more than twice the rate of hospital use of those under 65 years. Moreover, the use of hospital services by the elderly increases as they age. For example, the rate of hospital admissions of persons aged 75 and over is 51% higher than that of persons aged 65 to 74, and their rate of hospital days is 70% higher.

The elderly also are the principal users of nursing home services. The National Center for Health Statistics' most recent survey of nursing homes, conducted in 1977, found that almost 5% of persons aged 65 and over were in nursing homes, accounting for almost 90% of all nursing home residents. Again, use rises sharply with age: 21.6% of those aged 85 and over were in nursing homes, accounting for one third of all nursing home residents though constituting less than 1% of the total United States population.

Health Care Expenditures of the Elderly

In light of these health needs, it is hardly surprising that the elderly's share of total personal health care expenditures has risen faster than their proportion in the population, from 23.8% of total personal health care expenditures in 1965 to 29.4% in 1978 and 34.4% in 1984, based on a preliminary estimate. In 1965, average expenditures of persons aged 65 years and over were 5.7 times those of persons less than 19 years old and 2.2 times those of persons aged 19 to 64 years. By 1978, these figures had risen to 7.1 and 2.7 times the expenditures of persons in the two younger age groups, respectively.

A major reason for the steeper rise in average health care expenditures of the elderly compared to that of younger persons is the aging of the elderly population itself, that is, the increase to nearly 9% in the proportion of the old who are over 85 years old. Although there are no data on *total* health care expenditures by age for the 65-year and over population, Medicare data show that reimbursements increase with age. In 1982 average reimbursements *per person served* amounted to $2960 for Medicare beneficiaries aged 85 years and older, compared to $2172 for beneficiaries aged 65 to 74 years, or 36% more. The difference in average reimbursements *per enrollee* is even greater, with average reimbursements of the 85-year and older group being 66% higher than those of the younger group ($2170 versus $1303). This difference reflects both the higher medical care expenditures of the older beneficiaries who have some medical expenses and the greater proportion of older beneficiaries who use Medicare services. The difference between *total* health care expenditures of the "old old" and those of the "young old" is likely to be even greater than these figures indicate, because Medicare covers only a small fraction of nursing home expenditures and, as shown above, nursing home utilization rises sharply with age.

A dramatic change has also occurred in the source of payment for the care of the elderly. In 1965, the year the Medicare and Medicaid programs went into effect, public sources—federal, state and local government programs—accounted for just under 30% of the health care expenditures of the elderly. By 1978, the share of public funds had risen to 63.2% (and is estimated to have risen to 67.2% in 1984). There has also been a major shift from state and local government sources to federal sources. In 1965, public funding for health care of the elderly was about evenly divided between federal sources, on the one hand, and state and local sources, on the other. By 1978, 86% of total public funding of care for the elderly came from federal sources, representing 54% of the total expended on health care for the elderly. Estimates for 1984 suggest that the federal share today may even be slightly higher.

To sum up, the aging of the population, and especially the increase in the number and proportion of the very old, has been an important cause of the increase in national health care expenditures in the United States and is largely responsible for the financial difficulties of the Medicare program. Because

Medicare reimbursements increase with age, average annual reimbursements per enrollee have increased; and because elderly people live longer, Medicare payments per enrollee continue over a longer period of years than when the program was introduced in 1965.

THE ECONOMICS OF CARING FOR PATIENTS WHO DIE

Just as concern over the growing proportion of national expenditures devoted to health care often focuses on the major contribution made by the aging of the population, concern about the high cost of care for the elderly is heightened by the evidence from several studies that shows that a large part of these expenses is incurred in the last year or months of life. The most frequently cited statistic on this subject comes from a Health Care Financing Administration (HCFA) study by Lubitz and Prihoda, which found that the 5.9% of Medicare beneficiaries who died in 1978 accounted for 27.9% of Medicare expenditures. In fact, as Fuchs has pointed out, the high medical expenses of persons who die are the principal reason that medical care expenditures of the elderly rise with age. Using data on Medicare expenditures per enrollee by age and sex, he showed that adjusting for age-sex differences in survival status eliminates much of the age-related increase in expenditures, especially the very high expenditures of the 80-year and older group, for whom his figures actually show a decline rather than an increase in expenses. (It must be remembered, however, that the data on which these estimates are based are for Medicare reimbursements and thus do not include expenses for nursing home care, which are the heaviest for the oldest age group.)

To determine whether medical resources are being misused for the dying, a review and evaluation of the data on medical care use and expenditures at the end of life are essential.

Taken together the studies leave little doubt that medical care expenditures at the end of life are indeed high. From some of the earlier studies one can see that this is not a recent development: For at least 20 years, medical care costs of persons who died have been high compared to those of survivors. The greater concern about these costs today than 15 or 20 years ago is tied to the general concern over constantly rising medical care expenses which threaten to consume an ever larger share of the GNP and to sink the Medicare fund in red ink, as well as to the great public awareness of the details of high-technology medicine. As one public official opined, "We've got a duty to die and get out of the way with all our machines and artificial hearts and everything else like that and let the other society, our kids, build a reasonable life." However, although the studies establish that medical care costs at the end of life are high, this by no means proves that a "disproportionate" amount is being spent on terminally ill patients.

The assertion that the "dying elderly" are receiving "too much" health care could mean several different things. First, those concerned with controlling health care expenditures may mean that elderly patients who die absorb an "excessive" amount of the total public (and/or private) resources available for health care. Yet looking in the Lubitz-Prihoda study for decedents who probably received high-technology interventions in their last year of life — namely, those with Medicare reimbursements of $20,000 or more — reveals that only 3% of all elderly decedents (24,000 patients) fell into this category. Even going to a lower threshold figure of $15,000 yields only 56,000 decedents, or 6% of the total. Thus, the number of elderly patients who died who appear to have received aggressive, intensive medical care is very small. Had all medical care been withheld from them (a highly improbable step), the savings to the Medicare program would have been small: $644 million (3.5% of total Medicare reimbursements for the decedents and survivors included in Lubitz and Prihoda) if care had been withheld from those with reimbursements of $20,000 or more, or $1196 million (6.5% of total Medicare reimbursements) if the threshold had been $15,000. Thus, the bulk of Medicare reimbursements for all elderly patients who died is accounted for by patients other than those who received intensive medical care in their last year of life.

Alternatively, the claim of "too much" care may be that these patients are receiving care that is neither desired by, nor appropriate for, them. Rather than being an economic argument, this conclusion is explicitly framed in ethical terms. An analysis of the philosophical principles by which this assertion can be evaluated demonstrates, however, that the first version of the "disproportionality" claim also rests — and should be judged — on ethical as well as economic presuppositions.

CONCLUSION

In sum, although the available data are not conclusive, it appears unlikely that more than a relatively small part of the high medical expenses at the end of life, and of the elderly in general, are due to excessively aggressive care of terminally ill patients. Most of these expenses seem to be for the care of very ill but not necessarily dying patients, care that, especially in the case of the very old and chronically ill, is relatively conservative yet expensive.

This last group thus creates a double dilemma. On the one hand, the care of these patients is costly and probably accounts for far more than the costs of care of "terminally ill" patients, as that term is commonly used. On the other hand, the decision-making mechanisms (such as Durable Powers of Attorney) that are available to avoid unwanted or futile treatment in the case of the patients who maintain their vigor and powers of thought until near the time of their fatal illness, are less likely to be effective with chronically ill, debilitated patients, whose incapacity to participate in decisions is often of long standing, thus making it unlikely that they will have expressed their current wishes about the extent of care they desire.

Moreover, the fact that this second group of patients is not "dying" raises grave questions in the minds of many about the application to them of the substantive standards for withdrawal of "life-sustaining" treatment that have recently come to be widely accepted regarding more gravely ill patients. Many people may share the sentiments of the respected journalist Alan Otten, who publicly expressed concern over the fate of his 90-year-old mother and others like her in nursing homes, "enduring barren year after barren year, with chronic diseases that unfortunately do not kill but merely irrevocably waste the body and destroy the mind."

> Doctors, nursing homes and hospitals work to keep these old people alive with tube feeding, nutritional supplements, antibiotics at the first sign of infection. For what? Are we really doing these people any favor by fighting so hard to prolong their lives?

Yet, despite the prevalence of such views, society has only just begun to address this problem. Thus far, only one state's highest court has sanctioned the withdrawal of supportive care (including artificially provided nutrition and fluids) from debilitated elderly patients, based upon their previously expressed wishes or on an "objective" assessment of their "best interests," and respected ethicists remain troubled by the analogy drawn between artificial respirators and artificial feeding. Until firmer guidance emerges from professional bodies, the courts, and the legislatures for the treatment of these patients, including true alternatives to the "all-or-nothing" stance of most acute-care facilities, physicians may be left with a felt ethical compulsion to "do something"—even halfhearted and ineffective measures that make "no medical or ethical sense at all." Thus, until medical prognostic powers improve substantially and ethical and legal standards emerge to allay fears that any failure to "do everything possible" for these patients would send the country sliding into the abyss of active euthanasia, medical treatment will continue to be provided that possibly wastes resources and that may harm rather than help some patients.

Anne R. Somers/Victoria D. Weisfeld

Improving the Elderly "Healthspan" and Postponing "Old Age"

This statement addresses, with enthusiasm, Category XVI of the Public Health Service Institute of Medicine list of priority target areas for the year 2000: "Maintaining Health and Quality of Life in Older People." It builds on the discussion of "healthy older adults" in the 1979 Surgeon General's Report on Health Promotion and Disease Prevention. Our focus relates both to the quality of individual lives and to broad economic, ethical, and political issues that will become increasingly urgent in the 21st century.

RETHINKING U.S. POLITICS ON AGING

Although we are reluctant to admit it, most current U.S. policies on aging are increasingly obsolete and will probably be untenable by the year 2000. This is no one's fault. On the contrary, it is the price of phenomenal success.

In the 26 years between 1960 and 1986, average life expectancy at 65 increased by 2.6 years, more than during the previous 60 years, from 1900 to 1960. Average life expectancy at 65 is now almost 15 years for men and 19 years for women. Although people over 65 obviously suffer more illness and disability than their juniors, only 4.6% are in nursing homes. Of those aged 65 to 74, just a little more than 1% are nursing home residents.

Of all the noninstitutionalized people over 65, nearly 70% rank their health as "excellent" or "good," as opposed to "fair" or "poor." In 1986, fewer than 10% were unable to function independently — that is, could not perform one or more tasks on a defined list of activities of daily living such as feeding, dressing, or toileting without help. In 1976, 17% reportedly were in the category of the nearest comparable federal measure ("unable to carry on major activity").

Anne R. Somers, B.A., is adjunct professor in the Department of Environmental and Community Medicine at the University of Medicine and Dentistry of New Jersey, Robert Wood Johnson Medical School, Piscataway, New Jersey.

Victoria D. Weisfeld is senior communications officer with The Robert Wood Johnson Foundation, Princeton, New Jersey.

As for the unfortunate 10%, some of their problems, such as Alzheimer's disease, are currently beyond the reach of effective prevention. But a much greater proportion is amenable to preventive interventions at the primary (preventing the condition in the first place), secondary (early identification), or tertiary (preventing complications and minimizing dependency) levels. For example, heart disease is still the major single cause of severe disability among the noninstitutionalized elderly, and the major risks for heart disease are not only known but, in most cases, controllable.

Unfortunately, however, many or perhaps most older persons are still denied access to effective preventive services as a result of nonavailability, financial constraints, ignorance, or indifference (their own as well as that of many health professionals). The result is a great deal of unnecessary suffering and avoidable use of expensive acute care services.

The per capita costs of Medicare, Medicaid, and Social Security continue to grow dramatically while labor force participation by the elderly continues to fall. The recent cover story in *Time* (February 22, 1988) titled "And now for the fun years: Americans are living longer and enjoying it more—but who will foot the bill?" suggests the painful dilemma that lies ahead. Some 75 million baby boomers, about one-third of the population, will reach 65, retire, and expect to be supported by a shrinking proportion of younger workers.

The full implications of these developments go far beyond the health field and the focus of this discussion. Nevertheless, the health component is basic. The very concept of "old age" and all our protective policies and programs for the aged relate to the presumption of a sharp decline in physical and/or mental capacity, as well as life expectancy, after 65. This is now patently inaccurate, but as a nation we haven't decided how to adjust to the changed situation. We seem to be groping simultaneously in two diametrically opposed directions: one negative that offers a "rationing" solution, and the other a positive national commitment to "healthy and productive aging."

As to rationing, it may seem a long way from Medicare cutbacks and failure to provide adequate preventive, rehabilitative, and support services for the elderly to withholding treatment and eventual compulsory euthanasia, based on age, disability, or economic status. But the direction is clear—and tragic.

The alternative positive scenario is equally portentous. The concept of "healthy aging" has become the leading thrust of geriatric and gerontologic research. Starting with the 1979 Surgeon General's Report and its emphasis on "functional independence," numerous formulations have been described, including: "compression of morbidity," "preventive gerontology," extended "healthspan," "successful aging," "new roles" for older people, and "redefinition of aging."

We now need to push this approach one step further, emphasizing not only healthy but "productive aging," a term first coined by Dr. Robert Butler. It is no longer enough to say that older people have an equal right to good health care, including prevention and long-term care. The corollary is the obligation to take care of our own health insofar as possible, to learn to cope with various chronic conditions, and to continue working and contributing to society for as long as possible.

SUGGESTED GOAL FOR YEAR 2000

Looking to the year 2000, we suggest two broad and complementary goals: (1) Improve the "healthspan" or "active life expectancy" of older persons, including those with some chronic impairment. In other words, increase the number of years of independent functioning and capacity for productive activity. (2) Set the stage for upward redefinition of the concept of "old age," moving gradually from the obsolete figure of 65 toward a more realistic age of 75, with a target of at least 70 by 2000.

These actions would balance society's continuing commitment to the elderly, regardless of age, with the elderly's commitment to society to contribute as much as possible, regardless of age. The adjustment of social mores and legal entitlements to conform to such a redefinition is beyond the scope of this discussion. But we believe that progress toward these two goals would facilitate other changes.

SPECIFIC OBJECTIVES

Specific measurable objectives designed to move us in this direction might include several of the following. All percentages assume adjustment for the changing age composition of the over-65 population.

- By 2000 the proportion of those 65 and over in need of nursing home care will be reduced to 4%. (In 1985 4.6% were in nursing homes, down from 4.8% in 1977.)
- By 2000 the average annual number of bed-disability days for the noninstitutionalized will be reduced to 12. (This was the same 1990 goal, which we probably will not meet. The 1986 figure was 14.9 days.)
- By 2000 the proportion of the noninstitutionalized who cannot meet the federal definition of ability to function independently will be reduced to no more than 8.5%. (In 1986 the figure was 9.6%.)
- By 2000 the proportion of noninstitutionalized with self-reported health status of "excellent" to "good" will increase to 75%. (In 1985 the proportion was 68%.)
- By 2000 the labor force participation of those 65 and over will be at least 20%, defined as employed full- or part-time or looking for work. (In 1986 it was only 11%.)

- By 2000 at least another 30% will be engaged in some form of unpaid but productive activity, including care of disabled family members.

Many subsidiary objectives could and should be developed. For example, further reductions can be achieved in the number of elders with uncontrolled high blood pressure or high serum cholesterol, who are over- or underweight, or who suffer uncorrected dental, vision, or hearing problems. In addition, reductions can be made in the numbers who have alcohol or drug problems, still smoke, fail to exercise adequately, do not follow accepted nutrition guidelines, or do not receive periodic health checkups. In most of these areas, the results of good research undertaken over the past decade should be used to formulate and refine specific objectives.

IMPLEMENTING STRATEGIES

Continued progress toward the suggested goals and objectives will require commitment and much hard work by all of the primary components of U.S. society—government at all levels, the health professions, employers, labor, the insurance industry, the media, and, of course, the general public. Following are five major categories, but this is by no means a complete listing.

Government at All Levels

- Employment and pension policies need to be reviewed with the goals of (1) increasing employment of the elderly—full-time, part-time and/or voluntary—and (2) relating size of pension to age at retirement or disability.
- Health information and education materials should be developed at all levels of government and directed to both the general public and the health professions. Such materials should be frequently updated and widely disseminated through the media and senior citizen and professional organizations.

Federal

- The process already underway in the Public Health Service and Health Care Financing Administration to define effective primary, secondary, and tertiary preventive services for the elderly should be completed as quickly as possible. Provisions should be established for ongoing review and dissemination of findings to all relevant parties. This process is basic to most of the recommendations that follow.

- Packages of clinical preventive services, based on the previously mentioned studies and others, should be incorporated into Medicare, Medicaid, Veterans Administration, Older Americans, and other health programs for the elderly, along with financial incentives to both providers and consumers.

States

- State governments should strengthen their administrative and financial capacity for leadership in the area of health promotion, including greater attention to tertiary prevention and financial independence for the elderly.
- They should mandate approved basic packages of clinical preventive services in all private health insurance sold in their jurisdictions, including that for the elderly.
- They should consider mandating prevention programs in hospital outpatient units, HMOs, community health centers, and other institutions caring for ambulatory patients.

Health Professions

- Physicians, nurses, dentists, hospitals, HMOs, and others should devote more time, attention, and resources to prevention at all three levels as health care moves inevitably toward providing more care for the elderly.
- Institutional certifying bodies should require that programs of approved clinical preventive services be implemented as a condition of certification.
- Medical, nursing, and other schools of health professions should include, as a condition of professional certification, instruction in "clinical prevention" in all areas affecting the elderly.

Insurance Industry

- Health Insurance Association of America, Blue Cross Association, Group Health Association of America, and other leadership bodies should work closely with federal and state governments in the definition of approved packages of clinical preventive services for inclusion in all health insurance policies sold to the elderly, including new long-term care products.
- Individual carriers, companies, and plans should move voluntarily to cover such packages, as well as offer financial incentives encouraging their use. They should monitor both providers and policy holders for compliance.

Employers and Labor

- The current movement toward worksite wellness programs should be encouraged and rewarded with tax incentives as a means of helping people enter their older years in a healthier state.

- Employers/labor should be required to include basic clinical preventive services in employee and retiree health insurance programs as a condition of continued tax exemption.
- Employers/labor should be encouraged to adjust retirement and pension policies to reflect flexibility of retirement age and to encourage later retirement by adjusting hours, pay scales, and working conditions to meet the needs of older workers.

Media

- The media are extremely important to health promotion and disease prevention for the elderly. More adult Americans obtain information on good health practices from television, newspapers, books, and magazines than from their physicians. The quality of this information varies from irresponsible to excellent. Examples of the latter include the American Medical Association's *Family Medical Guide* and Jane Brody's nutrition column in the *New York Times*. Even responsible reporting can sometimes result in public confusion, which is inevitable as new research findings emerge and are confirmed or altered. On balance, the media contributions to the health of the elderly have been positive.
- The current trend toward more responsible and informative reporting on new medical developments and individual health maintenance should be encouraged and guided by well-designed information programs sponsored by governmental and professional organizations engaged in such activities.

Clearly, medicine in the 1990s will be different than it is today. However, considerable controversy and uncertainty exist as to the ultimate direction many of these changes will take.

ROBERT J. BLENDON
Harvard University, 1988

10

AIDS: The Human Immunodeficiency Virus

ACQUIRED IMMUNE DEFICIENCY SYNDROME (AIDS) came to the attention of public health officials in the United States in 1981. By December of that year, some 200 cases had been identified, and many of those stricken with *Pneumocystis carinii* and other opportunistic infections that are the hallmark of AIDS had already died. The number of cases reported in the United States has increased to epidemic proportions since that time, and the disease has now been reported in more than 113 countries on six continents. In 1983, the U.S. Department of Health and Human Services declared AIDS to be the nation's "number one health priority." The disease has gained prominence in research and public policy, as the nation and the international community grapple with its implications. Although the period from diagnosis to death may be several years, or even a decade, no one is known to have recovered from AIDS.

Although treatments have been developed in recent years that improve the quality of life for some of those infected, preventing transmission of the human immunodeficiency virus (HIV) is the only known means of preventing AIDS. This can be accomplished through avoidance of behaviors likely to transmit HIV—especially unprotected anal and vaginal intercourse and sharing needles used in intravenous drug injections—and assuring the safety of the blood supply.

The crisis caused by the HIV epidemic has stimulated responses from all levels of government as well as from the private sector to develop a variety of public health, medical, social, educational, and research resources. The nature of these responses determines what prevention programs are instituted from individuals at risk of HIV infection and what range of therapies and services persons with HIV disease receive; how successful communities, states, the nation, and other countries will be in quelling the spread of HIV infection; and how much HIV will cost.

The HIV epidemic has generated the need for a broad spectrum of public health, medical, social, and educational services in communities throughout the country. The financial impact has been felt by individuals stricken with the disease, by families and friends of persons with HIV disease, by nonprofit community-based health and social service agencies in areas with a concentration of high-risk groups, by hospitals and physicians caring for persons with HIV disease, by the private and commercial insurance industry, by employers, and by every level of government.

The economic costs of HIV disease are both direct and indirect. The major component of direct costs is the cost of care of patients in and out of the hospital, including physician services, drugs, ancillary services, home health and hospice care, and nursing home care. Other expenditures related to disease reporting and surveillance are for tracking the epidemic, establishing routes of HIV transmission, and for laying the epidemiologic groundwork to develop prevention strategies. Funds for prevention are for information and education directed toward the general public, particularly sexually active adults, as well as risk reduction programs aimed at changing high-risk behaviors in special populations — sexually active homosexual and bisexual men, intravenous drug users, sexual partners of IV drug users, and adolescents who may engage in such high-risk behaviors as IV drug use — and protecting the blood supply. Direct costs of care are high if hospital and nursing home care loom large in patient treatment. Indirect costs reflect the economic loss to society, generally measured by lost wages due to sickness and early death. Indirect costs are high if illness and death occur in young people at the peak of their earning power. Both of these circumstances are characteristic of HIV infection.

In the United States 50,000 AIDS cases were reported from 1981 to 1987; another 50,000 cases from 1987 to mid-1989, and at least 50,000 more cases are projected for 1990. The number of reported AIDS cases in January 1990 was nearly 120,000, and more than half of them had died. The World Health Organization estimated, at the same time, that there were 600,000 AIDS cases worldwide, with large numbers of unreported cases. The number of those infected with the HIV virus was estimated to be 50 to 10 million worldwide and 800,000 to 1.3 million in the United States.

Although AIDS became known in the early 1980s as a disease of homosexuals, patterns of the disease are shifting, and more and more it is manifesting as a disease of the disadvantaged — of poor, inner city blacks and Hispanics. Since the early 1980s, the transmission of HIV among homosexual men in cities such as San Francisco has declined dramatically, but this has not been the case among IV drug users, where the prevalence of HIV infection has continued to increase. This is because of the many complexities related to combatting the disease among drug addicts and their sex partners. An additional tragedy is that by the end of 1989, almost 2,000 infants and children had developed AIDS, nearly 60 percent of them the offspring of IV drug users or their sex partners.

The policy issues related to AIDS loom large; primary among them is the effort to curb the spread of HIV. Issues related to treatment, needle exchange for drug addicts, HIV drug treatment availability, costs, research, and ethics also pose great challenges. In this chapter, our authors explore these issues and the growing burden of HIV in our society.

In the opening article, Philip R. Lee examines the allocation of federal resources for AIDS research and patient care. He reports that the inadequate federal response has been in large part a result of the government's efforts to reduce spending on domestic programs and to shift fiscal responsibility to states and cities and to the private sector. These circumstances are compounded by the fact that a large proportion of those who contract AIDS are poorly insured or have no insurance, and the U.S. has no national policy for financing care for such people.

Allan M. Brandt provides the important historical prospective on AIDS as a public health issue. He draws parallels to previous epidemics and also illustrates the new problems posed by AIDS, and he draws four lessons from the social history of sexually transmitted diseases in the United States and assesses their relevance for the AIDS epidemic.

Health policy analyst John K. Iglehart diagrams the federal government's response to the AIDS epidemic in the mid-1980s during the Reagan administration and the profound impact it has had on the nation's health care system. He also discusses the delicate balance that must be struck between assuring humane care and treatment for those infected by HIV and the necessity of safeguarding the rest of the population.

Health economist Anne Scitovsky has been reporting on the costs of illnesses for a number of decades, and she has been examining the economic costs of AIDS since 1984 when it first became a major influence on the consumption of health care resources in the United States. In "The Economic Impact of AIDS in the United States" she and Mary Cline review the principal studies and estimates of health care costs for persons with AIDS, and they compare these costs with those of some other diseases. They also discuss the economic impact of AIDS on hospitals.

There could be no more profligate error than to have invested so deeply in the scientific insights of recent years and then fail to use them to meet the present crisis.

JUNE E. OSBORN
University of Michigan

Philip R. Lee

AIDS: Allocating Resources for Research and Patient Care

The epidemic of Acquired Immune Deficiency Syndrome (AIDS) has posed a dramatic challenge to medical investigators, clinicians, and policymakers. The problems have ranged from identifying the causative agent and determining the risk factors important in this disease to financing care for AIDS patients. Many public policy issues arising from the AIDS epidemic have yet to be resolved. These include how best to prevent the spread of AIDS; the appropriate use of antibody testing to identify possible carriers of the disease; the closure of bathhouses and the effective use of public education programs; the civil rights of AIDS victims; and the respective roles of the federal, state, and local governments in dealing with the epidemic. Although it would be useful to address all of these issues, the purpose here is to examine those issues specifically related to the allocation of resources for research and patient care.

The U.S. AIDS epidemic broke out just as the Reagan administration was moving to adopt policies designed to reduce the role of the federal government, particularly its role in domestic social programs. Thus, the federal response to AIDS was shaped by a new set of national policy goals that called for reduced federal spending for domestic social programs; decentralization of program responsibility and the transfer of authority to state and local governments through block grants—the so-called new federalism; federal deregulation; increased competition; and a greater role for the private sector in meeting the needs of the poor. The policies adopted in the Omnibus Budget Reconciliation Act of 1981 and the Tax Equity and Fiscal Responsibility Act of 1982, as well as the recession of 1981–82, resulted in new intergovernmental relationships and conditions that were to shift the focus of concern and debate about a range of social issues, including AIDS.

The most important factor influencing the federal policy response to the AIDS epidemic was the dramatic reduction in revenues the federal government needed to fund domestic social programs. The tax reductions adopted in 1982

Philip R. Lee, M.D., is professor of social medicine and director of the Institute for Health Policy Studies, School of Medicine, University of California, San Francisco, California.

[398]

contributed significantly to the huge federal budget deficit that set the framework for broad policy decisions and that had a major impact on many government programs.

Although funding for biomedical research has not been as adversely affected as other areas of health policy, there is considerable uncertainty about the future availability of federal funds. In early October 1985 the Senate Appropriations Committee recommended $227 million for research and treatment of AIDS in fiscal year 1986, more than doubling the fiscal year 1985 appropriation. However, the Senate Budget Committee and then the full Senate adopted the so-called Gramm-Rudman amendment to eliminate the federal budget deficit by 1991. This amendment (appended to a resolution raising the federal debt ceiling) or a similar deficit-reduction measure could significantly reduce AIDS appropriations in future years and also sharply curtail funding for other domestic programs, particularly those serving the poor.

The new federalism policies have also been key in shaping the federal role in domestic social programs. Introduced in the early 1970s by President Nixon and revived by President Reagan, these policies are designed to eliminate or curtail many of the Great Society programs developed during the 1960s. For anyone closely associated with state or local government, the new federalism has meant a reduction of federal funds and the added burden of increased responsibilities for social welfare.

Federal deregulation has also had an impact—one that has been greater in some states than in others and in some program areas than in others. The effects of federal deregulation are evident in the discretion given states to reduce eligibility for a variety of social programs, to cut costs, to reduce or eliminate any direct state role in planning for health care facilities, and to relax affirmative action and civil rights requirements.

The federal government vigorously advocates greater competition and an expanded role for the private sector in health care. This has often meant greater choice in health plans for consumers, but has also meant that individuals must bear increased financial responsibility for the costs of their own medical care. In addition, encouraging participation by the private sector has meant the rapid expansion of proprietary corporations in health care, particularly in the areas of hospital care and community-based and in-home health services.

It is small wonder that within this new policy climate the leadership of the U.S. Public Health Service has found itself in an extremely difficult position when asked to respond to a new and baffling disease. While agents of the Public Health Service's Centers for Disease Control (CDC) have maintained surveillance of AIDS, and the National Cancer Institute has successfully isolated the causative retrovirus, the overall federal response has been cautious and measured.

Total appropriations for AIDS research and public education in fiscal year 1982 were only $5.5 million. In 1984 the U.S. Department of Health and Human Services designated AIDS as its number one health priority, and much of the research into the biology of AIDS was federally sponsored. At the insistence of the White House, however, the department has consistently argued that funds for AIDS activities should be transferred from other federal health programs rather than be raised by new appropriations. Furthermore, the Department of Health and Human Services has failed to give firm direction to the efforts to understand and control the disease, and it has provided no overall strategy or program to guide physicians in how best to care for AIDS patients.

The federal government's hesitant response to AIDS has been echoed by the states and local communities. With few exceptions the initial reaction of state and local authorities to AIDS has been either to ignore the epidemic or to pass the buck to some other level of government or to the private sector. In California, for example, state health officials initially left it up to local governments to respond. As a result San Francisco spent $7 million on community-based programs for AIDS victims in fiscal year 1985. The city will spend $9 million in the 1986 fiscal year. State officials are only now considering providing some state funds for AIDS antibody testing programs. In New York, support services for AIDS victims are almost entirely dependent on volunteers and private donations rather than local government services and funding.

Because of the popular view that medical research can conquer any disease, and because of the very real public health concerns about the AIDS epidemic, the initial failure of the federal government to quickly allocate new funds for AIDS research provoked sharp criticism from Congress, scientists, public health officials, and the gay community.

The Reagan administration's first budget proposals for fiscal year 1986 called for a reduction in funding for AIDS research. The Public Health Service, however, subsequently proposed to increase funding to $199 million. That the Public Health Service was able to convince the Office of Management and Budget and the White House that more AIDS research money was essential was a significant turnaround.

Support for biomedical, social science, and behavioral sciences research has long been a primary responsibility of the federal government. The private sector, including the pharmaceutical industry and private foundations, has played a significant but lesser role. State governments have not been primary supporters of health sciences research, even in states with major research universities.

Not only has the Department of Health and Human Services submitted AIDS-related funding requests lower than those requested by individual Public Health Service agencies, but it has called for reduced personnel ceilings. There has been intense competition for funding among the agencies, and members of Congress have justifiably questioned the adequacy of the resources devoted to vaccine development, research on the role of cofactors such as drug abuse on the transmissibility of AIDS, the treatment of patients, and prevention through public education.

A major portion of federal AIDS research funding has been aimed at the search for factors affecting the development of AIDS. After the discovery of the HTLV-III retrovirus as the causative agent in AIDS, the Public Health Service increased funding for cofactor research (to 14.9 percent of total AIDS resources in fiscal year 1985) and epidemiologic studies (to 26 percent). About 14.8 percent of the AIDS budget for fiscal 1985 is for research on treatment, and about 2.1 percent is for research on psychosocial factors related to AIDS, such as stress, depression, and the loss of social support. No federal funds are available for the treatment of AIDS patients except those at the Clinical Center of the National Institutes of Health (NIH).

Although research efforts directed toward treatment of AIDS and the accompanying opportunistic infections are urgently required, the federal government has given this area inadequate support and relatively low priority. The problems are exceedingly complex, and it is now clear that drugs need to be developed that are effective against a retrovirus that both destroys the body's immune system and infects the brain.

Development of new therapeutic drugs to treat AIDS has been delayed by a lack of funding for the laboratories required to culture the AIDS virus used to develop the drugs tested in those trials and by a shortage of funds for computer-based information systems to manage the trials efficiently. Funding is needed to create interdisciplinary research teams to conduct large-scale clinical trials, including the development of common protocols and data systems, supervision of clinical investigators in multiple sites, and prompt data analysis.

Several major questions need to be addressed with respect to research policies. The first of these is the establishment of appropriate goals for the continuing effort to cope with the AIDS epidemic. At a minimum these goals should include the development of accurate tests to determine if a person is infected with the AIDS virus; vaccines; specific therapeutic agents for the treatment of AIDS; and finally, other effective preventive measures, particularly in the social and behavioral sciences area.

The second major policy question is the appropriate level of federal funding in the face of other competing demands. In the early years of the AIDS epidemic (1982–83), the Centers for Disease Control supported AIDS activities by shifting funds and personnel from surveillance of hepatitis, studies of influenza, and studies of chlamydial infections and pelvic inflammatory diseases. The same was true of the Food and Drug Administration, where staff and funds were redirected from work on various other viruses, the improvement of pertussis vaccines, and hepatitis vaccine research. A third policy question is the optimum distribution of limited research dollars for basic research related to causative agents, cofactors, and disease mechanisms; for research related to vaccine development; for epidemiologic studies of risk-factors and the natural history of AIDS; for clinical trials; and for social and behavioral science studies.

A fourth policy question is the appropriate level of funding for intramural and extramural research, and how best to expedite the review of AIDS research proposals without undermining the normal processes of scientific review and peer review. Initially, most federally funded AIDS research was intramural — being carried out within NIH and CDC. Little was extramural — that is, made available for university-based research or other investigators outside the federal government. Also, the use of the standard NIH peer review process meant that the review, approval, and funding of a research proposal often took a full year — hardly an appropriate response in view of the lethal and fast-growing nature of the epidemic.

A fifth policy question is the issue of what is the best mechanism within NIH to oversee drug screening and to expedite the clinical testing of new drugs. Certainly, a committee with members from NIH and the Food and Drug Administration, as well as extramural scientists, could play a critically important role in hastening the development of effective therapeutics. An NIH drug information clearinghouse to maintain up-to-date information on drugs currently being tested is also needed. Such a clearinghouse will become increasingly important as more investigators become involved, more patients are treated, and more drugs are studied.

NIH, CDC, and other segments of the Public Health Service should consider other steps to facilitate the kind of international cooperation and collaboration among basic scientists, clinical investigators, epidemiologists, and social and behavioral scientists that is so essential in dealing with a worldwide epidemic. New policies that would give the Public Health Service more discretion in funding research outside the United States could help foster truly collaborative research with foreign investigators.

The private sector has made important contributions in the fight against AIDS. One example is the rapid development of test kits for the detection of HTLV-III antibodies and the use of these tests to screen and thereby protect the safety of the nation's blood supply. However, certain policy areas related to the role of the private sector require study. For example, commercial development of AIDS-related technologies (for example, the antibody test) or antiviral drugs in the private sector, including technologies derived from federally funded or conducted biomedical research, are considered proprietary by the Food and Drug Administration and cannot be made public unless voluntarily released by the companies involved. Thus, important information about clinical investigations of new drugs is not always disseminated promptly to researchers outside of industry.

Urgent attention must be devoted to finding adequate resources for the care of the growing number of AIDS patients. The failure of the Reagan administration and Congress to examine openly and explicitly this financial issue is related to the lack of national health insurance and the lack of any coherent national policy for financing health care. Health care financing today is a hodgepodge of third-party coverage (Medicare, Medicaid, employer-provided nonprofit and commercial health insurance), self-insurance by employees, and out-of-pocket payments by individuals.

AIDS patients with little or no health insurance are quickly impoverished by the catastrophic medical costs. They do not qualify for government programs until they have exhausted enough of their own resources to meet the income or asset requirements for Medicaid or local government services. In contrast, every other western industrialized country has funding mechanisms to assist patients with AIDS or other serious health problems requiring medical care and social services.

Although AIDS poses special challenges for biomedical, behavioral, and social science researchers, the financing of medical care for AIDS patients poses no unique or special problems. The problems are shared by a growing number of Americans who are either uninsured or underinsured—anywhere from 30 to 50 million people. It is small wonder that federal policymakers have chosen not to take on the burden of 14,000 AIDS patients—some of whom have little or no health insurance—when there are at least 30 million people who are also unable to pay for health care.

What the policymakers may define as a problem of the uninsured or underinsured, the individual defines as a problem of catastrophic costs leading to bankruptcy, and it can be catastrophic whether a person has AIDS, cancer, or injuries from an auto accident. Hospitals and other health care providers define this as a problem of uncompensated care. However it is defined, financing health care is an issue that federal policymakers have chosen to ignore as they have focused instead on cost containment in health care delivery.

As the burden of financing health care for the poor has shifted increasingly to the states in recent years, the state governments have introduced various methods to contain costs while continuing to ensure access to an adequate level of care. The four states with the largest number of AIDS cases—New York, Florida, California, and New Jersey—have taken quite different approaches. New York, for example, has established special revenue pools to reimburse hospitals in financial trouble because of charity cases and bad debts. Florida has expanded its Medicaid program to assist uninsured or underinsured patients, and also created a pool to reimburse hospitals carrying a heavy burden of indigent patients. California, on the other hand, has reduced access to services for nonemergency care, particularly elective surgery, and transferred the state-funded program for medically indigent adults to the counties. These policies were adopted prior to a general awareness of the dimensions of the AIDS epidemic.

Many other states have begun to reexamine the issues related to financing health care for the poor, the uninsured, and the underinsured. The states now vary widely in access to care, the scope of services available, and the degree of cost sharing required of sick patients when they seek or receive health care. For these reasons, access to care for AIDS patients varies from state to state, from community to community, and, in some cases, from patient to patient.

The bill for the treatment of victims of the AIDS epidemic is rising steadily. Despite dramatic research findings into the causative factor in AIDS in the last four years, the AIDS epidemic is not going away. Furthermore, the epidemic is spreading geographically. From the initial major outbreaks in New York, San Francisco, Newark, Miami, and Los Angeles, AIDS has spread to 47 states, the District of Columbia, Puerto Rico, and the Virgin Islands. There is little doubt that AIDS is a national problem in terms of patient care and the allocation of resources for patient care, and the federal government should recognize it as such.

As with access to care, the financial resources for treatment of AIDS vary from state to state, from community to community, and from patient to patient. In California, private health insurance, including group-practice pre-payment plans, have been very important in paying for the care of AIDS patients. In addition, Kaiser Permanente provides a significant percentage of coverage for AIDS patients who have health insurance. As a result a large number of AIDS victims are treated in Kaiser hospitals in northern and southern California, as well as in community hospitals. Medicaid is also critically important for those AIDS patients who are uninsured or who lose their health insurance after they become ill. In New York, Blue Cross, which is the dominant third-party insurer, plays the most important role, but Medicaid also is important.

Many AIDS victims have lost their jobs and perhaps their health insurance, and have faced social isolation and catastrophic medical expenses. AIDS patients who have inadequate health insurance or lose their coverage because of losing their jobs must turn to charity or apply for supplemental security income as disabled persons under Social Security. A diagnosis of AIDS is a presumptive qualification for eligibility for supplemental security income, and this in turn qualifies a person for Medicaid. However, state Medicaid offices often refuse to pay hospital costs for AIDS patients who are being treated with experimental drugs. A national policy is urgently needed to ensure that AIDS patients receiving experimental drug treatment are not denied coverage by Medicaid.

Unless suffering from the most acute aspects of the disease, the great majority of AIDS patients are ambulatory. Probably less than one-third, however, are employed. Many require intensive medical care, both inpatient and outpatient, as well as psychological and social support. New York City, Newark, Jersey City, and Miami face an additional problem in that many of their AIDS patients are also suffering from heroin addiction, thereby compounding the difficulty of providing needed medical, social, and other support services.

The AIDS epidemic raises serious questions for policymakers about the appropriate mix of services (inpatient, outpatient, home care, hospice, etc.) to ensure adequate care while also controlling costs. Estimates of the average direct lifetime cost of caring for an AIDS patient range from $21,000 to $140,000. Preliminary findings from a study in San Francisco indicate that the lifetime in-hospital treatment costs for an AIDS patient in that city are between

$25,000 and $32,000. The costs of in-hospital care for AIDS patients in San Francisco are well below those in most cities because fewer AIDS patients present the costly problem of drug addiction and because the comprehensive range of ambulatory and in-home services makes hospital stays shorter. At San Francisco General Hospital the average length of stay has been 11.5 days, while in Los Angeles it has averaged 17 days, and in New York City it has been 25 days or more.

The AIDS epidemic has sharply delineated the current policy issues in both health services delivery and health care financing. In the face of federal strategies of decentralization, deregulation, and competition in health care, the major question for those concerned with the care of AIDS patients is the adequacy of the resources at the state and local levels.

The failure of the federal government to meet its responsibilities in providing for an equitable system of health care financing does not eliminate the high costs of health care. Rather, it simply shifts those costs to other levels of government or to the private sector and to the individual citizen. If the AIDS epidemic does nothing else, it must underscore the urgent need for an adequate and just system of national health insurance.

Although the problem of finding resources for the treatment of AIDS patients remains unresolved, funding for research now appears adequate, assuming that the money appropriated by Congress is finally distributed and spent. A number of research policy questions, however, require attention. Federal health officials must provide strong leadership in setting specific goals for the AIDS research effort and determining how research funds should be distributed. They should give the highest priority to clinical trials of antiviral drugs, particularly those that are effective against a virus that infects the brain, to studies related to cofactors, such as other infections, and to behavioral and social sciences research related to prevention strategies.

In the health care area, federal officials should give the highest priority to the development of nonhospital services such as hospice care, in-home services, psychological counseling, social services, and other office- or clinic-based physician and nursing services. In addition, they should concentrate on community education programs and other measures designed to reduce the risk of AIDS and to slow its spread.

The lethality of AIDS has been its most impressive and dismaying feature.

AMERICAN COLLEGE OF PHYSICIANS

Allan M. Brandt

AIDS in Historical Perspective: Four Lessons from the History of Sexually Transmitted Diseases

INTRODUCTION

It has become abundantly clear in the first six years of the AIDS (acquired immunodeficiency syndrome) epidemic that there will be no simple answer to this health crisis. The obstacles to establishing effective public health policies are considerable. AIDS is a new disease with a unique set of public health problems. The medical, social, and political aspects of the disease present American society and the world community with an awesome task.

The United States has relatively little recent experience dealing with health crises. Since the introduction of antibiotics during World War II, health priorities shifted to chronic, systemic diseases. We had come to believe that the problem of infectious, epidemic disease had passed—a topic of concern only to the developing world and historians.

In this respect, it is not surprising that in these first years of the epidemic there has been a desire to look for historical models as a means of dealing with the AIDS epidemic. Many have pointed to past and contemporary public health approaches to sexually transmitted diseases (STDs) as important precedents for the fight against AIDS. And indeed, there are significant similarities between AIDS and other sexually transmitted infections which go beyond the mere fact of sexual transmission. Syphilis, for example, also may have severe pathological effects. In the first half of the twentieth century, it was both greatly feared and highly stigmatized. In light of these analogues, the social history of efforts to control syphilis and other STDs may serve to inform our assessments of the current epidemic.

But history holds no simple truths. AIDS is not syphilis; our responses to the current epidemic will be shaped by contemporary science, politics, and culture. Yet the history of disease does offer an important set of perspectives on current proposals and strategies. Moreover, history points to the range of variables that will need to be addressed if we are to create effective and just policies.

Allan M. Brandt, Ph.D., is associate professor of history, medicine and science at Harvard Medical School, Boston, Massachusetts.

In these early years of the AIDS epidemic, there has been a tendency to use analogy as a means of devising policy. It makes sense to draw upon past policies and institutional arrangements to address the problems posed by the current crisis. But we need to be sophisticated in drawing analogues; to recognize not only how AIDS is like past epidemics, but the precise ways in which it is different. This article draws four "lessons" from the social history of sexually transmitted disease in the United States and assesses their relevance for the current epidemic.

LESSON #1. Fear of disease will powerfully influence medical approaches and public health policy.

The last years of the nineteenth century and first of the twentieth witnessed considerable fear of sexually transmitted infection, not unlike that which we are experiencing today. A series of important discoveries about the pathology of syphilis and gonorrhea had revealed a range of alarming pathological consequences from debility, insanity, and paralysis, to sterility and blindness. In this age of antibiotics, it is easy to forget the fear and dread that syphilis invoked in the past.

Theories of casual transmission reflected deep cultural fears about disease and sexuality in the early twentieth century. In these approaches to venereal disease, concerns about hygiene, contamination, and contagion were expressed, anxieties that reflected a great deal about the contemporary society and culture. Venereal disease was viewed as a threat to the entire late Victorian social and sexual system, which placed great value on discipline, restraint, and homogeneity. The sexual code of that era held that sex would receive social sanction only in marriage. But the concerns about venereal disease and casual transmission also reflected a pervasive fear of the urban masses, the growth of the cities, and the changing nature of familial relationships.

Today, persistent fears about casual transmission of AIDS reflect a somewhat different, yet no less significant, social configuration. First, AIDS is strongly associated with behaviors which have been traditionally considered deviant. This is true for both homosexuality and intravenous drug use. After a generation of growing social tolerance for homosexuality, the epidemic has generated new fears and heightened old hostilities. Just as syphilis created a disease-oriented xenophobia in the early twentieth century, AIDS has today generated a new homophobia. AIDS has recast anxiety about contamination in a new light. Among certain social critics, AIDS is seen as "proof" of a certain moral order.

Second, fears are fanned because we live in an era in which the authority of scientific expertise has eroded. This may well be an aspect of a broader decline in the legitimacy of social institutions, but it is clearly seen in the areas of science and medicine. Despite significant evidence that HIV (human immunodeficiency virus) is not casually transmitted, medical and public health experts have been unable to provide the categorical reassurances that the public would like. But without such guarantees, public fear has remained high.

Third, as a culture, we Americans are relatively unsophisticated in our assessments of relative risk. How are we to evaluate the risks of AIDS? How shall social policy be constructed around what are small or unknown risks? The ostracism of HIV-infected children from their schools in certain locales, the refusal of some physicians to treat AIDS patients, job and housing discrimination against those infected (and those suspected of being infected) all reveal the pervasive fears surrounding the epidemic. Clearly, then, one public health goal must be to address these fears. Addressing such fears means understanding their etiology. They originate in the particular social meaning of AIDS — its "social construction." We will not be able to effectively mitigate these concerns until we understand their deeper meaning. The response to AIDS will be fundamentally shaped by these fears; therefore, we need to develop techniques to assist individuals to distinguish irrational fears of AIDS from realistic and legitimate concerns. In this respect, many have focused on the need for more education.

LESSON #2. Education will *not* control the AIDS epidemic.

Early in the twentieth century, physicians, public health officials, and social reformers concerned about the problem of syphilis and gonorrhea called for a major educational campaign. They cogently argued that the tide of infection could not be stemmed until the public had adequate knowledge about these diseases, their mode of transmission, and the means of prevention. They called for an end to "the conspiracy of silence" — the Victorian code of sexual ethics — that considered all discussion of sexuality and disease in respectable society inappropriate. Physicians had contributed to this state of affairs by hiding diagnoses from their patients and families, and upholding what came to be known as the "medical secret."

Educational efforts may have actually contributed to the pervasive fears of infection, to the stigma associated with the diseases, and to the discrimination against its victims. Indeed, educational materials produced throughout the first decades of the twentieth century emphasized the inherent dangers of all sexual activity, especially disease and unwanted pregnancy. In this respect, such educational programs, rather than being termed sex education were actually anti-sex education. Pamphlets and films repeatedly emphasized the "loathsome" and disfiguring aspects of sexually transmitted disease; the most drastic pathological consequences (insanity, paralysis, blindness, and death); as well as the disastrous impact on personal relations.

There are, nonetheless, some precedents for successful educational campaigns. During World War II, the military initiated a massive educational campaign against sexually transmitted disease. But unlike prior efforts, it reminded soldiers that disease could be prevented through the use of condoms, which were widely distributed. The military program recognized that sexual behaviors could be modified, but that calls for outright abstinence were likely to fail. Given the need for an efficient and healthy army, officials maintained a pragmatic posture that separated morals from the essential task of prevention. As one medical officer explained, "It is difficult to make the sex act unpopular."

Today, calls for better education are frequently offered as the best hope for controlling the AIDS epidemic. But this will only be true if some resolution is reached concerning the specific content and nature of such educational efforts. The limited effectiveness of education which merely encourages fear is well-documented. Moreover, AIDS education requires a forthright confrontation of aspects of human sexuality that are typically avoided. To be effective, AIDS education must be explicit, focused, and appropriately targeted to a range of at-risk social groups. As the history of sexually transmitted diseases makes clear, we need to study the nature of behavior and disease. If education is to have a positive impact, we need to be far more sophisticated, creative, and bold in devising and implementing programs.

Education is not a panacea for the AIDS epidemic, just as education did not solve the problem of other sexually transmitted diseases earlier in the twentieth century. It is one critical aspect of a fully articulated program. As this historical vignette makes clear, we need to be far more explicit about what we mean when we say "education." Certainly education about AIDS is an important element of any public health approach to the crisis, but we need to substantively evaluate a range of educational programs and their impact on behavior for populations with a variety of needs.

Because the impact of education is unclear and the dangers of the epidemic are perceived as great (see lesson #1), there has been considerable interest in compulsory public health measures as a primary means of controlling AIDS.

LESSON #3. Compulsory public health measures will *not* control the epidemic.

Given the considerable fear that the epidemic has generated and its obvious dangers, demands have been voiced for the implementation of compulsory public health interventions. The history of efforts to control syphilis during the twentieth century indicates the limits of compulsory measures which range from required premarital testing to quarantine of infected individuals.

Next to programs for compulsory vaccination, compulsory programs for premarital syphilis serologies are probably the most widely known of all compulsory public health measures in the twentieth-century United States. The development of effective laboratory diagnostic measures stands as a signal contribution in the history of the control of sexually transmitted diseases. With the development of the Wassermann test in 1906, there was a generally reliable way of detecting the presence of syphilis. The achievement of such a test offered a new series of public health potentials. No longer would diagnosis depend on strictly clinical criteria. Diagnosis among the asymptomatic was now possible, as was the ability to test the effectiveness of treatments. The availability of the test led to the development of programs for compulsory testing.

Significantly, calls for compulsory screening for syphilis predated the Wassermann exam. Beginning in the last years of the nineteenth century, several states began to mandate premarital medical examinations to assure that sexually transmitted infections were not communicated in marriage. But without a definitive test, such examinations were of limited use. With a laboratory test, however, calls were voiced for requiring premarital blood tests.

Legislation is currently pending in 35 state legislatures that would require premarital HIV serologies. The rationale for such programs is often the historical precedent of syphilis screening. The logic seems intuitively correct: We screen for syphilis. AIDS is a far more serious disease; we should therefore screen for AIDS. In this respect it is worth reviewing the effectiveness of premarital syphilis screening as well as those factors that distinguish syphilis from AIDS.

Mandatory premarital serologies never proved to be a particularly effective mechanism for finding new cases of syphilis. First, physicians and public health officials recognized that there was a significant rate of false positive tests which occurred because of technical inadequacies of the tests themselves or as a result of biological phenomena (such as other infections).

As many physicians pointed out, a positive serology did not always mean that an individual could transmit the disease. Because the tests tended to be mandated for a population at relatively low risk of infection, their accuracy was further compromised. Some individuals reportedly avoided the test altogether.

Many of the difficulties associated with the high numbers of false positives were alleviated as new, more specific tests were developed in the 1940s and 1950s, but the central problem remained. Premarital syphilis serologies failed to identify a significant percentage of the infected population. In 1978, for example, premarital screening accounted for only 1.27 per cent of all national tests found to be positive for syphilis. The costs of these programs were estimated at $80 million annually. Another study in California projected costs per case found through premarital screening to be $240,000.

Compulsory premarital syphilis serologies thus offer a dubious precedent for required HIV screening. The point, of course, is *not* that the test is inaccurate. ELISA (enzyme-linked immunosorbent assay) testing coupled with the Western blot *can be* quite reliable, but only when applied to populations which are likely to have been infected. Screening of low-prevalence populations, like premarital couples, is unlikely to have any significant impact on the course of the epidemic. Not only will such programs find relatively few new cases, they will also reveal large numbers of false positives. A recent study concluded that a national mandatory premarital screening program would find approximately 1,200 new cases of HIV infection, one-tenth of 1 per cent of those currently infected. But it would also incorrectly identify as many as 380 individuals — actually free of infection — as infected, even with supplementary Western blot tests. Such a program would also falsely reassure as many as 120 individuals with false negative results. Moreover, the inability to treat and render non-infectious those individuals who are found to be infected severely limits the potential benefits of such mandatory measures. With syphilis serologies, the rationale of the program was to treat infected individuals.

This, of course, is *not* to argue that testing has no role in an effective AIDS public health campaign. During the late 1930s, a massive voluntary testing campaign heightened consciousness of syphilis in Chicago, bringing thousands of new cases into treatment. AIDS testing, conducted voluntarily and confidentially, targeted to individuals who have specific risk factors for infection, may have significant public health benefits. Compulsory screening, however, could merely discourage infected individuals from being tested. This makes clear the need to enact legislation guaranteeing the confidentiality of those who volunteer to be tested and prohibiting discrimination against HIV-infected individuals.

As a mandatory measure, premarital screening is a relatively modest proposal. During the course of the twentieth century, more radical and intrusive compulsory measures to control STDs, such as quarantine, have also been attempted. These, too, have failed. During World War I, as hysteria about the impact of STDs rose, Congress passed legislation to support the quarantine of prostitutes suspected of spreading disease. The Act held that anyone suspected of harboring a venereal infection could be detained and incarcerated until determined to be non-infectious. During the course of the War, more than 20,000 women were held in camps because they were suspected of being "spreaders" of venereal disease.

The program had no apparent impact on rates of infection, which actually climbed substantially during the War. In sexually transmitted infections, the reservoir of infection is relatively high, modes of transmission are specific, and infected individuals may be healthy. In the case of AIDS, where there is no medical intervention to render individuals non-infectious, quarantine is totally impractical because it would require life-long incarceration of the infected.

Compulsory measures often generate critics because such policies may infringe on basic civil liberties. From an ethical and legal viewpoint, the first question that must be asked about any potential policy intervention is: Is it likely to work? Only if there is clear evidence to suggest the program would be effective does it make sense to evaluate the civil liberties implications. Then it is possible to evaluate the constitutional question: Is the public health benefit to be derived worthy of the possible costs in civil liberties? Is the proposed compulsory program the least restrictive of the range of potential measures available to achieve the public good?

In this respect, it is worth noting that compulsory measures may actually be counterproductive. First, they require substantial resources that could be more effectively allocated. Second, they have often had the effect of driving the very individuals that the program hopes to reach farther away from public health institutions. Ineffective draconian measures would serve only to augment the AIDS crisis. Nevertheless, despite the fact that such programs offer no benefits, they may have substantial political and cultural appeal (see lesson #1).

Because compulsory measures are controversial and unlikely to control the epidemic, there is considerable hope that we will soon have a "magic bullet" — a biomedical "fix" to free us of the hazards of AIDS.

LESSON #4. The development of effective treatments and vaccines will *not* immediately or easily end the AIDS epidemic.

As the history of efforts to control other sexually transmitted diseases makes clear, effective treatment has not always led to control. In 1909, German Nobel laureate Paul Ehrlich discovered Salvarsan (arsphenamine), an arsenic compound which killed the spirochete, the organism which causes syphilis. Salvarsan was the first effective chemotherapeutic agent for a specific disease. Ehrlich called Salvarsan a "magic bullet," a drug which would seek out and destroy its mark. He claimed that modern medicine would seek the discovery of a series of such drugs to eliminate the microorganisms which cause disease. Although Salvarsan was an effective treatment, it was toxic and difficult to administer. Patients required a painful regimen of injections, sometimes for as long as two years.

Unlike the arsphenamines, penicillin was truly a wonder drug. In early 1943, Dr. John S. Mahoney of the U.S. Public Health Service found that penicillin was effective in treating rabbits infected with syphilis. After repeating his experiments with human subjects, his findings were announced and the massive production of penicillin began.

With a single shot, the scourge of syphilis could be avoided. Incidence fell from a high of 72 cases per 100,000 in 1943 to about 4 per 100,000 in 1956. As rates reached all-time lows, it appeared that venereal diseases would join the ranks of other infectious diseases that had come under the control of modern medicine.

Although there is no question that the nature and meaning of syphilis and gonorrhea underwent a fundamental change with the introduction of antibiotic therapy, the decline of venereal diseases proved short-lived. Rates of infection began to climb in the early 1960s. By the late 1950s much of the machinery, especially procedures for public education, case-finding, tracing and diagnosis had been severely reduced.

In 1987, the Centers for Disease Control (CDC) reported an increase in cases of primary and secondary syphilis. The estimated annual rate per 100,000 population rose from 10.9 to 13.3 cases, the largest increases in 10 years. These figures are particularly striking in that they come in the midst of the AIDS epidemic, which many have assumed has led to a substantial decline in sexual encounters. Moreover, after an eight-year decline, rates of congenital syphilis have also reportedly risen since 1983. The CDC concluded that individuals with a history of sexually transmitted infection are at increased risk for infection with the AIDS virus.

Despite the effectiveness of penicillin as a cure for syphilis, the disease has persisted. The issue, therefore, is not merely the development of effective treatments but the *process* by which they are deployed; the means by which they move from laboratory to full allocation to those affected. Effective treatments without adequate education, counseling, and funding may not reach those who most need them. Even "magic bullets" need to be effectively delivered. Obviously effective treatments should be a priority in a multifaceted approach to AIDS and will ultimately be an important component in its control; but even a magic bullet will not quickly or completely solve the problem.

No doubt, new and more effective treatments for AIDS will be developed in the years ahead, but their deployment will raise a series of complex issues ranging from human subject research to actual allocation. And while effective treatments may help to control further infection, as they do for syphilis and gonorrhea, treatments which prolong the life of AIDS patients may have little or no impact on the rates of transmission of the virus, which occurs principally among individuals who have no symptoms of disease.

This suggests certain fundamental flaws in the biomedical model of disease. Diseases are complex bio-ecological problems that may be mitigated only by addressing a range of scientific, social, and political considerations. Nosingle intervention—even an effective vaccine—will adequately address the complexities of the AIDS epidemic.

CONCLUSIONS

As these historical lessons make clear, in the context of fear surrounding the epidemic (lesson #1), the principal proposals for eradicating AIDS (lessons #2–4) are unlikely to be effective, at least in the immediate future. These lessons should not imply, however, that nothing will work; they make evident that no single avenue is likely to lead to success. Moreover, they suggest that in considering any intervention we will require sophisticated research to understand its potential impact on the epidemic. While education, testing, and biomedical research all offer some hope, in each instance we will need to fully consider their particular effectiveness as measures to control disease.

Simple answers based upon historical precedents are unlikely to alleviate the AIDS crisis. History does, however, point to a range of variables which influence disease, and those factors which require attention if it is to be effectively addressed. Any successful approach to the epidemic will require a full recognition of the important social, cultural, and biological aspects of AIDS. A public health priority will be to lead in the process of discerning those programs likely to have a beneficial impact from those with considerable political and cultural appeal, but unlikely to positively affect the course of the epidemic. Only in this way will we be able to devise effective and humane public policies.

Although we are confronted by a public health problem of potentially catastrophic dimensions, it is essential to appreciate that unwarranted fears of HIV transmission have compounded the suffering of young men, women, and children infected with HIV and have blunted an appropriate societal response aimed at reduction of transmission.

GERALD H. FRIEDLAND and ROBERT S. KLEIN
Albert Einstein College of Medicine

John K. Iglehart

Financing the Struggle Against AIDS

The federal government, propelled by the first widely publicized indications of serious presidential and congressional concern over the spread of the acquired immunodeficiency syndrome (AIDS), is moving rapidly to increase the resources it allocates to fighting the disease. But it has only begun to address how the war on AIDS will be waged, who will command it, and how government and the private sector will finance it.

These difficult questions lie ahead for the federal government as it steps up the drive against AIDS, an infectious disease that has spread throughout most parts of the world but whose current victims live predominantly in the United States. As of June 1 (1987), 113 countries had reported 51,535 cases of AIDS to the World Health Organization (WHO). On that same date, the Centers for Disease Control (CDC) said that 36,058 of that total had been reported by the United States and that the number is doubling every 12 to 15 months. Of the U.S. patients, 20,849 had died.

The first cases of AIDS were identified in 1981. Since that time, federal spending for biomedical research, public health measures, and patient care has risen from $5.5 million to an estimated current level of $416 million in fiscal 1987 at the Department of Health and Human Services (DHHS) alone. During this period, the way the DHHS arrives at decisions related to AIDS has also evolved, and it remains in flux.

Although the agency has said that combating the disease is its most important health-related activity, Secretary Otis R. Bowen has remained in the background with respect to the department's AIDS policies, preferring to let the Public Health Service take the lead. The uncertain nature of AIDS decision making at the DHHS stems in part from sharp ideological conflicts between public health professionals and the administration's more conservative political appointees, both within the agency and throughout the executive branch.

In this report, I will cover issues relating to the financing of medical care for patients with AIDS, noting that more of the burden will fall on state Medicaid programs and public hospitals, which provide most of the inpatient services for

John K. Iglehart, is editor of *Health Affairs*, Project HOPE, Millwood, Virginia.

patients with the disease. I will begin by noting the evolutionary manner in which the United States has recognized AIDS—an approach characteristic of the way it addresses most new major problems.

As a nation committed to limited government, the United States has a particular style of moving to recognize a new problem. In the case of AIDS, the process—one of growing concern—has developed gradually over the past five years, not only because of the pluralism of American society but because the problem presented itself most forcefully among groups (principally homosexuals and intravenous drug users) whose plight attracted less attention from most policy makers than if the disease had initially struck the heterosexual middle class. But the rising number of cases of AIDS and its gradual spread to the heterosexual population, the absence of a cure or effective treatment, and the financial strain it is placing on the health care delivery system have accelerated the concern of governments (and obviously many private interests as well) at every level.

Reflections of this growing social concern abound. But for most Americans, the most important signal that a problem has become a national priority comes when a president speaks out on that problem in a highly, visible fashion. President Reagan sent such a signal on May 31, 1987, when he expressed his concern about AIDS at a fund-raising dinner sponsored by the American Foundation for AIDS Research. The problem has achieved presidential importance in other respects, as well. Every major entrant in the 1988 contest for the White House addressed the subject of AIDS in one way or another.

Another important recent development has been more rapid congressional and executive action in appropriating more money for the fight against AIDS. In all likelihood, the DHHS will spend $1 billion for AIDS-related activities in fiscal 1987, divided among biomedical research, public health measures, and payment for medical services, mostly through Medicaid. And now federal officials are estimating that AIDS-related government spending will rise to $10 to $15 billion by 1991.

Although conflicting philosophies produce disagreement between political factions over the issue of testing people for antibodies to the AIDS virus and the design of an educational campaign, there is little disagreement among policy makers of whatever stripe that resources must be increased substantially to mount an effective fight against the disease. In recent months, action in that direction has been taken in supplemental budget exercises whose message, in essence, is that the need for additional support is too great to await the normal appropriating processes. Indeed, Congress appears ready to begin throwing money at the problem, with hopes, but no guarantees, that it will be well spent.

Increasingly, AIDS is penetrating the consciousness of every medical care provider and hospital, as its profound consequences to the health care system become more apparent to a broader cross section of America. Although AIDS will remain a serious and growing problem in the cities where it is now concentrated, it is outside New York City, San Francisco, Los Angeles, Miami, and Houston that the greatest increases are projected by the CDC. The number of cases outside New York City and San Francisco is predicted to increase sevenfold, from 17,094 to 116,290 by 1991.

The organizations representing physicians, dentists, nurses, and allied health professionals that were not attending fully to the implications of AIDS before May 20, 1987, were compelled to do so then, because on that day the CDC announced that three health care workers had contracted the disease after being exposed to blood from infected patients. The issue has become a matter of serious concern among medical residents at the large teaching hospitals, because they provide much of the care to AIDS patients. At the Johns Hopkins Hospital, for example, a former resident has sued the institution, claiming he was infected with the AIDS virus when he cut his finger on a tube of a patient's blood. Dr. Hacib Aoun, a 32-year-old cardiologist, charged that hospital officials spread rumors that he must have been infected through sex or drug abuse, obscured test results, and broke a promise to provide income and death benefits to his wife and daughter.

While the national response to AIDS has demonstrated the diversity of reaction to a new health crisis, it has also underscored the weaknesses of a system of combined private and public medical care financing that requires patients with AIDS to become impoverished before they are eligible for Medicaid and leaves many more people at risk financially, because when they become too sick to work, they lose their jobs and health insurance coverage. And of course, there are many more people who are vulnerable because they neither fit Medicaid's arbitrary definitions nor work for employers who offer insurance to their employees.

Finally, although expressions of public and private concern about AIDS have been increasing, there will inevitably be increased conflict over issues of resource allocation. If the federal government and private organizations increase spending for AIDS, that money will obviously not be available for other, perhaps equally worthy, purposes.

Estimates of the costs associated with AIDS vary widely. Reports of hospital costs over the lifetime of a patient with AIDS range from a low of $24,517 to $147,000. Studies that seek to determine how care is financed also range widely in their estimates. Studies have estimated that Medicaid pays for the care of from 12 to 65 percent of patients with AIDS, depending on the type of hospital and scope of benefits. Medicare has covered the expenses of from 1 to 3 percent of patients. The figures are low, because patients with AIDS do not become eligible for coverage until they have survived a 24-month waiting period required of persons under 65 to qualify for disability payments and Medicare. Commercial insurers and Blue Cross and Blue Shield plans have covered 13 to 65 percent of patients. Economist Jane Sisk of the Office of Technology Assessment recently completed a useful review of all the recognized studies that have estimated the cost of AIDS.

There is no question that financing AIDS-related care will become a more prominent issue, because private health insurers are striving to tighten the restrictions on whom they will cover, leaving more of the burden to the federal-state Medicaid program and other public programs.

Approximately half of all insurance companies use AIDS-antibody tests for individual health and life policies. Employed persons who are insured under a group policy (some 85 percent of all people with private health insurance who are not elderly) are not subject to an AIDS-antibody test in order to be eligible for coverage. But persons who contract AIDS eventually become too sick to work, and thus lose not only their jobs but their employment-related health insurance as well. Most states still permit insurance carriers to employ the AIDS-antibody tests to assess the health status of applicants for individual policies, but their use has been barred in California and the District of Columbia. The New York State Department of Insurance is considering a proposed regulation, supported by Governor Mario Cuomo, that would prohibit blood tests for the AIDS virus for health insurance. However, the department has no plans to prohibit the same tests for life insurance.

The extent of Medicaid coverage for inpatient care and other medical services needed by patients with AIDS varies widely according to geographic region, a recent survey conducted by the National Association of Public Hospitals found. Nationally, 43 public hospitals that responded to the survey reported the following payment sources for the medical care of patients with AIDS: Medicaid, 61.8 percent; payment by the patient and "other," 25.2 percent; private insurance, 7.7 percent; and government support for prisoners, 4.1 percent. When these figures were broken down regionally, though, the importance of Medicaid as a payment source ranged from a high of 68.8 percent in the Northeast to 16.4 percent in the South. The category of payment by the patient and "other" constituted 73.6 percent of the payments received by 15 public hospitals in the South that reported treating 1,113 patients with AIDS.

The DHHS has been dealing with such issues on an incremental basis. The administration has encouraged states to provide AZT to patients who become eligible for Medicaid coverage, but it has resisted efforts by Waxman and other legislators to extend federal payment for the drug to other persons with the disease. It is quite likely that Congress will authorize such federal payments for AZT, but this will become a more difficult policy question as other palliative drugs become available.

The CDC favors such testing, but on a largely voluntary basis. Ironically, top officials in an administration whose President has long held the view that states should be preeminent in a federal system are now leaning on those very jurisdictions to carry out policies that reflect their strong personal beliefs in the efficacy of mandatory testing.

However, the administration position on testing articulated by President Reagan on May 31 represented a carefully worded compromise between the factions within his administration battling over whether or not testing should be mandatory. Reagan called for mandatory testing of federal prisoners and said that he had approved the addition of the AIDS virus to the list of contagious diseases for which immigrants and aliens can be denied entry. Reagan also urged that states conduct "routine" testing of couples applying for marriage licenses, people who visit venereal-disease clinics and drug-abuse clinics, and persons imprisoned in state and local facilities.

Reagan's policy was based on CDC recommendations that were embraced by his Domestic Policy Council on May 28, 1987, but its meaning was clouded because many did not recognize that people could refuse to take what Reagan characterized as routine tests. The Domestic Policy Council has become the battleground on which administration officials struggle over the AIDS issues that divide them.

Meanwhile, the DHHS is in the process of studying ways to improve its own decision-making structure. One change that seems inevitable is the establishment of the position of Public Health Service AIDS coordinator as a permanent rather than a rotating assignment held for only one year. The issue of whether there should be a permanent coordinator raises sensitive questions of bureaucratic turf, which have historically been of greatest concern perhaps to the National Institutes of Health. The House Appropriations Committee report (99–289) on the fiscal 1986 appropriation bill for the DHHS, dated September 26, 1985, called for a "permanent coordinator over the AIDS effort, who shall exercise oversight over the funds appropriated for the national effort against AIDS." The department never took the action, however, largely because "a cabal of NIH directors eviscerated the idea of central control," a congressional aide said.

In the coming months, attention to AIDS will only grow. The House and Senate have approved fiscal 1988 budget resolutions that set AIDS spending ceilings well above the levels sought by the administration. Although the administration favors less spending on AIDS in fiscal 1988, Bowen recently sent to the Office of Management and Budget a supplemental budget request calling for additional spending of $283 million—a change that would bring Public Health Service spending on AIDS to $817 million next year.

Interestingly, Congress generally uses the budget resolution as a mechanism for applying restraint in federal spending. In this instance, the House and Senate budget committees, by setting higher spending thresholds for AIDS, were encouraging the appropriations panels to increase federal resources in the fight against the disease. When asked why the committees took this action, a professional staff member of the Senate Budget Committee said in an interview: "Everybody keyed on the recommendation of the Institute of

Medicine–National Academy of Sciences AIDS report that called for federal spending of $1 billion by 1990." Actually, the study calls for an appropriation of $1 billion for biomedical research and "significant federal contributions toward the $1 billion annually required for the total costs of education and public health measures."

Appropriating more money for AIDS-related research and public health measures will be among the easier tasks facing the government. The more difficult policy issues that the federal government – and indeed all of society – must confront will concern striking an appropriate balance between caring for patients with AIDS and safeguarding them from discrimination on the one hand, and public health measures deemed necessary to secure the well-being of the population on the other. Physicians will be at the center of this struggle, because they are in commanding positions of responsibility within the government, in organized medicine, and at the patient's bedside. When the history of this medical generation is written, certainly one of the important criteria in measuring the social responsibility of physicians will be how well they reacted to the tragic new disease called AIDS.

AIDS exposes the underbelly of many enduring social problems – lack of access to health care, prostitution, drug use, discrimination, and poverty.

MERVYN F. SILVERMAN
President
American Foundation for AIDS Reserach

Anne A. Scitovsky

The Economic Impact of AIDS in the United States

Nearly ten years have passed since the first cases of acquired immunodeficiency syndrome (AIDS) were reported in the United States. Because of the virulence and deadliness of the disease, which has generally required acute hospital care, serious concerns about its impact on health care costs were raised almost from the beginning. Yet only in the past three or four years have some data on its costs become available from a number of studies that have estimated the economic impact of AIDS. Even now, serious data gaps remain.

Because we appear to have reached the end of the first phase of the medical management of AIDS, with its heavy reliance on inpatient hospital care, it is timely now to review the studies and estimates relating to the costs of the epidemic and its economic impact that have been made to date. Although the evidence is not yet conclusive, new methods of medical treatment, notably the use of drugs such as zidovudine (AZT), appear to make it possible to treat many persons with AIDS (PWAs) on an ambulatory basis. In addition, providers of care, third-party payers, and some local communities are making concerted efforts to find ways of managing the care of PWAs in an ambulatory setting. To evaluate the effect of both the new medical tools available for the treatment of PWAs and the new methods of managing their care, it is useful to review past studies and estimates so that these data can be used as a kind of benchmark against which to set the costs of AIDS in this new phase of providing medical care to PWAs.

In this article I review the principal studies and estimates to date of the personal health care costs of PWAs, how these costs compare with the costs of some other diseases, and the expected impact of the epidemic on hospitals. After very brief sections on estimates of direct nonpersonal costs of the epidemic (that is, for research; screening for human immunodeficiency virus, or HIV, infection; blood screening and replacement; education; information; and various support services) and of indirect costs (that is, the value of lost output due to illness and premature death), I discuss the limitations of the

Anne A. Scitovsky is chief of Health Economics at the Palo Alto Medical Foundation/ Research Institute, Palo Alto, California, and lecturer at the Institute for Health Policy Studies, School of Medicine, University of California, San Francisco.

estimates of personal health care costs of PWAs made to date and the major data gaps that make better estimates difficult. I conclude with some suggestions regarding the type and contents of future studies of the costs of AIDS.

THE PERSONAL HEALTH CARE COSTS OF PEOPLE WITH AIDS

Empirical studies and estimates.   All the empirical studies of the personal health care costs of PWAs made to date have been retrospective and based on patients' medical and/or financial records. Seage and colleagues in Boston, Scitovsky and colleagues in San Francisco, and Berger in Maryland conducted studies in which data were collected and analyzed for a number of cohorts of PWAs. The California State Department of Health Services, using MediCal (Medicaid) claims data, has made two estimates of the lifetime costs of PWAs in California in 1984–1985 and 1985–1986. A study published in summer 1987 by Andrulis and colleagues reports on a survey of 169 metropolitan public and private teaching hospitals that treated PWAs in 1985. They collected and analyzed data on hospital utilization (that is, number of patients and admissions, length of stay, and total inpatient days) by risk group, and, for smaller subsamples, data on costs, revenues, and sources of payment. In addition, a dozen or so other empirical studies are currently being conducted or have been completed but have not yet been published. Additional data on costs of treating PWAs can be found in unpublished reports by state and local health departments, hospital associations (such as the Hospital Council of Southern California and the New York Health and Hospital Corporation), and some individual hospitals.

Useful as these studies and data are, none of them covers all medical services used by PWAs, many of the studies being limited to inpatient services or at best to inpatient and outpatient services provided by hospitals. In addition, many of them report data for relatively small numbers of cases. The Boston study by Seage, for example, included forty-five cases; the Maryland study by Berger, twenty-six cases. The San Francisco study by Scitovsky had inpatient and outpatient data for 201 cases, data on 445 hospital admissions of PWAs, and data on lifetime hospital costs of eighty-five cases.

Despite this scarcity of data, five estimates have been made of the medical care costs of PWAs in the United States. The first (which received a great deal of publicity at the time) was made in early 1985 by Ann Hardy and colleagues at the Centers for Disease Control (CDC). They estimated the lifetime hospital costs of the first 10,000 patients with AIDS reported in the United States at about $1.5 billion, or $147,000 per AIDS patient.

In early 1986, Scitovsky and Rice, at the request of the CDC, made estimates of the direct and indirect costs of AIDS in the United States in 1985, 1986, and 1991. Because of the uncertainty of much of the data, three estimates of the direct personal costs of PWAs were made for each of the three years — low, medium, and high. However, for each of the three years they used the CDC estimates of the number of PWAs alive at any time during the year, increased at the suggestion of the CDC by 20 percent to take into account under-reporting. They consider their medium estimates the best possible at the time: $630 million in 1985, $1.1 billion in 1986, and $8.5 billion in 1991, all in current dollars.

More recently, an estimate was made by Anthony Pascal, of The RAND Corporation. In connection with estimating the impact of the AIDS epidemic on the Medicaid program for the Health Care Financing Administration (HCFA), he made three estimates of the total costs of treating PWAs in the five-year period 1986 to 1991. His estimates range from a low of $15.4 billion to an intermediate estimate of $37.6 billion (which he regards as the most likely) and a high of $112.5 billion. Another recent estimate, by Andrulis and colleagues for 1985, based on their findings from the hospital survey mentioned earlier, put total hospital inpatient costs of PWAs in the United States at $380 million.

The latest estimate has been made by Hellinger, who states that it takes account of "the wider use of AZT," although he gives no details regarding his assumptions about the effect of the use of AZT on costs. He forecasts the personal medical care costs of PWAs to be $2.2 billion in 1988 and $4.5 billion in 1991.

There are several reasons for the wide differences in these estimates. One source of difference is the fact that some of the estimates are incidence-based (Hardy, Pascal, and Hellinger) while others are prevalence-based (Scitovsky and Rice, Andrulis). Incidence-based estimates attribute all the medical care costs incurred over a person's lifetime to the year when the patient was diagnosed; while prevalence-based estimates cover the costs of all medical care received by persons with the disease in a given year, regardless of when the condition was diagnosed and of whether they lived the full twelve months, died during this period, or were newly diagnosed in the course of the year. This source of difference, however, is not a major obstacle to comparisons when average life expectancy is relatively short, as it has been in the case of AIDS at least until very recently (about thirteen months from diagnosis to death).

The principal reasons for differences between the estimates are differences in the underlying assumptions regarding (1) medical care costs per PWA and (2) the projected number of cases with AIDS. Hardy's estimate of average lifetime hospital costs of $147,000 for the first 10,000 cases of AIDS reported in the United States (with an average life expectancy of thirteen months) compares with Pascal's estimate of lifetime costs of $94,000 in the period 1986–1991 (assuming an average life expectancy of twelve months) and Hellinger's estimate of $61,800 in 1991 (assuming an average life expectancy of twenty-four months). The medium estimate by Scitovsky and Rice for 1991 can be converted to an estimated lifetime cost of about $70,000 (assuming an average life expectancy of thirteen months). The latter two estimates are in 1985 prices, that by Pascal apparently in 1986 prices.

Differences in the projected number of cases of AIDS parallel the differences in estimated lifetime costs per case of AIDS. Scitovsky and Rice used the projections of the CDC, increased by 20 percent to take account of under-reporting. Pascal, using a different forecasting model, arrived at an estimate of cumulative cases by 1991 that is about 50 percent higher than the CDC estimate and about 23 percent higher than the adjusted CDC estimate used by Scitovsky and Rice. By contrast, Hellinger, using yet another forecasting model, estimated about 18 percent fewer newly diagnosed cases for 1991 than the CDC estimates indicate, allowing for a 20 percent increase in both his and the CDC's estimate for underreporting.

The Hardy estimate of lifetime hospital costs is now generally regarded as much too high. It was based on very fragmentary data, and there is consid-erable evidence that the medical care costs of treating PWAs have declined since the early days of the epidemic. For example, Kizer (in the studies cited earlier) found that average lifetime costs (over an eighteen-month average life span) for PWAs in California declined from $91,000 in 1984–1985 to $70,000 in 1985–1986. But statistically sound estimates of lifetime costs of PWAs are currently not possible, and all we can say is that they range somewhere between $60,000 and $90,000, with a strong possibility that they are closer to the lower range since all (with the possible exception of Hellinger's) are based on data from retrospective studies that do not yet reflect more recent changes in treatment, which may be cost-saving to some extent. With regard to the projections of the number of AIDS cases in the next five or more years there is also considerable uncertainty, and any cost estimates therefore must be based on a range of estimates of the number of future cases.

Because the estimates of the national costs of AIDS by Scitovsky and Rice lie about halfway between the high estimates of Pascal and the low estimates of Hellinger, I use them for comparing the costs of AIDS with other health care expenditures and for evaluating the impact of AIDS on the nation's hospitals.

Comparing the costs of AIDS with other health care expenditures.   Scitovsky and Rice's medium estimate of $8.5 billion represents 1.4 percent of estimated total personal health care costs in 1991. By comparison, their medium estimate for 1985 represents a mere 0.2 percent and that for 1986, 0.3 percent of personal health care expenditures in these two years. In 1985 and 1986, their estimated annual medical care costs of PWAs, high as they are, are consider-ably lower than those of patients with some other diseases. For example, based on 1980 data, they have estimated that persons with end-stage renal disease had total expenses of about $2.2 billion; persons injured in automobile acci-dents, $5.6 billion; with cancer of the digestive system, $3.4 billion; cancer of the lungs, $2.7 billion; and cancer of the breast, $2.2 billion.

Comparing their estimates for 1991 with estimates of the medical care costs of some other diseases in 1991 is rather problematic since the base year for other diseases is 1980, and the prevalence of these conditions is bound to change over this eleven-year period. But assuming neither drastic changes in the prevalence nor in the treatment of other conditions, they believe that it is likely that the medical care costs of PWAs will exceed those of patients with cancer of the digestive system, cancer of the lung, and cancer of the breast, and be exceeded only by the costs of persons injured in automobile accidents.

Data on the lifetime costs of other diseases are not available. However, Scitovsky and Rice estimated, on the basis of Medicare data, that the lifetime costs of persons with end-stage renal disease who are on dialysis are about $158,000, assuming an average lifetime of four years for these patients. Thus, the lifetime costs of these patients are considerably higher than those of PWAS.

The Impact of AIDS on Hospitals

Because inpatient hospital care has been and continues to be the driving force behind the costs of AIDS, it is important to examine the likely impact of the epidemic on hospitals. Scitovsky and Rice's $8.5 billion estimate of total medical care costs of PWAs in 1991 assumes 5.9 million hospital days. This is equivalent to 2.6 percent of all hospital days used in 1985, almost four times the number of hospital days used in 1985 by patients with cancer of the colon (1.6 million) or cancer of the breast (1.5 million), and twice the number of hospital days used by patients with cancer of the lung (2.8 million). Only patients with acute myocardial infarction (7.2 million days), pneumonia (6.8 million days), and normal infant deliveries (12.6 million days) used more inpatient days in 1985 than their estimate for AIDS patients in 1991.

Their estimate of 5.9 million hospital days needed by AIDS patients translates into a requirement of just over 16,000 beds in 1991, which represents 1.2 percent of all hospital beds available in 1985. Although there is an excess of hospital beds in the United States (possibly as much as 20 percent), the AIDS epidemic will impose a serious strain on hospitals, especially public hospitals, in metropolitan areas with large numbers of PWAs. On the basis of Scitovsky and Rice's assumptions regarding hospital use by PWAs and the CDC estimates of the prevalence of AIDS in New York and San Francisco in 1991, increased again by 20 percent to account for underreporting, I have estimated that in 1991 AIDS patients would require about 2,100 beds in New York, or about 5 percent of all hospital beds in the New York metropolitan area in 1985, and 648 beds in San Francisco, or about 9.5 percent of all hospital beds in that city in 1985. Other metropolitan centers such as Los Angeles, Washington, D.C., Miami, Houston, and Newark would face similar demands on their hospital systems.

Public hospitals in these centers, however, will face the most serious problems if they continue to provide inpatient care for the same percentage of

PWAs they currently care for and if they have the same number of hospital beds as they do now. I have estimated (again using Scitovsky and Rice's assumptions regarding hospital use) that under these conditions PWAs in 1991 would require between 10 percent and 13 percent of all public hospital beds in New York City and about one-third of all beds in San Francisco General Hospital. In fact, according to a report presented at the Fourth International Conference on AIDS in Stockholm in June 1988, 30 percent of all acute care beds in one public hospital in New York already are occupied by patients suffering from HIV-related illnesses. Clearly there is a limit to the number of beds that public hospitals can provide for PWAs because they have an obligation to provide many other essential medical services to their cities' populations.

In addition to the strain on their physical resources, the public hospitals also face the most serious financial problems posed by the AIDS epidemic because of the high percentage of their AIDS patients either who are covered by Medicaid, which generally reimburses the hospitals for less than their costs, or who are self-pay, which frequently turns into uncollectible bills. According to a 1987 report, of the PWAs hospitalized in the public hospitals of the New York Health and Hospital Corporation, 70 percent were covered by Medicaid, 6 percent by Blue Cross, 1 percent by Medicare, less than 1 percent by commercial insurance, and 12 percent were self-pay.

While these data clearly indicate the need for community hospitals to play a greater role in providing inpatient services to PWAs, it is equally clear that in view of the financial and insurance situation of PWAs currently being treated by public hospitals, private hospitals may not be eager to treat large numbers of AIDS cases. Moreover, there is some evidence that the proportion of PWAs covered by private insurance has been declining, with payment responsibilities shifting to the public sector, primarily Medicaid and local communities. This highlights the increasingly urgent need for comprehensive planning on how to finance medical care for PWAS. One way or another, the medical care costs of PWAs will be met. But unless the present piecemeal system is drastically reformed, the AIDS epidemic will cause severe economic hardships for and place disproportionate financial burdens on not only many PWAs and their families but also public hospitals and local communities.

THE DIRECT NONPERSONAL COSTS OF THE HIV EPIDEMIC

To date, Scitovsky and Rice have made the only estimates of the direct nonpersonal costs of the HIV epidemic—that is, the costs of research; blood screening and replacement; screening of individuals for HIV infection; and health education, information, and support services. Their medium estimates, in current dollars, range from $319 million in 1985 to $542 million in 1986 to $2.3 billion in 1991. However, these estimates should be regarded with great caution. The data available to estimate current costs of these services are even more fragmentary than those available for estimating the direct medical care costs of PWAs. It is virtually impossible to project these costs because of the uncertainties of future policy regarding the provision of these services. For example, costs will differ enormously depending on the extent of screening for HIV infection, the breadth of educational programs, and the funds made available for research of all types.

THE INDIRECT COSTS OF THE HIV EPIDEMIC

Both Hardy and colleagues and Scitovsky and Rice have made estimates of the indirect costs of the HIV epidemic—that is, the value of lost output due to illness and premature death. Hardy estimated the indirect costs of the first 10,000 cases of AIDS in the United States at $4.8 billion, or more than three times her estimate of health care costs. Scitovsky and Rice's estimates range from $3.9 billion in 1985 to $7.0 billion in 1986 to $55.6 billion in 1991, or more than six times their estimates of personal health care costs. Most of the indirect costs (93 percent) represent losses due to premature death. While their estimates of indirect costs represent only 1.2 percent and 2.1 percent of the estimated total indirect costs of all illness in 1985 and 1986, they rise to close to 12 percent of the estimated total costs of all illness in 1991.

These estimates, too, should be regarded as very tentative because there are no data on the earnings of PWAs. There is some evidence that of the two major risk groups, homosexual and bisexual males and intravenous (IV) drug abusers, the former have above-average earnings, while the majority of the latter are likely to have either no or below-average earnings or earnings from illegal sources such as drug dealing, theft, and prostitution. We assumed that PWAs had the same average earnings as others in their age and sex group. But this assumption is not based on any hard data.

RECOMMENDATIONS FOR FUTURE STUDIES

Currently available data do not permit reliable estimates and projections of the personal health care costs of persons infected with HIV. Because they come from retrospective studies, they do not reflect more recent changes in the treatment and management of the disease. Moreover, they are generally limited to data on inpatient hospital care or at best inpatient and outpatient hospital care and shed little light on the costs of ambulatory care. Finally, they come primarily from a few geographic areas, which may not be representative of costs in other areas and the nation as a whole. To make plans for meeting the medical resource and financial needs of persons infected with HIV, better and more comprehensive data on their use and costs of medical care are essential. What follows are my recommendations regarding the type and content of future studies of the costs of AIDS and HIV infection in general.

Prospective Studies

First and foremost, future studies should be prospective studies in which patients are followed for at least one year but preferably longer. These studies should be conducted in geographically representative areas and obtain detailed data on the use and costs of all services used rather than only of data on hospital services. Only prospective studies can reflect the changes that are occurring in the medical treatment of PWAs.

Similarly, only prospective studies can capture the effect on costs of new methods of managing the care of PWAs. The experience with AIDS in San Francisco has shown that medical care costs can be held down when appropriate community support systems exist that enable patients to be treated at home. However, I fear that the extent to which this "San Francisco model" can be exported to other areas is limited. PWAs in San Francisco are predominantly male homosexuals; San Francisco's well-organized gay community rallied to the epidemic. Whether similar community services can be organized in centers such as New York City, where more than one-third of PWAs are IV drug abusers, is questionable.

Finally, prospective studies should include not only persons with full-blown AIDS but also those with less severe manifestations of HIV infection, such as patients with ARC and even asymptomatic seropositive persons.

Data on Payers for Care of PWAs

It is essential that future studies obtain data on the insurance coverage of PWAs and other HIV-infected persons. This is increasingly important as the percentage of PWAs who are IV drug abusers continues to increase as it has done in recent years (from 15.3 percent of all reported cases in the year ending July 11, 1987, to 22.2 percent in the year ending July 11, 1988). These patients are less likely to have private insurance than homosexual and bisexual males, and thus the costs borne by public programs and local communities may rise. Similarly, if life expectancy of PWAs increases, more of them may qualify for Medicare, which in the past has paid very little of the costs of PWAs because most patients did not live the two years it takes to qualify under the Medicare disability program; or they may become dependent on Medicaid as they lose their private insurance coverage. Alternatively, if their quality of life improves so that they can continue to work longer, more of them may retain their private insurance.

Finally, if HIV-infected persons other than those with full-blown AIDS become heavier users of medical care than they have been to date, this will raise serious financing problems. If drugs become a relatively important item in their costs (as seems likely), many of these patients may have difficulties paying for them since private insurance generally does not pay for out-of-hospital drugs and prescriptions. At the same time, unless such persons are automatically declared disabled for purposes of Medicare coverage, their costs are also not paid by Medicaid.

Prevalence of HIV Infection

To make possible better projections of the number of persons with AIDS, better data on the prevalence of HIV infection are urgently needed. As mentioned earlier, the CDC is planning a series of surveys to obtain data on the extent of HIV infection in different geographic areas and among the different population groups at risk of HIV infection. It is to be hoped that despite the difficulties of conducting these surveys — difficulties due largely to the problems of confidentiality that this particular disease raises — they will be successful.

In centuries past, societies have dealt poorly with plagues. Despite all our high-tech know-how, our society is responding the same as in the past. We still are manifesting unwarranted fears, calling for repressive legislation to compromise civil rights, calling for quarantine of those infected despite every evidence that this would be ineffective and inhumane, and some physicians and other health care workers are refusing to care for those infected with the virus. People with AIDS are modern-day lepers.

MERVYN F. SILVERMAN
President
American Foundation for AIDS Research

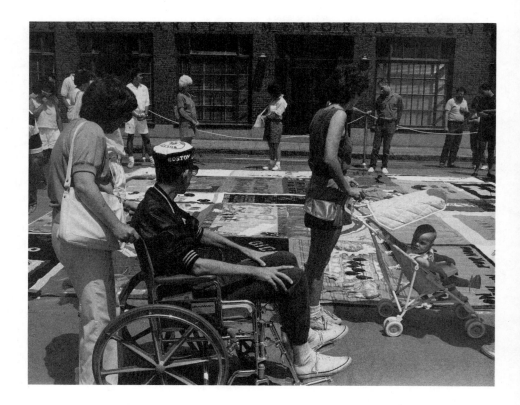

Suggested Readings

Chapter One: Health Status and Its Determinants

Banister E W et al. *Contemporary Health Issues*. Jones and Bartlett Publishers: Boston, 1988.

Cousins N. *Anatomy of an Illness as Perceived by the Patient*. Norton: New York, 1979.

Dubos R. *Mirage of Health*. Harper & Row: New York, 1979.

Health Insurance Association of America. 1986–1987 *Source Book of Health Insurance Data*. Washington, DC, 1987.

Kasper J D. Health status and utilization: Differences by Medicaid coverage and income. *Health Care Financing Review* 7(4): 1–17, 1986.

Lewis T. *The Lives of a Cell*. Viking Press: New York, 1974.

McKeown T. *The Role of Medicine*. Basil Blackwell Publisher: Oxford, England, 1979.

McKinlay JB. A case for refocussing upstream: The political economy of illness. In Conrad P and Kern R (eds) *The Sociology of Health and Illness: Critical Perspectives* (2nd edition). St. Martin's Press: New York, pp 484–498, 1986.

Mechanic D and Aiken LH. Improving the care of patients with chronic mental illness. *The New England Journal of Medicine* 317(26): 1634–1638, 1987.

Chapter Two: Shaping the Health Care System

Dickman RL, Ford AB, Liebman J, Milligan S and Schorr AL. An end to patchwork reform of health care. *The New England Journal of Medicine* 317(17): 1086–1089, 1987.

Ellwood PM Jr. and Paul BA. But what about quality? *Health Affairs* 135–140, Spring 1986.

Fein R. History of efforts in the past 75 years to bring about a national health program in the U.S. and analysis of why these efforts failed. In Smith MW and Labrie V (eds). *Options for a National Health Program: A Public Forum* (Proceedings). National Health Program Coalition: Berkeley, 7–27, 1987.

Ginzberg E. *From Physician Shortage to Patient Shortage*. Westview Press: Boulder, 1986.

Gornick M, Greenberg JN, Eggers PW and Dobson A. Twenty years of Medicare and Medicaid: Covered populations, use of benefits, and program expenditures. *Health Care Financing Review* Annual Supplement: 13–59, 1985.

Health Care USA: 1984. The National Citizens Board of Inquiry into Health in America. Washington, DC, 1984.

Rosenthal G. The federal health structure. In Mechanic D (ed) *Handbook of Health, Health Care, Health Professions*. Free Press: New York, pp 379–393, 1983.

Visotsky HM. The great American roundup. *The New England Journal of Medicine* 317(26): 1662–1663, 1987.

Williams SJ and Torrens PR (eds) *Introduction to Health Services* (3rd edition). John Wiley & Sons: New York, 1988.

Winkenwerder W and Ball JR. Transformation of American health care: The role of the medical profession. *The New England Journal of Medicine* 318(5): 317–319, 1988.

Chapter Three: The Politics of Health

Alford RR (ed) *Health Care Politics: Ideological and Interest Group Barriers to Reform*. The University of Chicago Press: Chicago, pp 249–266, 1975.

Conrad P and Kern R (eds) *The Sociology of Health and Illness: Critical Perspectives* (2nd edition). St. Martin's Press: New York, pp 484–498, 1986.

Dickman RL et al. An end to patchwork reform of health care. *The New England Journal of Medicine* 317(17): 1086–1089, 1987.

Downs A. *An Economic Theory of Democracy*. Harper & Row: New York, 1957.

Falk SI. Proposal for national health insurance in the USA: Origins and evolution, and some perceptions for the future. *Milbank Memorial Fund Quarterly/Health and Society* 161–191, Spring 1977.

Feldstein PJ. National Health Insurance: An approach to the redistribution of medical care. Health Care Economics (2nd edition). John Wiley & Sons: New York, pp 525–553, 1983.

Fox DM. The consequences of consensus: American health policy in the twentieth century. *The Milbank Quarterly* 64(l): 76–99, 1986.

Jain SC and Paul JE (eds) *Policy Issues in Personal Health Services*. Aspen Systems Corporation: Rockville, Maryland, pp 289–342, 1983.

Luft HS and Arno P. Impact of increasing physician supply: A scenario for the future. *Health Affairs* 5(4): 31–46, 1986.

Mechanic D. Correcting misconceptions in mental health policy: Strategies for improved care of the seriously mentally ill. *The Milbank Quarterly* 65(2): 203–230, 1987.

Public Health Service, Office of Disease Prevention and Health Promotion, U.S. Department of Health and Human Services. Strategies for promoting health for specific populations. *Journal of Public Health Policy* 8(3): 369–423, 1987.

Roth JA and Ruzek SB (eds) *Research in the Sociology of Health Care: The Adoption and Social Consequences of Medical Technologies*. Volume 4. JAI Press Inc.: Greenwich, Connecticut, pp 147–183, 1986.

Tarlov AR. The rising supply of physicians and the pursuit of better health. *Journal of Medical Education* 63: 94–107, 1988.

Chapter Four: The Critical Role of Nurses

Aiken LH and Gortner SR (eds) *Nursing in the 1980s*. Lippencott: Philadelphia, 1982.

Fitzpatrick JJ, Taunton RL and Benoliel JQ (eds) *Annual Review of Nursing Research* Volume 6. Springer Publishing Company: New York, pp 85–109, 1988.

Friss L. The nursing shortage: Do we dislike it enough to cure it? *Inquiry* 25: 232–242, 1988.

Harrington C. Nursing home reform: Addressing critical staffing issues. *Nursing Outlook* 35(5): 208–209, 1987.

Iglehart JK. Problems facing the nursing profession. *The New England Journal of Medicine* 317(10): 646–651, 1987.

Jameton A. Duties to self: Professional nursing in the critical care unit. In Fowler M and Levine-Ariff J. *Ethics at the Bedside: A Source Book for the Critical Care Nurse*. J.B. Lippincott Co.: Philadelphia, pp 115–135, 1987.

Moskowitz S. Strategies for ending wage discrimination in nursing. *Nursing Economic$* 2: 25–32, 1984.

Muyskens JL. The role of the nurse. *Moral Problems in Nursing*. Rowman and Littlefield: Totowa, New Jersey, pp 30–40, 1982.

Vance C, Talbott SW, McBride AB and Mason DJ. Coming of age: The women's movement and nursing. *Political Action Handbook for Nurses: Changing the*

Workplace, Government, Organizations, and Community. Addison-Wesley Publishing
   Company: Menlo Park, California, pp 23–37, 1985.
Winslow GR. From loyalty to advocacy: A new metaphor for nursing. The *Hastings
   Center Report* 14(3): 32–40, 1984.

Chapter Five: The Rising Costs of Health Care

Christensen S, Long SH and Rodgers J. Acute health care costs for the aged
   Medicare population: Overview and policy options. *The Milbank Quarterly* 65(3):
   397–425, 1987.
Doubilet P, Weinstein MC, McNeil BJ. Use and misuse of the term "cost effective"
   in medicine. *The New England Journal of Medicine* 314(4): 253–256, 1986.
Fein R. *Medical Care, Medical Costs: The Search for a Health Insurance Policy.* Harvard
   University Press: Cambridge, 1986.
Fry ST. Rationing health care: The ethics of cost containment. *Nursing Economic$* 1:
   165–169, 1983.
Fuchs VR. Has cost containment gone too far? *The Milbank Quarterly* 64(3): 479–488,
   1986.
Fuchs WR. *Who Shall Live? Economics and Social Choice.* Basic Books: New York, 1974.
Harrington C. Catastrophic health insurance: What is needed? *Nursing Outlook* 35(6):
   254–255, 1987.
Hentoff N. The rationing of human life in Oregon. *The Village Voice* XXXIII(21): 44,
   1988.
Hicks LL and Boles KE. Why health economics? *Nursing Economic$* 2: 175–180, 1984.
Iglehart JK. The recommendations of the Physician Payment Review Commission.
   New England Journal of Medicine 320(17): 1156, 1989.
Lee PR and Ginsburg PB. Building a consensus for physician payment reform in
   Medicare: The Physician Payment Review Commission. *The Western Journal of
   Medicine* 149(3): 352–358, 1988.
Newacheck PW and McManus MA. Financing health care for disabled children.
   Pediatrics 81(3): 385–394, 1988.
Newacheck PW. The costs of caring for chronically ill children. *Business and Health*
   pp 18–24, January 1987.
Physician Payment Review Commission. *Annual Report to Congress 1989.* 2120 L St.,
   NW, Washington, DC 20037.
Reagan MD. Physicians as gatekeepers: A complex challenge. *The New England
   Journal of Medicine* 317(27): 1731–1734, 1987.
Robinson JC. Philosophical origins of the economic valuation of life. *The Milbank
   Quarterly* 64(1): 133–155, 1986.
Thurlow LC. Medicine versus economics. *The New England Journal of Medicine*
   313(10): 611–614, 1985.
Vladeck BC. The limits of cost-effectiveness (editorial). *American Journal of Public
   Health* 74(7): 652–653, 1984.
Weissert WG. The cost-effectiveness trap. *Generations* pp 47–50, Summer 1985.

Chapter Six: Competition vs. Regulation

Enthoven AC. *Health Plan: The Only Practical Solution to the Soaring Cost of Medical Care.*
   Addison-Wesley: Reading, 1980.
Enthoven AC. Managed competition: An agenda for action. *Health Affairs* 7(3): 25, 1988.
Fuchs VR. The competition revolution in health care. *Health Affairs* 7(3): 5, 1988.
Ginzberg E. *American Medicine: The Power Shift.* Rowman & Allanheld Publishers:
   Totawa, New Jersey, 1985.

434

Ginsberg PB and Hammons GT. Competition and the quality of care. *Inquiry* 25(l): 108–115, 1988.

Goldsmith JC. Competitions impact: A report from the front. *Health Affairs* 7(3): 162, 1988.

Kinzer D. The decline and fall of deregulation. *The New England Journal of Medicine* 318(2): 112–116, 1988.

Luft HS. Competition and regulation. *Medical Care* 23(5): 383–400, 1985.

Reinhardt UE. Resource allocation in health care: The allocation of lifestyles to providers. *The Milbank Quarterly* 65(2): 153–176, 1987.

Salmon JW. Profit and health care: Trends in corporatization and proprietization. *International Journal of Health Services* 15(3)395–418, 1985.

Chapter Seven: Inequities in Access to Health Care

Bachrach LL. Homeless women: A context for health planning. *The Milbank Quarterly* 65(3): 371–396, 1987.

Blendon RJ et al. Uncompensated care by hospitals or public insurance for the poor: Does it make a difference? *The New England Journal of Medicine* 314(18): 1160–1163, 1986.

Cohodes DR. America: The home of the free, the land of the uninsured. *Inquiry* 23: 227–235, Fall 1986.

Davis K. What about the poor? *Generations* pp 13–15, Summer 1985.

Dutton DB. Social class, health, and illness. In *Applications of Social Science to Clinical Medicine and Health Policy*, New Brunswick: Rutgers University Press, pp 31–62, 1986.

Farley R. The quality of life for black Americans twenty years after the civil rights revolution. *The Milbank Quarterly* 65(Sl): 9–34, 1987.

Harrington C and Lempert L. Medicaid: A public program in distress. *Nursing Outlook* 36(l): 6–8, 1988.

James G. Poverty as an obstacle to public health progress in our cities. *American Journal of Public Health* 55: 1757–1771, 1965.

Manton KG, Patrick CH, and Johnson KW. Health differentials between blacks and whites: Recent trends in mortality and morbidity. *The Milbank Quarterly* 65(Sl): 129–199, 1987.

Mundinger MO. Health services funding cuts and the declining health of the poor. *The New England Journal of Medicine* 313(l): 44–47, 1985.

Newacheck PW and Halfon N. Access to ambulatory care services for economically disadvantaged children. *Pediatrics* 78(5): 813–819, 1986.

Reinhardt UE. Health insurance for the nation's poor. *Health Affairs* 6(1): 101–112, 1987.

Rossi PH and Wright JD. The determinants of homelessness. *Health Affairs* pp 19–32, Spring 1987.

Schlesinger M et al. The privatization of health care and physician's perceptions of access to hospital services. *The Milbank Quarterly* 65(l): 25–58, 1987.

Chapter Eight: Quality, Effectiveness, and Appropriateness of Care

Caper P. The epidemiologic surveillance of medical care. *American Journal of Public Health* 77: 669–670, 1987.

Eisenberg JM. *Doctors' Decisions and the Cost of Medical Care.* Ann Arbor: Health Administration Press, 1986.

Elwood PM. Outcomes management: A technology of patient experience. *New England Journal of Medicine* 318: 1549–1556, 1988.

Luft HL. HMOs and the quality of care. *Inquiry* 25(l): 147–156, 1988.

Measuring Quality of Care: A Resource Guide. Chicago: American Medical Association, 1987.

Relman AS. Assessment and accountability: The third revolution in medical care. *New England Journal of Medicine* 319: 1220–1222, 1988.

Roper WL et al. Effectiveness in health care. *New England Journal of Medicine* 319(18): 1197–1202, 1988.

Wyszewianski L. Quality of care: Past achievements and future challenges. *Inquiry* 25(l): 13–22, 1988.

Chapter Nine: Chronic Illness, Aging, and Long-Term Care

Ball RM. Medicare: A strategy for protecting and improving it. *Generations* pp 9–12, Summer 1985.

Blumenthal D, Schlesinger M, Drumheller PB, and The Harvard Medicare Project. The future of Medicare. *The New England Journal of Medicine* 314(11): 722–728, 1986.

Christensen S, Long SH, and Rodgers J. Acute health care costs for the aged Medicare population: Overview and policy options. *The Milbank Quarterly* 65(3): 397–425, 1987.

Densen PM. The elderly and the health care system: Another perspective. *The Milbank Quarterly* 65(4): 614–638, 1987.

Doty P. Family care of the elderly: The role of public policy. *The Milbank Quarterly* 64(l): 34–75, 1986.

Estes CL and Binney EA. Toward a transformation of health and aging policy. *International Journal of Health Services* 18(l): 69–81, 1988.

Fox PJ. Alzheimer's disease: An historical overview. The *American Journal of Alzheimer's Care* pp 18–24, Fall 1986.

Greenberg JN et al. The social/health maintenance organization and long term care. *Generations* pp 51–54, Summer 1985.

Harrington C and Newcomer RJ. Social health maintenance organizations: New policy options for the aged, blind, and disabled. *Journal of Public Health Policy* 6(2): 204–222, 1985.

Holahan J and Palmer JL. Medicare's fiscal problems: An imperative for reform. *Journal of Health Politics, Policy and Law* 13(l): 53–81, 1988.

Lipton HH. Drug economics and the elderly: Prescriptions for change. *Business and Health* pp 8–11, March 1988.

Manton KG and Soldo BJ. Dynamics of health changes in the oldest old: New perspectives and evidence. *Health and Society* 63(2): 206–285, 1985.

Olshansky SJ and Ault AB. The fourth stage of the epidemiologic transition: The age of delayed degenerative diseases. *The Milbank Quarterly* 64(3): 355–391, 1986.

Rice DP and LaPlante MP. Chronic illness, disability, and increasing longevity. In Sean Sullivan and Marion Ein Lewin (eds) *The Economics and Ethics of Long Term Care and Disability.* Washington, DC: American Enterprise Institute for Public Policy Research, pp 9–55, 1988.

Stone R, Cafferata GL, and Sangl J. Caregivers of the frail elderly: A national profile. *The Gerontologist* 27(5): 616–626, 1987.

Chapter Ten: AIDS

Arno PS and Hughes RG. Local policy responses to the AIDS epidemic: New York and San Francisco. *New York State Journal of Medicine* 87: 264–272, 1987.

Beck-Sague CM, Alexander ER and Jaffe HW. Coping with AIDS: The special problems of New York City. *The New England Journal of Medicine* 317(23): 1469–1473, 1987.

Corless IB and Pittman-Lindeman M (eds) *AIDS: Principles, Practices and Politics.* Reference edition. Hemisphere Publishing: New York, 1989.

Friedland GH and Klein RS. Transmission of the Human Immunodeficiency Virus. *The New England Journal of Medicine* 317(18): 1125–1135, 1987.

Gong V and Rudnick N (eds) *AIDS: Facts and Issues.* New Brunswick: Rutgers University Press, pp 167–178, 1986.

Griggs J. (ed) *AIDS: Public Policy Dimensions.* New York: United Hospital Fund, pp 3–20, 1987.

Health and Public Policy Committee, American College of Physicians and the Infectious Diseases Society of America. The Acquired Immunodeficiency Syndrome (AIDS) and the Human Immunodeficiency Virus (HIV). *Annals of Internal Medicine* 108: 460–469, 1988.

Health and Public Policy Committee, American College of Physicians. Financing the care of patients with Acquired Immunodeficiency Syndrome (AIDS). *Annals of Internal Medicine* 108: 470–473, 1988.

Institute of Medicine. *Mobilizing Against AIDS.* Harvard University Press: Cambridge, 1989.

National Research Council. *AIDS: Sexual Behavior and Intravenous Drug Use.* National Academy Press: Washington, DC, 1989.

Osborn JE. AIDS: Politics and science. *The New England Journal of Medicine* 318(7): 444–447, 1988.

Rogers DE and Ginzberg E (eds) *The AIDS Patient: An Action Agenda.* Westview Press: Boulder, 1988.

Scitovsky AA and Rice DP. Estimates of the direct and indirect costs of Acquired Immunodeficiency Syndrome in the United States, 1985, 1986, and 1991. *Public Health Reports* 102(l): 5–17, 1987.

Shilts R. *And the Band Played on.* St. Martin's Press: New York, 1988.

Sisk JE. The costs of AIDS: A review of the estimates. *Health Affairs* pp 5–21, Summer 1987.

Weinberg DS and Murray HW. Coping with AIDS: The special problems of New York City. *The New England Journal of Medicine* 317(23): 1469–1473, 1987.

Index